Textbook of
Voice and Laryngology

Textbook of
Voice and Laryngology

KK Handa
MBBS DNB MNAMS MS
Director and Head
Department of ENT and Head Neck Surgery
Medanta—The Medicity
Gurugram, Haryana, India

Foreword

Markus Hess

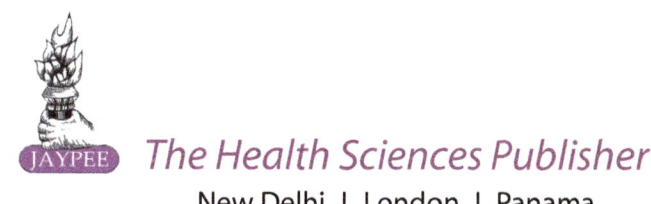

The Health Sciences Publisher
New Delhi I London I Panama

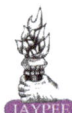 **Jaypee Brothers Medical Publishers (P) Ltd.**

Headquarters

Jaypee Brothers Medical Publishers (P) Ltd.
4838/24, Ansari Road, Daryaganj
New Delhi 110 002, India
Phone: +91-11-43574357
Fax: +91-11-43574314
E-mail: jaypee@jaypeebrothers.com

Overseas Offices

J.P. Medical Ltd.
83, Victoria Street, London
SW1H 0HW (UK)
Phone: +44-20 3170 8910
Fax: +44(0) 20 3008 6180
E-mail: info@jpmedpub.com

Jaypee Brothers Medical Publishers (P) Ltd.
17/1-B, Babar Road, Block-B, Shaymali
Mohammadpur, Dhaka-1207
Bangladesh
Mobile: +08801912003485
E-mail: jaypeedhaka@gmail.com

Jaypee-Highlights Medical Publishers Inc.
City of Knowledge, Bld. 235, 2nd Floor, Clayton
Panama City, Panama
Phone: +1 507-301-0496
Fax: +1 507-301-0499
E-mail: cservice@jphmedical.com

Jaypee Brothers Medical Publishers (P) Ltd.
Bhotahity, Kathmandu, Nepal
Phone: +977-9741283608
E-mail: kathmandu@jaypeebrothers.com

Website: www.jaypeebrothers.com
Website: www.jaypeedigital.com

Textbook of Voice and Laryngology

First Edition: **2017**

ISBN: 978-93-86322-92-0

Printed at

Dedicated to

My patients

Medical Institutions: Medanta—The Medicity, Gurugram, where I currently work; and, AIIMS, New Delhi, where I worked PGIMER, Chandigarh, where I did my residency; and, Armed Forces Medical College, Pune, my medical school

My wife, Dr Aru; and, sons, Karan and Ishaan, who let me use the family time for professional and academic pursuits

Contributors

Aliza P Cohen
Otolaryngologist
Department of Pediatrics
Otolaryngology–Head and Neck Surgery
Cincinnati Children's Hospital Medical
Center
University of Cincinnati College of
Medicine
Cincinnati, Ohio, USA

Anup Singh Yadav
Senior Resident
Department of ENT and
Head Neck Surgery
Medanta—The Medicity
Gurugram, Haryana, India

Aru Chhabra Handa
Senior Consultant
Department of ENT and
Head Neck Surgery
Medanta—The Medicity
Gurugram, Haryana, India

Ashu Seith Bhalla
Professor
Department of Radiodiagnosis
All India Institute of Medical Sciences
New Delhi, India

Ashutosh Hota
Senior Resident
Department of ENT and
Head Neck Surgery
Medanta—The Medicity
Gurugram, Haryana, India

Claudio Vicini
Otolaryngologist
Department of Otolaryngology–
Head and Neck Surgery,
Stomatology and Oral Surgery Unit
GB Morgagni–L Pierantoni Hospital
Forlì, Romagna
Infermi Hospital
Department of Head and Neck Surgery
Faenza, Romagna, Italy

Dhananjay Kumar
Senior Resident
Department of ENT and
Head Neck Surgery
Medanta—The Medicity
Gurugram, Haryana, India

Divya Chandrasekhar
Voice and Swallow Therapist
Department of ENT and Head Neck
Surgery
Medanta—The Medicity
Gurugram, Haryana, India

Fabiola Incandela
Otolaryngologist
Department of Otorhinolaryngology–
Head and Neck Surgery
University of Genoa
Genoa, Liguria, Italy

Filippo Montevecchi
Otolaryngologist
Department of Otolaryngology–
Head and Neck Surgery,
Stomatology and Oral Surgery Unit
GB Morgagni–L Pierantoni Hospital
Forlì, Romagna
Infermi Hospital
Department of Head and
Neck Surgery
Faenza, Romagna, Italy

Giorgio Peretti
Otolaryngologist
Department of Otorhinolaryngology
Head and Neck Surgery
University of Genoa
Genoa, Liguria, Italy

Jaya Kumar Menon
Consultant Laryngologist
Kerala Institute of Medical Sciences
Thiruvananthapuram, Kerala, India

Joseph P Bradley
Assistant Professor
Department of Otolaryngology
Head and Neck Surgery
Washington University School of
Medicine
St Louis, Missouri, USA

J Paul Willging
Otolaryngologist
Department of Pediatrics
Otolaryngology–Head and Neck Surgery
Cincinnati Children's Hospital Medical
Center
University of Cincinnati College of
Medicine
Cincinnati, Ohio, USA

Karan Aggarwal
Fellow in Laryngology
Department of ENT and
Head Neck Surgery
Medanta—The Medicity
Gurugram, Haryana, India

KK Handa
Director and Head
Department of ENT and Head Neck
Surgery
Medanta—The Medicity
Gurugram, Haryana, India

Marco Barbieri
Otolaryngologist
Department of Otorhinolaryngology–
Head and Neck Surgery
University of Genoa
Genoa, Liguria, Italy

Mausumi N Syamal
Fellow
Head and Neck Institute
The Cleveland Clinic
Cleveland, Ohio, USA

M Haq
Attending Consultant
Department of ENT and
Head Neck Surgery
Medanta—The Medicity
Gurugram, Haryana, India

Michael M Johns
Associate Professor and
Director
Emory Voice Center
Emory University
Atlanta, Georgia, USA

Michael S Benninger
Professor
Department of Surgery
Lerner College of Medicine
The Cleveland Clinic
Cleveland, Ohio, USA

Mohamed Rashwan
Faculty
Department of Otorhinolaryngology–
Head and Neck Surgery
Suez Canal University
El Salam, Ismailia, Egypt

Ravindhra G Elluru
Associate Professor
Department of Pediatric Otolaryngology
Cincinnati Children's Hospital Medical
Center
University of Cincinnati College of
Medicine
Cincinnati, Ohio, USA

Smita Manchanda
Assistant Professor
Department of Radiodiagnosis
All India Institute of Medical Sciences
New Delhi, India

Usha Rani
Voice Therapist
Medanta—The Medicity
Gurugram, Haryana, India

Valeria Roustan
Otolaryngologist
Department of Otorhinolaryngology
Head and Neck Surgery
University of Genoa
Genoa, Liguria, Italy

Foreword

Just in time when world experts in laryngology and phonosurgery meet in India at Phonocon–2017, Dr KK Handa managed to publish a superb textbook on pearls within our field—*Textbook of Voice and Laryngology*. The editor has chosen outstanding and experienced experts on laryngology to elaborate on chapters ranging from anatomy, physiology, and voice assessment up to laryngotracheal reconstruction. This texbook also covers the important topics such as pediatric laryngology, swallowing, singers and their special attention to voice, aging larynx, and, rare but important disorders, such as papillomatosis and spasmodic dysphonia—just to mention a few highlights of the book. I am sure that this textbook will be a helpful guide in the hands of beginners as well as the advanced laryngologists.

Markus Hess
MD
Professor and Director
Department of Voice, Speech and Hearing Disorders
University Medical Center of Hamburg-Eppendorf
University of Hamburg
Hamburg, Germany

Preface

The field of voice and laryngology has made rapid strides in the past decade. This has been possible due to the advancement in technology and our better understanding of the basics of laryngology. Larynx is an area that was difficult to visualize at one time; but, today, not only it can be examined in detail but also every associated condition can be treated either conservatively or surgically. In each subarea of laryngology, such as laryngeal framework surgery, laser phonomicrosurgery, swallowing, office-based procedures, spasmodic dysphonia, laryngopharyngeal reflux, and airway, there has been a lot of progress both in diagnosis and management.

The clinical work, which is behind the writing of this book, involves my experience in ENT department of Medanta—The Medicity, Gurugram, Haryana, India, from 2009 till date; and, before that, in All India Institute of Medical Sciences, New Delhi, from September 1996 to October 2009. It was the wide spectrum of patients of laryngology who were presented in these institutions that inspired me to take the task of writing this book. The first stroboscope which came to the department in the year 1996 provided a detailed visualization of the free edge of the vocal cords, which helped in improving diagnosis of laryngeal conditions. Traveling and lecturing with my colleagues in voice and laryngology workshops, nationally and internationally, has further provided the stimulation after mutual exchange of ideas and learning from one another.

The book also has significant contributions from international and national experts in the fields of voice and laryngology. They were very kind in agreeing to write for the book and sending the chapters in time.

KK Handa

Acknowledgments

It is very satisfying to see this book finally take shape. The idea was there for a long time since the running of voice clinic in the All India Institute of Medical Sciences, New Delhi; and later, Medanta—The Medicity, Gurugram.

My first thanks go to the contributors and their coauthors, including Michael S Benninger, Mausumi N Syamal, Michael M Johns, Ravindhra G Elluru, J Paul Willging, Claudio Vicini, Filippo Montevecchi, Jaya Kumar Menon, Divya Chandrasekhar, Usha Rani, and Ashu Seith Bhalla, for providing the chapters.

My special thanks go to Professor Marcus Hess, an eminent laryngologist from Hamburg, Germany, for writing the Foreword.

My co-authors in the chapters written by me, especially Dr Dhananjay Kumar, deserve a special mention. My wife Dr Aru, who has been of direct and indirect help in a number of ways, also needs to be thanked.

I would also like to thank Shri Jitendar P Vij (Group Chairman), Mr Ankit Vij (Group President), Ms Chetna Malhotra Vohra (Associate Director–Content Strategy) of Jaypee Brothers Medical Publishers (P) Ltd., New Delhi, India, for publishing the book; and, also Ms Heena Gogia, Development Editor, for constantly nudging me to send the chapters on time, when I was busy with my clinical work.

Last but not least, my thanks go to the voice therapists, along all these years, who have helped to complete the treatment of the patients.

Contents

1. Clinical Anatomy   1
KK Handa, Dhananjay Kumar
Anatomy of the Larynx   *1*
Laryngeal Cartilages   *2*
Laryngeal Ligaments   *3*
Laryngeal Musculature   *4*
Laryngeal Joints   *5*
Laryngeal Innervation   *6*

2. Voice Evaluation   9
KK Handa, Karan Aggarwal
Problems in Voice Evaluation   *9*
Voice Test Battery   *9*
Voice Material   *9*
Voice Testing in Detail   *10*
Acoustic and Electrolaryngographic Voice Evaluation   *14*
Aerodynamic Measures   *15*

3. Imaging of Benign Laryngeal Pathology: Expanding Horizons   17
Smita Manchanda, Ashu Seith Bhalla
Imaging Techniques in the Study of the Larynx   *17*
Laryngeal Obstruction in the Pediatric Age Group   *18*
Stenosis (Noncongenital)   *19*
Cysts and Laryngoceles   *20*
Benign Tumors or Mass Lesions of Larynx   *20*
Vocal Cord Paralysis   *23*
Trauma   *24*

4. Laryngopharyngeal Reflux   27
KK Handa, Aru Chhabra Handa, Ashutosh Hota
Pathophysiology   *27*
Mechanism of Symptoms   *28*
Signs and Symptoms   *29*
Effects of Reflux in Aerodigestive Tract   *30*
Investigations   *31*
Diagnosis   *34*
Treatment   *34*

5. Spasmodic Dysphonia   39
KK Handa
Etiopathogenesis   *39*
Management   *40*
Surgery for Spasmodic Dysphonia   *41*

6. Care of Singing Voice 45

Jaya Kumar Menon

Voice Production 45
Assessing the Breath Support 46
Assessment of Singing Voice 47
Management 47
Vocal Hygiene 48

7. The Aging Voice 50

Joseph P Bradley, Michael M Johns

Geriatric Dysphonia 50
History and Examination 51
Rejuvenation of the Aging Voice 51
Professional Vocalist 52
Future Directions 52
Case Studies 53

8. Voice Therapeutic Approaches 56

Usha Rani

Symptomatic Voice Therapy 56
Physiological or Holistic Voice Therapy 59

9. Voice and Medicines 65

KK Handa

Steroids in Acute Laryngeal Conditions 65
Sex Hormones 65
Drugs Used for Gastroesophageal and Laryngopharyngeal Reflux 65
Drugs Used for Cough and Thick Mucus 66
Drugs Used In Allergic Rhinitis 66
Drugs Acting on Autonomic Nervous System 67
Psychotropic Agents 67

10. Vocal Fold Immobility 69

Mausumi N Syamal, Michael S Benninger

Etiology 69
Clinical Presentation 70
Evaluation or Workup 71
Unilateral Vocal Fold Immobility Management 72
Bilateral Vocal Fold Immobility Management 75

11. Laryngeal Framework Surgery 80

KK Handa

Advantages of the Laryngeal Framework Surgery 80
Procedures under Local Anesthesia 80

12. Pediatric Voice Disorders 84

KK Handa, M Haq

Pediatric Larynx   *84*
Specific Disorders   *85*

13. Office-based Laryngeal Procedures 91

KK Handa

Anesthesia and Patient Selection for Office Procedures   *91*
Airway Evaluation   *92*
Vocal Cord Injections   *94*
Laryngeal Biopsy   *95*
Secondary Tracheoesophageal Puncture   *95*
Superficial Vocal Cord Injection   *96*
Botox Injection   *96*
Transnasal Esophagoscopy   *96*

14. Recurrent Respiratory Papillomatosis 99

KK Handa, Anup Singh Yadav

Epidemiology   *99*
Etiology   *99*
Pathophysiology   *100*
Mode of Transmission and Risk Factors of Disease   *101*
Presenting Symptomatology   *101*
Tracheostomy in Recurrent Respiratory Papillomatosis   *102*
Extralaryngeal Spread   *102*
Patient Evaluation   *102*
Management   *103*
Surgical Techniques   *105*
Adjuvant Treatment Modalities   *106*
Antireflux Therapy in Recurrent Respiratory Papillomatosis   *109*
New Frontiers in Recurrent Respiratory Papillomatosis   *110*
Recurrent Respiratory Papillomatosis Resources   *111*

15. Lasers in Phonosurgery and Laryngology 116

KK Handa

Laser Safety Protocol   *116*
Vocal Cord Cysts and Polyps   *117*
Abductor Cord Paralysis   *117*
Leukoplakia and Keratosis   *117*
Recurrent Respiratory Papillomatosis   *117*
Early Laryngeal Cancer   *118*
Vocal Cord Polyps   *119*
Vascular Lesions   *119*
Laryngotracheal Stenosis   *119*

16. Adult Laryngotracheal Stenosis   **121**

KK Handa, Dhananjay Kumar

Etiology *121*

Classification of Laryngotracheal Stenosis *122*

Diagnosis *123*

Management *124*

Various Operative Techniques for Laryngotracheal Stenosis *126*

17. Reconstruction Techniques for the Treatment of Anatomical Upper Respiratory Tract Anomalies in Children   **133**

Ravindhra G Elluru

Overview *133*

Pediatric versus Adult Upper Airway Anatomy *133*

Laryngomalacia *134*

Vocal Cord Paralysis *134*

Posterior Laryngeal Clefts *137*

Vascular Compression *139*

Tracheomalacia *139*

Complete Tracheal Rings *139*

18. Pediatric Dysphagia   **142**

J Paul Willging, Aliza P Cohen

Maturational Changes in Swallowing *142*

Normal Swallowing Physiology *143*

Mechanics of Swallowing *144*

Clinical Presentation *144*

Etiologies *144*

Overall Evaluation *145*

Diagnostic Workup *146*

Management Approaches *149*

19. Effects of Swallow Therapy in Oropharyngeal Dysphagia   **151**

Divya Chandrasekhar

Indirect Therapeutic Strategies *151*

Direct Therapeutic Strategies *154*

20. Laryngeal Management in Sleep Apnea Patients   **160**

Claudio Vicini, Filippo Montevecchi, Mohamed Rashwan, Marco Barbieri, Valeria Roustan, Fabiola Incandela, Giorgio Peretti

Drug-induced Sedation Endoscopy *160*

Surgical Treatment Options *161*

Postoperative Management *164*

Index   *165*

1

Clinical Anatomy

KK Handa, Dhananjay Kumar

INTRODUCTION

Detailed knowledge of laryngeal anatomy and its clinical significance can help an otolaryngologist to understand the laryngeal pathology and its possible management to a great extent.

ANATOMY OF THE LARYNX

The anatomical location is from third to sixth cervical vertebra. This position may be slightly higher in females. The laryngeal skeleton is formed by cartilages which are joined by ligaments and membranes.

The cartilages are as follows:
- Unpaired cartilages namely thyroid, cricoid, and epiglottis
- Paired cartilages namely arytenoid, corniculate, and cuneiform.

An important associated part is the hyoid bone. It is connected with thyroid cartilage by the thyrohyoid membrane.

The average length of adult larynx is about 44 mm in males and 36 mm in females, transverse diameter is approximately 43 mm in males and 41 mm in females, anteroposterior (AP) diameter is 36 mm in males and 26 mm in females and circumference is 136 mm in males, and 112 mm in females (Fig. 1).[1]

Internal Anatomy

Larynx is divided into three regions:[2]
1. Supraglottis
2. Glottis
3. Subglottis.

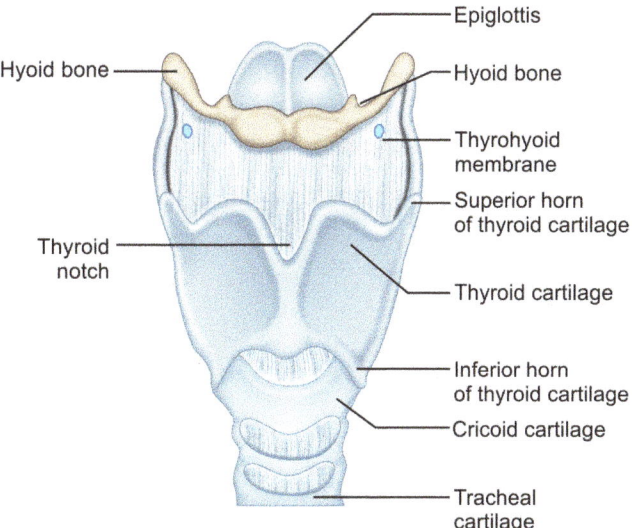

Fig. 1 Larynx anterior view

Supraglottis

Supraglottis has five segments or subsites (Fig. 2):
1. Suprahyoid epiglottis
2. Infrahyoid epiglottis
3. Laryngeal surface of aryepiglottic fold
4. Arytenoids
5. False vocal cords.

The inferior level of supraglottis is horizontal plane through lateral margins of ventricle.

Glottis

It comprises of true vocal cords, anterior commissure, and posterior commissure. The space between true vocal folds

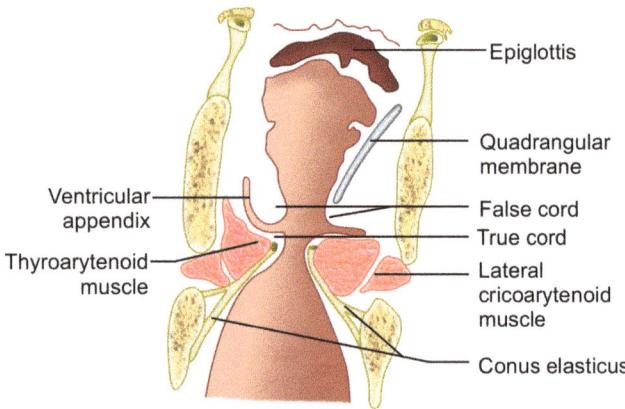

Fig. 2 Coronal section of larynx

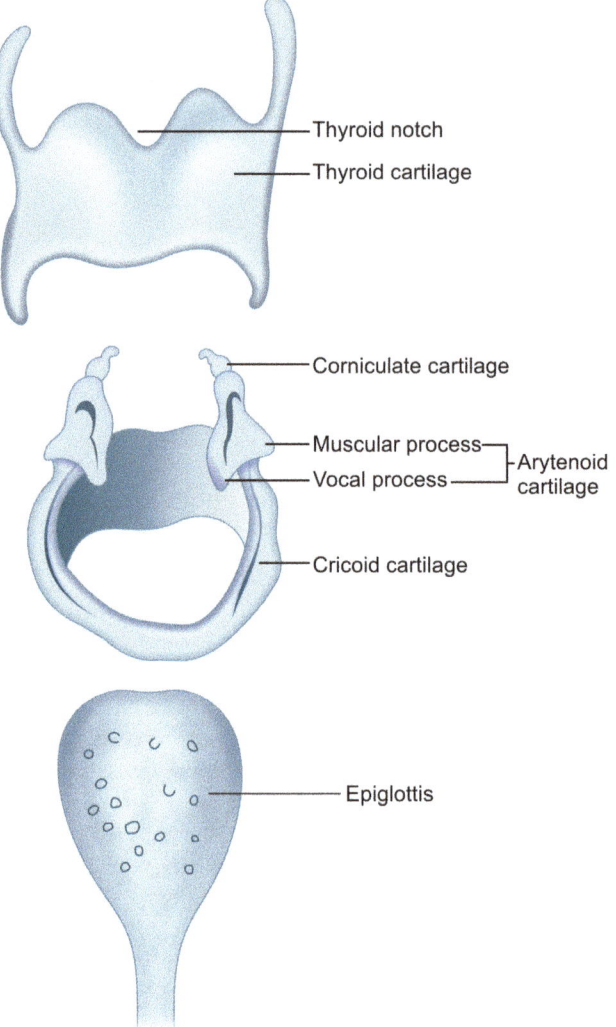

Fig. 3 Cartilages of the larynx

is called Rima glottis. It continues approximately 1 cm caudally.

Subglottis

It starts at the lower end of the glottis and continues till inferior border of the cricoid cartilage.[3]

LARYNGEAL CARTILAGES

Larynx is a framework of cartilages. It has three unpaired and three paired cartilages (Fig. 3). A brief description is given below:

Unpaired Cartilages

Thyroid

Thyroid is the largest laryngeal cartilage. It is made up of two rectangular laminae which are fused in midline anteriorly and forms a laryngeal prominence which is also called as Adam's apple. Thyroid notch is formed superiorly by meeting of the two laminae. The angle between the two thyroid laminae is more acute in males causing a more prominent Adam's apple. The angle is 90° in males and 120° in females. The superior cornu of thyroid cartilage articulates with greater horn of the hyoid bone. Superior tubercle is the prominence on the cartilage at the junction between superior cornu and thyroid lamina. Superior laryngeal artery and vein pierce the thyrohyoid membrane 1 cm above the superior tubercle. Oblique line on the thyroid lamina has insertions of sternothyroid and sternohyoid muscles. Inferior constrictor is inserted slightly posteriorly on the edge of the thyroid lamina.

In thyroplasty, vertical levels of vocal cords in relation to external landmarks of thyroid cartilage are very important. The vocal fold is more toward the lower border of the thyroid lamina not at its midpoint. The window is made about 3 mm from the lower border of the thyroid cartilage. So, window placement should be at proper site to avoid medialization of the false vocal folds or ventricles.[4]

Cricoid

This is a complete ring of cartilage at level of C6. Its shape resembles a signet ring. It articulates with inferior cornua of thyroid over facets of cricothyroid (CT) joint. Inferiorly, it is attached with first tracheal ring. The posterior arch is broader than anterior arch and superiorly articulate with the arytenoid cartilages. There is a marked difference in the vertical height of anterior and posterior arch which forms the gap between thyroid cartilage and cricoid arch anteriorly in which CT membrane lies.

Sellick's maneuver[5] is used to prevent aspiration. It consists of putting pressure over the cricoid which is able to press the esophagus as cricoid is a complete ring.

A cadaveric study by Rajan et al. reported that there is wide range of racial variations in inner AP and transverse diameter, and this is half in Indians as compared with European, Nigerian, and German population. It has clinical significance regarding the size of endotracheal tube use for intubation.[6]

Epiglottis

Epiglottis is the feather-shaped structure which is made from fibroelastic cartilage. It is attached inferiorly to the thyroid cartilage just above the anterior commissure through thyroepiglottic ligament. Its anterosuperior attachment to the hyoid bone is through hyoepiglottic ligament. The aryepiglottic fold attaches the epiglottis to the arytenoid cartilages. The attachment to the base of tongue is through lateral and median glossoepiglottic fold. The epiglottis helps to prevent aspiration during swallowing. The laryngeal part of epiglottis is perforated with multiple holes, so epiglottis has little or no resistance to the tumor invasion.

Paired Cartilages

Arytenoids

Arytenoids are paired cartilages and pyramidal in shape. Posteroinferiorly, it articulates with the cricoid cartilage at cricoarytenoid joint. The shape is pyramidal type with a vocal process medially and a muscular process laterally. There are three surfaces, a base, and apex. The apex of the arytenoid articulates with the corniculate cartilage. The base articulates with the upper border of the cricoid lamina.

Accessary Cartilages: Cuneiform and Corniculate

Cuneiform are *also* called cartilages of Santorini which articulate with apices of arytenoid cartilage. The cuneiform cartilages are also known as cartilages of Wrisberg and are placed in the margin of the aryepiglottic fold. Both these cartilages provide extra structural support to the aryepiglottic fold.

LARYNGEAL LIGAMENTS

Extrinsic Ligaments

These are connecting ligament between laryngeal cartilages with hyoid bone and trachea.

Thyrohyoid Membrane

This lies between hyoid bone superiorly and upper border of thyroid cartilage inferiorly. It is made of fibroelastic

tissue and medial part is called medial thyrohyoid ligament while the posterior part is called the lateral thyrohyoid ligament. The superior laryngeal arteries and nerves pass through the lateral thyrohyoid ligament. There is often a small nodule in the ligament called cartilage triticea. The membrane helps in upward movement of the larynx during swallowing. A triticeal cartilage (cartilage triticea) is located in the thyrohyoid membrane. This cartilage is calcifying frequently and mimics a foreign body on plain radiographic films.

Hyoepiglottic Ligament

This connects epiglottic anterior surface to the upper body of the hyoid bone.

Cricotracheal Ligament

This forms connection between cricoid cartilage and first ring of trachea.

Intrinsic Ligaments

These form connection between different cartilages of the laryngeal framework. They strengthen the inside of the framework by forming broadsheet of the fibroelastic tissue lying under the mucus membrane.

Conus Elasticus or Triangular Membrane

It is also cricovocal ligament or CT ligament. This is fibroelastic and provides support for glottis and subglottis.[4] The free upper border constitutes the vocal ligament and the framework of the vocal cord. It is attached below to the upper border of the cricoid cartilage and extends to inferior border of the thyroid cartilage anteriorly and behind to the vocal processes of the arytenoid. It is in continuation with the CT membrane in anterior part.

It consists of two parts: (1) laterally it forms lateral CT ligament and also called as cricovocal membrane, and (2) anteriorly it forms the anterior CT ligament. The entire structure with fibers of both parts is also called conus elasticus.

Just lateral to the median CT ligament, there is a gap where paraglottic space is in continuation with the extralaryngeal tissue. This is a likely route of extralaryngeal spread of laryngeal cancer.

Quadrangular Membrane

This forms the support of the upper part of the larynx.[4] The upper quadrilateral membrane extends between border of epiglottis and the arytenoid. The upper margin forms the framework of the aryepiglottic inlet while the lower margin is thickened to form the vestibular ligament. It also forms the medial limit of the paraglottic space.

LARYNGEAL MUSCULATURE

Intrinsic Laryngeal Muscles

These are very important as they not only affect the position and shape of vocal cords but also the tension. These are classified as adductor muscles, abductor muscles, and tensor muscles.

Adductor Muscles

Thyroarytenoid muscles (TA): Origin is from lower half of the angle of the thyroid cartilage and middle CT ligament. TA is responsible for most of the bulk of the true cords. It is a broad muscle with two bellies: (1) externus and (2) internus. The externus (lateral portion) extends from anterior commissure to lateral surface of arytenoid. The internus (medial portion) arises from anterior commissure and attached to vocal process of arytenoid, parallel to the vocal ligament and is also called vocalis muscle. The lateral portion forms the main bulk and thus the true cord (Fig. 4).

To the radiologist, this muscle is important because it is the landmark for the level of true vocal fold.

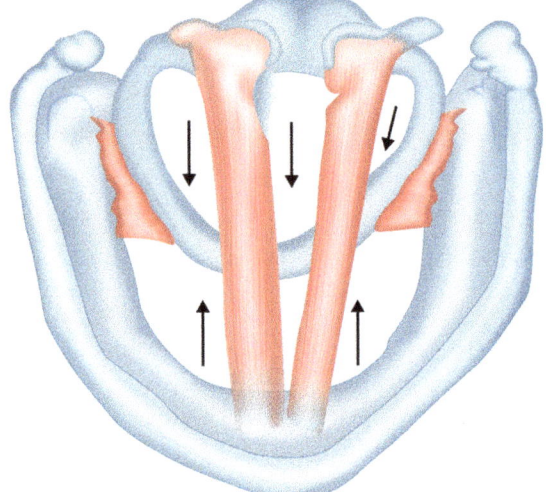

Fig. 4 Action of thyroarytenoid muscle

Lateral cricoarytenoid (LCA): This is paired laryngeal muscle extend laterally from the arch of the cricoid to insert onto the muscular process of the arytenoid cartilage medially. It is lateral and parallel to the TA muscle. Contraction in this muscle results the downward and medial movement of vocal process with anterolateral movement of muscular process.

Therefore, it causes the adduction and lengthening of the vocal fold (Fig. 5).

Interarytenoid muscle: This is unpaired muscle. It consists of oblique and transverse fibers. The transverse fibers are horizontal in direction and attached on posterior face of the arytenoid. The oblique fibers extends from the apex to the face of opposite arytenoids.

The functions of this muscle are arytenoids adduction, narrowing of laryngeal inlet, and closure of posterior glottis (Fig. 6).

Abductor Muscle

Posterior cricoarytenoid (PCA) muscle: PCA muscle is the only muscle with function to open the glottis aperture. Origin is from lower surface of the back of the cricoid lamina and inserts into the back of the muscular process of the arytenoid cartilage of the ipsilateral side. PCA muscle has two separate muscle bellies namely—(1) medially, the horizontal belly and (2) laterally, the vertical belly. There is slight difference in

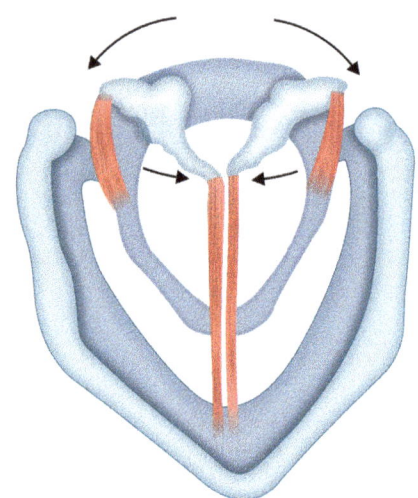

Fig. 5 Action of lateral cricoarytenoid muscle

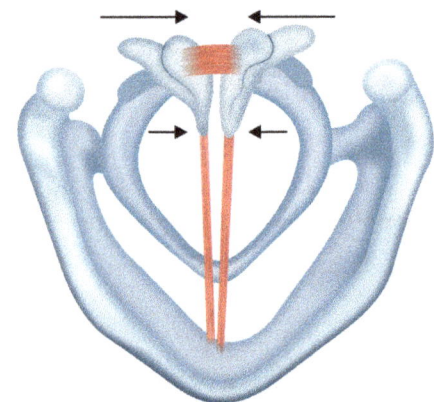

Fig. 6 Action of transverse arytenoid muscle—abduction of vocal folds

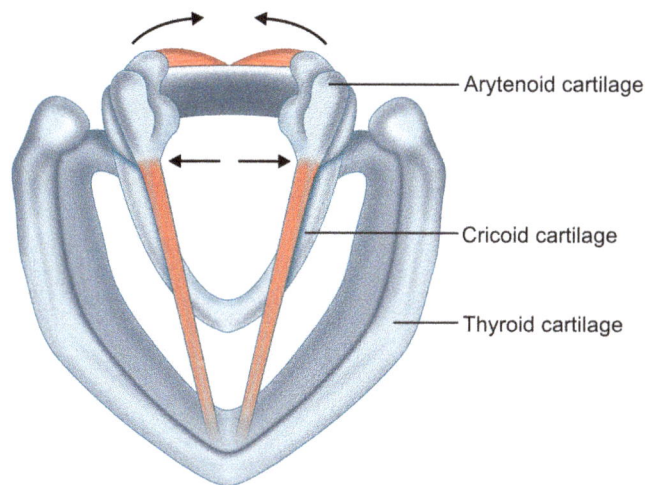

Fig. 7 Action of posterior cricoarytenoid muscle—abduction of vocal folds

Arytenoid cartilage

Cricoid cartilage

Thyroid cartilage

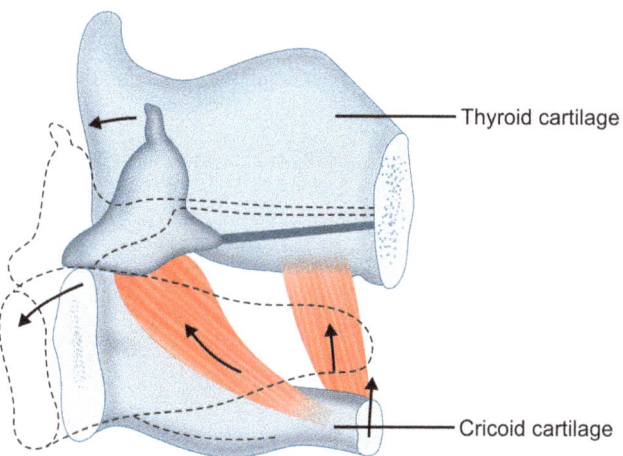

Fig. 8 Action of cricothyroid muscle—tension (lengthening) of vocal folds

Thyroid cartilage

Cricoid cartilage

position, orientation, and contraction of these bellies which results in motion of cricoarytenoid joint motion in different oblique axis (Fig. 7).

The horizontal action causes rotation of arytenoids and draws the muscular process of two sides towards each other. The vertical fibers causes the arytenoids to move down the slope of cricoid cartilage hence separating the arytenoids from each other.

Tensor Muscle

Cricothyroid muscle: The origin is from lateral surface of the anterior arch of the cricoid. There are two types of fibers namely—(1) the anterior vertical ones which insert into inferior border of the thyroid cartilage and (2) the lower oblique ones which go obliquely and backwards to insert into lower border of the thyroid lamina. This is the only intrinsic muscle of the larynx which is supplied by external branch of superior laryngeal nerve (SLN). This muscle affects the movement at the CT joint. The contraction of CT muscle also causes increase in length and tension of the vocal cords. Hence in type 4 thyroplasty, an attempt is made to simulate the action of CT muscle and increase the pitch of voice (Fig. 8).

Extrinsic Laryngeal Muscles

These are divided as suprahyoid and infrahyoid.

The infrahyoid muscles are:
- *Thyrohyoid:* It elevates larynx if hyoid is fixed
- *Sternothyroid:* It depresses the larynx
- *Sternohyoid:* It depresses the larynx
- Omohyoid.

Main role of infrahyoid muscle is to oppose the action of suprahyoid muscles in elevating the larynx.

The suprahyoid muscles are:
- Geniohyoid
- Stylohyoid
- Digastric
- Stylopharyngeus
- Palatopharyngeus
- Salpingopharyngeus
- Suprahyoid muscle.
  The main action is to elevate the larynx.

LARYNGEAL JOINTS

Cricothyroid Joint

It is the articulation of inferior cornu of thyroid cartilage with the facets of cricoid lamina. It is a synovial type of joint. The AP sliding and rotation of the inferior thyroid cornu over cricoid is the action at this joint. Manipulation of the joint can be helpful to control the pitch in paralytic dysphonia cases (Fig. 9).

During medialization procedures, the subluxation at this joint can aids and provide vocal fold tightening.

Cricoarytenoid Joint

This is the multiaxial joint between cricoid and arytenoid at the angle of 45° with horizontal plane. It forms the primary moving structure of the intrinsic larynx and allows the sliding, rocking, and twisting motions. Its movement changes the distance between two vocal process and between vocal process and anterior commissure (Fig. 10).

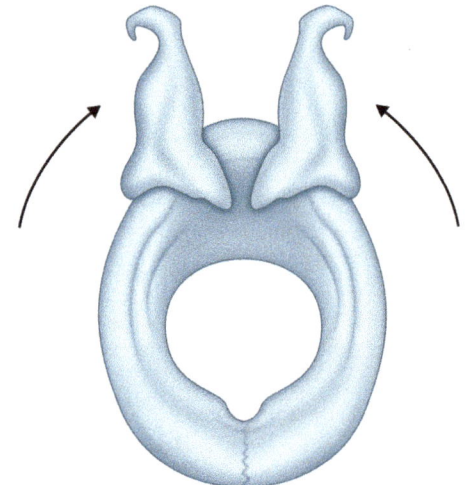

Fig. 9 Cricoarytenoid joint—adduction movement

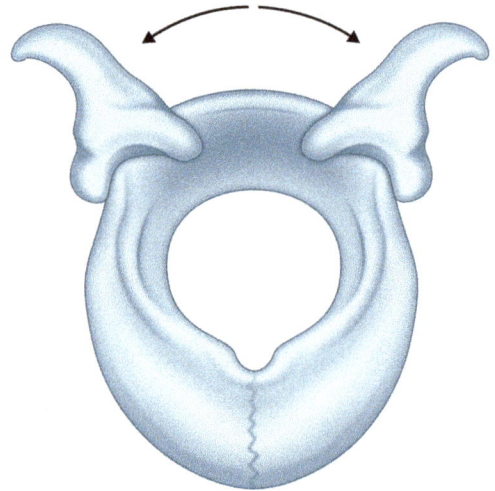

Fig. 10 Cricoarytenoid joint—abduction movement

LARYNGEAL INNERVATION

Superior Laryngeal Nerve

Superior laryngeal nerve (SLN) arises from the inferior vagal ganglion and divides into an internal and external branch. The internal branch goes through the thyrohyoid to enter the laryngeal lumen (Fig. 11).

The *internal branch* is further divided into three branches supplying:
1. Epiglottis mucosa and part of anterior vallecular
2. Aryepiglottic folds
3. Interarytenoid muscles.[7]

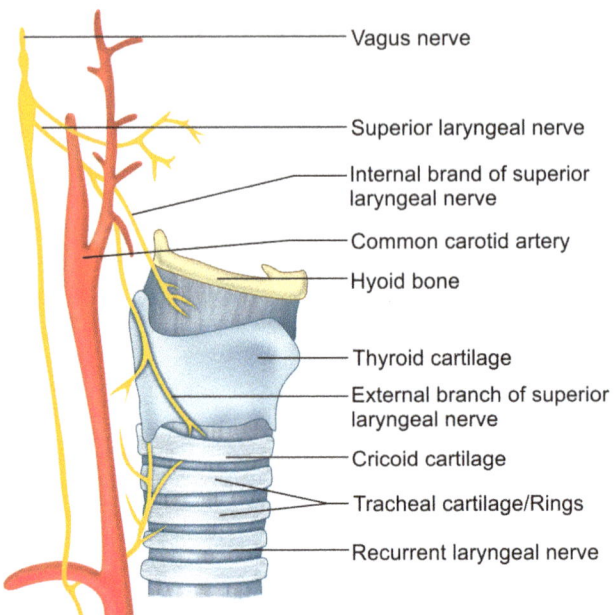

Fig. 11 Anatomy of superior laryngeal nerve

The internal branch is responsible for the laryngeal cough reflex and is prone to injury during conservational laryngeal surgeries. It can be preserved by identifying it in the viscerovertebral angle medial to the carotid bifurcation.[8]

The *external branch* of the SLN (EBSLN, also called *Galli-Curci* nerve) goes more superficially along the inferior constrictor muscle and superior thyroid artery. It then curves anteromedially near the inferior thyroid cartilage edge to pierce the CT muscle. This nerve lies in the triangle which is bounded on the side by the superior thyroid vessels, medially by the midline and superiorly by the attachment of the strap muscles and deep fascia to the hyoid bone. The relation between the superior thyroid pole and the EBSLN is of paramount importance during tying of superior laryngeal vessels in thyroid surgery.[9] There are four types of relationships of the nerve with superior thyroid vessels and superior thyroid pole.
1. *Type 1*: Nerve crosses the superior thyroid vessels at least 1 cm above the superior thyroid pole.
2. *Type 2a*: Nerve crosses the superior thyroid vessels within 1 cm of the superior thyroid pole.
3. *Type 2b*: Nerve crosses the superior thyroid vessels below of the superior thyroid pole.
4. *Type Ni*: EBSLN not identified (subfascial/intramuscular course)

The maximum chance of nerve injury is with the type 2b configuration owing to the course of the nerve behind the thyroid.

Recurrent Laryngeal Nerve

The recurrent laryngeal nerve (RLN) takes origin from vagus nerve in the thorax and goes up in tracheoesophageal groove before entering the voice box. Right-sided RLN runs a more oblique path while left-sided nerve runs in a vertical direction. There can also be a variable relationship of RLN with inferior thyroid artery (ITA) with nerve lying behind, in front or between branches of the ITA. The difference in the paths of the right and left RLNs and also their different surrounding relations hold importance during thyroidectomies and especially in cases of thyroid malignancies with neck nodes. The left RLN is being juxtaposed over the esophagus directly, results in no nodes being present between the nerve and the esophagus, however, because the right RLN is more obliquely placed, the paraesophageal gutter can be involved with nodes leading to more extensive dissection and thereby placing the right RLN at a higher risk of injury. The RLN can have extralaryngeal branching proximal to the nerve's entry into the larynx in approximately 50% of cases, therefore it is imperative to identify full course of the nerve in the neck during anterior neck procedures such as thyroidectomies or conservational laryngeal surgeries. In a majority of situations, the nerve bifurcates approximately 2–3 cm proximal to the CT joint.

The location of bifurcation can be classified as follows:
- Arterial—at or just adjacent to the ITA-RLN crossing.
- Postarterial—between the ITA-RLN crossing and laryngeal entry.
- Prearterial—proximal to the ITA-RLN crossing.[10]

The anterior branch is considered to carry the motor fibers and the posterior branch carries the sensory fibers. In a minority of cases, the nerve can trifurcate or produce multiple branches proximal to its laryngeal entry.

The RLN provides motor supply to all the intrinsic laryngeal muscles except the CT; however, a recent study has showed CT muscle innervation by the RLN also.[11] The RLN also provides sensory supply to the glottis and subglottic mucosa.

Nonrecurrent Laryngeal Nerve

The right-sided non-RLN (NRLN) is more common. There is an association with abnormal right subclavian artery running behind the esophagus, in this situation the inferior laryngeal nerve does not get pulled down during embryogenesis, therefore remaining nonrecurrent.[12]

The NRLN can be classified according to its course:[13]
- Type 1—NRLN arises high in the neck from the tenth nerve along with superior thyroid vessels

- Type 2A—NRLN arises a little below than type 1 but stays horizontal and parallel to the course of ITA
- Type 2B—NRLN arises at the same level as in type 2A but has a more ascending path and stays inferior to ITA.

Galen's Anastomosis

This is the anastomosis between inferior laryngeal branch of RLN and internal laryngeal branch of SLN.

Human Communicating Nerve

This is a small twig that originates from the external branch of the SLN and anastomoses with the RLN. It mainly remains intralaryngeal but can be present as an extralaryngeal variant.

Different Laryngeal Nerve Blocks

Superior Laryngeal Nerve Block

The SLN block is a useful technique for awake endotracheal intubation and increases patient comfort with inhibition of coughing and laryngospasm.[14] It is local infiltration of lidocaine in the piriform fossa via just anteroinferior to the greater cornu of the hyoid beneath which it pierces the thyrohyoid membrane.

An alternative method can be used when the hyoid bone is difficult to locate. In this technique, needle is inserted along the superior border of thyroid cartilage through thyrohyoid membrane where the anterior one-third meets the posterior two-thirds. This is comparatively safe method.[15]

Recurrent Laryngeal Nerve Block

The RLN is the motor nerve of all intrinsic laryngeal muscles except CT. It also gives sensory supply to mucosa of larynx. These nerves should never be directly anesthetized as it may induce a closed glottis and an airway emergency. However, the sensory function of these nerves can be blocked by infiltrating LA through the CT membrane upon which cough is induced and the spray is dispersed in the larynx.

Position of the Larynx and Its Clinical Implications

Framework of the larynx is suspended behind by the constrictor muscles and is suspended anteriorly by the hyoid and mandible with their related muscles.

In infants, the thyrohyoid membrane is short in vertical dimension and therefore the thyroid notch is positioned just behind or just below the hyoid bone. Thus, a laryngeal release procedure does not cause swallowing difficulties or aspiration in children.

The cervical trachea also has a variable length which changes with age. There are about 10 tracheal rings above the sternal notch in infants whereas in the elderly they get reduced to six or less.[16]

The laryngeal position also varies with age, with it being higher up at the level of third or fourth cervical vertebra in infants. It starts descending down after the age of 2 years reaching the sixth or seventh cervical vertebra by adulthood.[17] Also, the epiglottis tip stays at or just posterior to the soft palate in infants, explaining the ability to suckle and breathe simultaneously. It also explains why infants are obligatory nasal breathers.

The infant larynx is differing from adult larynx in many ways:[17]
- Thyrohyoid membrane in the infant is of less length than adult and the thyroid notch is positioned just behind the hyoid
- In adults, the thyroid cartilage is well formed and shaped sharply while in children it is round
- Infant arytenoid cartilages makes up for more than half of the AP glottis till 3 years of age. In adults, it is one-fifth of the total glottis
- In newborns, 60% of the inner subglottic diameter is represented by the interarytenoid distance
- Cuneiform cartilages are of relatively bigger size in infants and there is no direct connection with the arytenoid cartilages
- Laryngeal mucosa in children and infants is laxer and more likely to swell up with any injury or trauma
- During open surgery on laryngotracheal framework, e.g. laryngofissure or cricotracheal resection the thyrohyoid membrane should be cut along the thyroid cartilage's upper border
- As the larynx is round-shaped getting the anterior commissure splitting incision exactly through anterior commissure is difficult. Hence, a vertical incision should be given through epiglottis especially when the anatomy is further deformed, e.g. in a case of web
- Endotracheal intubation is more likely to injure arytenoids and cricoid in a child because of different anatomy as described above[18]
- During laser vaporization in laryngomalacia along with mucosa part of cuneiform cartilage should also be removed
- Children are more likely to have postoperative edema in the glottis and subglottis. Hence, postoperative intubation is required after one stage laryngotracheal reconstruction.[19]

REFERENCES

1. Henry Gray. Anatomy of the Human Body. Philadelphia: Lea & Febiger; 1918.
2. Mor N, Blitzer A. Functional anatomy and oncologic barriers of the larynx. Otolaryngol Clin N Am. 2015;48:533-45.
3. Cooper H. Anatomy of the larynx. In: Blitzer A, Brin MF, Ramig LO (Eds). Neurologic disorders of the larynx. New York: Thieme Publishers; 2009. p. 3.
4. Rosen CA, Simpson B. Anatomy and physiology of larynx. Operative Techniques in laryngology. Verlag Berlin Heidelberg: Springer; 2008. XXVI, p. 312.
5. Ovassapian A, Salem MR. Sellick's maneuver: to do or not do. Anesth Analg. 2009;109(5):1360-2.
6. Singla RK, Kaur R, Laxmi V. Morphology and morphometry of adult human cricoid cartilage. A cadaveric study in North Indian population. Int J Anat Res. 2015;3(1):910-14.
7. Kiray A, Naderi S, Ergur I, et al. Surgical anatomy of the internal branch of the superior laryngeal nerve. Eur Spine J. 2006;15(9):1320-5.
8. El-Guindy A, Abdel AM. Superior laryngeal nerve preservation in peri-apical surgery by mobilization of the viscerovertebral angle. J Laryngol Otol. 2000;114(4):268-73.
9. Cernea CR, Ferraz AR, Nishio S, et al. Surgical Anatomy of the External Branch of the Superior Laryngeal Nerve. Head & Neck. 1992;14(5):380-3.
10. Cetin F, Gürleyik E, Dogan S. Morphology and Functional Anatomy of the Recurrent Laryngeal Nerve with Extralaryngeal Terminal Bifurcation. Anat Res Int. 2016;2016:9503170.
11. Henry BM, Vikse J, Graves MJ, et al. Extra laryngeal branching of the recurrent laryngeal nerve: a meta-analysis of 28,387 nerves. Langenbecks Arch Surg. 2016;401:913-23.
12. Kamani D, Potenza AS, Cernea CR, et al. The nonrecurrent laryngeal nerve: anatomic and electrophysiologic algorithm for reliable identification. Laryngoscope. 2015;125(2):503-8.
13. Toniato A, Mazzarotto R, Piotto A, et al. Identification of the non-recurrent laryngeal nerve during thyroid surgery: 20-year experience. World J Surg. 2004;28:659-61.
14. Monso A, Riudeubàs J, Palanques F, et al. A new application for superior laryngeal nerve block: treatment or prevention of laryngospasm and stridor. Reg Anesth Pain Med. 1999;24:186-7.
15. Thomas JL. Awake intubation. indications, techniques and e review of 25 patients. Anaesthesia. 1969;24:28-35.
16. Grillo H.C. Anatomy of the trachea. In: Grillo HC (Ed). Surgery of the trachea and bronchi. BC Decker Incorporation, Hamilton: London; 2004. pp. 40-59.
17. Hollinger LD, Lusk RP, Green CG. Pediatric Laryngology and bronchoesophagoscopy. Philadelphia, New York: Lippincott-Raven; 1997. pp. 1-17.
18. Benjamin B, Hollinger LD. Laryngeal complications of endotracheal intubation. Ann Otol Rhinol Laryngol. 2008;117:2-20.
19. Williams PL, Bannister LH. Gray's Anatomy- The anatomical basis of medicine and surgery. New York: Churchill-Livingstone; 1995.

Voice Evaluation

KK Handa, Karan Aggarwal

INTRODUCTION

Voice is produced not only by vibrations from vocal cords but also by contributions from the lower airway and the oropharyngeal resonance systems. Voice evaluation helps laryngologists to document the status of not only the vocal cords but also the status of the voice generators, i.e. lungs which are the bellows and the resonators. It helps to characterize the type and severity of the voice disorder. It also helps to correlate voice quality and findings on stroboscopy. All these test measures help to capture pitch, loudness, and quality which are basic parameters in voice evaluation.

Voice is the acoustic output from the vocal tract that depends on vibrations of the vocal cord.[1] Dysphonia is impaired voice while aphonia is the absent voice.[2] Phonation means how the voice is produced. Impaired phonation can have either rough voice or noisy voice.

Adequate energy is also needed to produce a good quality voice. Other factors contributing to quality of voice include good functioning of the vibratory units, i.e. vocal folds and the resonance centers, i.e. supraglottic and oropharyngeal airway.

PROBLEMS IN VOICE EVALUATION

Visual assessment in all cases of impaired voice remains mandatory. Assumptions that acoustic analysis and other measures may obviate the need for visual assessment have not been possible. The best assessment is by endoscopic visualization and it cannot be replaced by any parameter of voice evaluation. Different workers have tried to standardize measurement and assessment protocols for voice testing.[3-5]

VOICE TEST BATTERY

Commonly following measures are used to assess voice are:
- Visual assessment
- Patient scales and quality-of-life measures
- Acoustic measurements
- Electrolaryngography or electroglottography
- Perceptual evaluation of voice
- Aerodynamic measures
- Tests of vocal loading
- Combined measures.

VOICE MATERIAL

Sustained vowels have been traditional favorites in the voice measurement for the following reasons:
- Vowels are simplest separable speech components
- Parameters such as loudness, pitch, timber, etc. can be controlled easily
- Stable mid-portion of the sustained vowel is independent of language[6,7]
- Easy to measure.

Fluent speech is also being used commonly as:
- It is more relevant to patient's day-to-day use.
- More in tune with normal voice production and also to listener's comprehension of the speaker voice.

VOICE TESTING IN DETAIL

Visual Assessment

Stroboscopy

Today stroboscopy is one of the standard and accepted methods of assessing voice. It is used to study the vibration of the vocal cord and also behavior of the free-edge of the vocal fold. Synchronized light flashes are generated from a strobe light source. These are synchronized with vibration of vocal cords to produce illusion of slow motion or standstill of the vocal cords. This flashing light is used through a flexible scope or a rigid scope to assess the full vibration cycle of the vocal folds.

The advantages of stroboscopy are:
- Assessment of the free-edge of vocal fold
- Image of the vocal fold and of the present lesion
- Real-time assessment of the nature of the vibration.

Mechanism of stroboscopy: According to Talbot's law, if any image is presented to human retina it stays on the retina for 0.2 second more. If successive images are presented to the retina less than 0.2 second apart they give illusion of a continuous image which can be either shown as slow motion or standstill.

Strobe light produces intermittent light flashes close to vocal cord frequency of vibration. Patient's voice is picked by a microphone and which in turn triggers the strobe source of light. A flash of light with frequency same as vocal cord produces a standstill image of the vocal cord. However, if the frequency of the flash is slightly different from that of the vocal fold it causes an illusion of slow motion. In reality, stroboscopy produces a pattern which is an average of few cycles.

Instrumentation for stroboscopy: A stroboscope unit (Fig. 1) consists of:
- Strobe light source
- Video camera
- Microphone
- Printer
- Rigid or flexible laryngoscope can be used to perform stroboscopy.

Strobe evaluation can be objectivized despite some clinician bias. Stroboscopic signs are associated with different lesions and can be given a score. Stroboscopy is able to subtly assess the free vocal cord edge, abnormalities of structure, vibratory parameters including pliability of vocal fold after surgery.

Different parameters evaluated in stroboscopy:[8]
- Fundamental frequency (F_0)
- *Periodicity*: It refers to how regular successive vocal vibratory cycles.

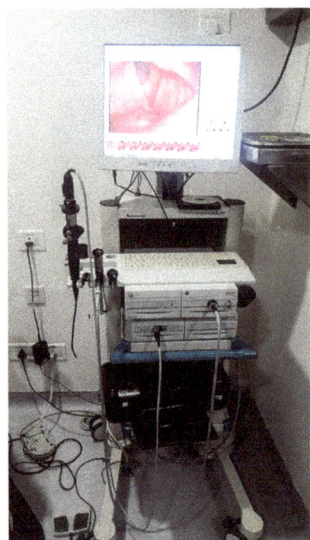

Fig. 1 Modern video stroboscope (make XION) being used in our department consisting of a strobe light source, microphone, camera, telescope, capture software, monitor and a printer

- *Amplitude*: It refers to the lateral excursion of the vocal folds during their movement away from the midline during vibration. It is graded as:
  - Normal
  - Below normal
  - More than normal.
- *Symmetry*: This pertains to comparing movements of the two sides
- *Glottic closure*: This is the measurement of the glottic chink or phonatory gap
- *Mucosal wave*: This is the wave-like motion of the vibrating layer of the vocal fold. Mucosal wave presence and interpretation of its motion is one of the most important parameters during stroboscopy (Figs 2 to 5).

Limitations of stroboscopy:
- Inter- and intrajudge variation
- It is an optical illusion
- Assumption that vocal fold vibrations are always stable and regular which is not always true
- Cannot assess voice breaks and vocal tremors
- Cannot assess suitably diplophonia and very rough voice
- Sources of voice production other than vocal cords.

However, this limitation has been overcome by use of digital high-speed video camera technology[9] that can produce color images at high rates, i.e. 4,000 images/second.

Videokymography

Many pathological conditions are not adequately diagnosed by stroboscopy as it is based on periodic voice. It is not useful in vocal tremor, diplophonia, voice breaks, and short vocal

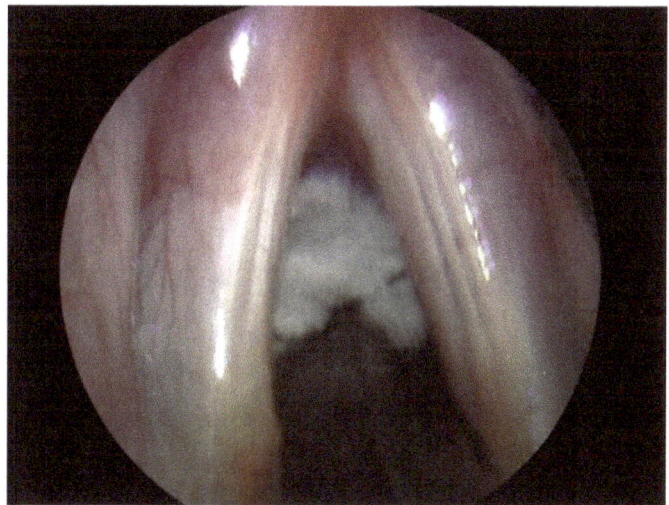

Fig. 2 Sulcus vocalis

gestures. Assessment of voice cannot be adequately done by stroboscopy when the performer is changing vocal register as going from falsetto-to-modal voice. These shortcomings of stroboscopy lead to description of kymography for the first time in clinical practice by Schutte 1998.[10]

It is a line-scan imaging digital technique which has proven to be an efficient way for studying high-speed assessment of the vocal fold vibratory patterns. Two different modes can be used during videokymography:
1. High speed (8,000 images/sec)
2. Standard (50 images/sec).

Both normal and videokymographic images are recorded and displayed. It displays the pattern of vocal cord vibration in one image that summarizes all the vibratory cycles at the line of interest. It is possible by videokymography to trace vocal cord vibration in very hoarse and very breathy voice which may not be possible by stroboscopy. By being able to see

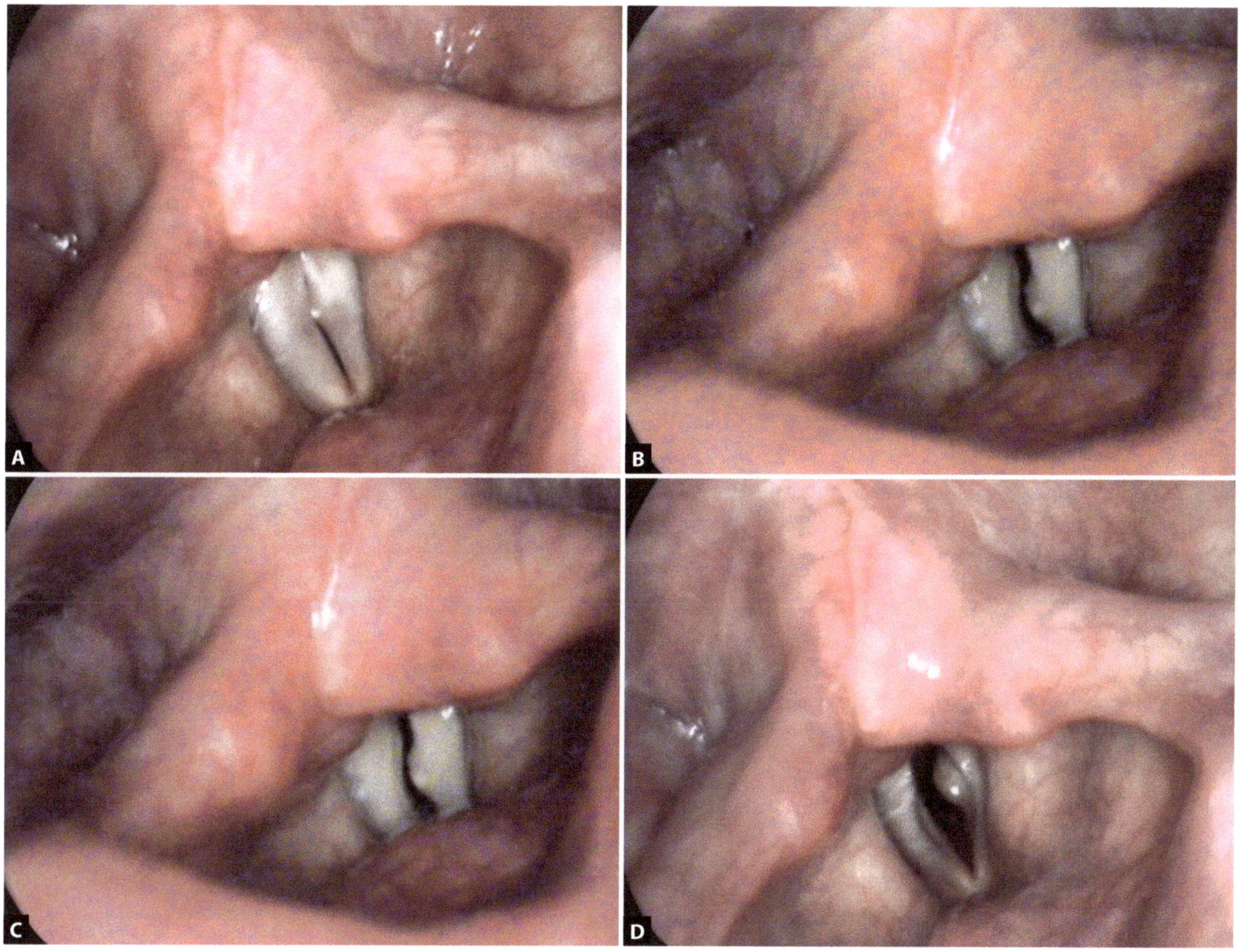

Figs 3A to D Mucus retention cyst of vocal cord in different phases of stroboscopy

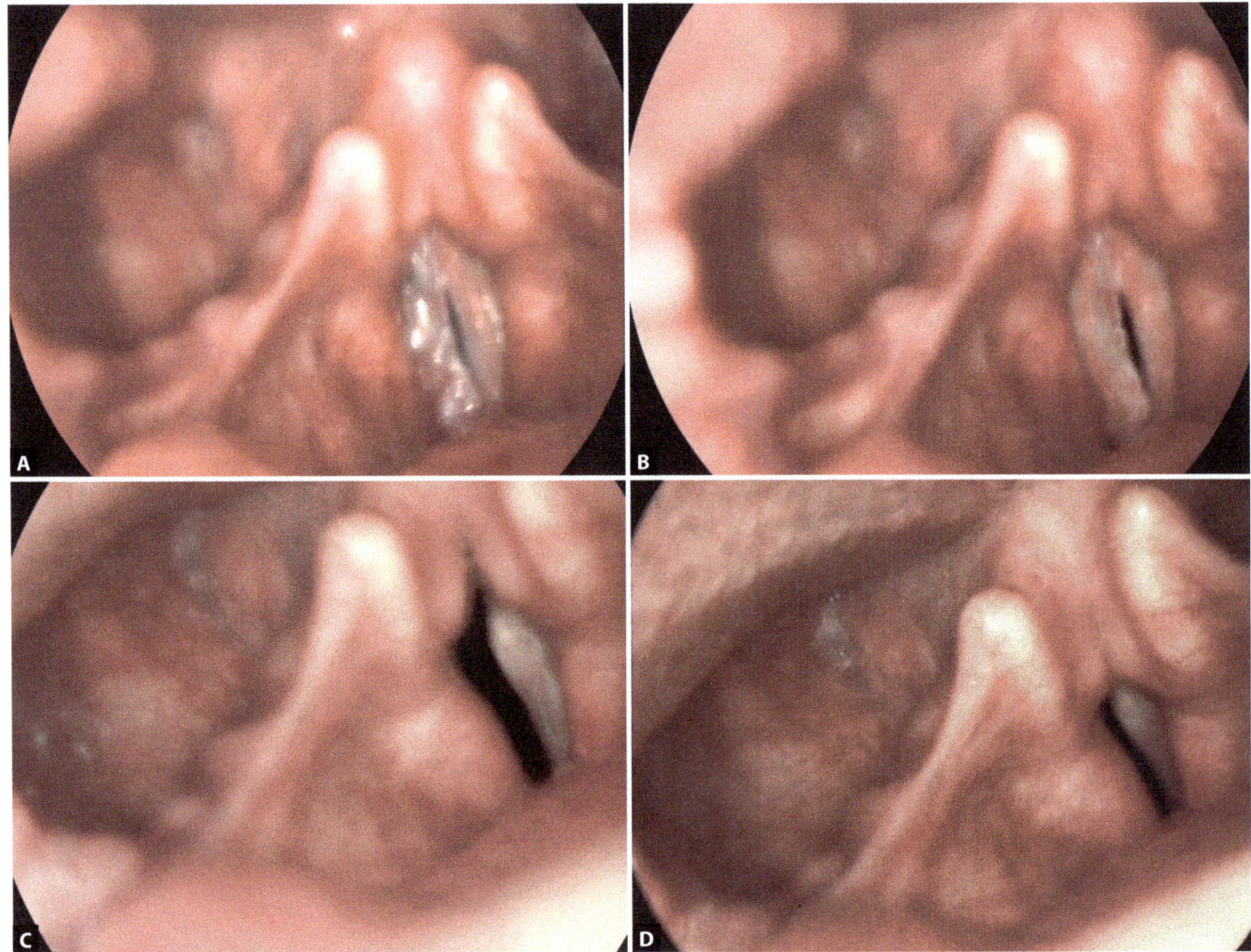

Figs 4A to D Early cancer larynx; stroboscopic images before and after transoral laser resection

every glottal cycle during phonation much more information may be obtained than by stroboscopy. However, some workers established that the two modalities stroboscopy and videokymography are complementary.[11]

Kymography[10] can help in:
- Studying symmetries between the two sides
- Mucosal waves properties
- Movement of the margins of the vocal folds.

High-speed Digital Imaging

High-speed digital imaging[12] is a new technology which enables the recording and study of the detailed vocal fold movements (frame rate up to 2,000 frames/sec) by using slow motion play back and frame-by-frame analyzing tools. Furthermore, it allows capturing and studying of the actual

aperiodic vocal fold vibrations, as those in patients of hoarseness.

The first report was by Hirose and coworkers.[13] This was not an advanced system and was limited to 100 × 100 pixels with poor resolution. The first commercially available system became available in 2000. It had 256 × 256 pixel resolution (black and white). However today the standard is 512 × 512 pixel advanced color system. It allows taking of unlimited pictures of vibrating vocal cords to be clicked every second. A maximum of 4,000 images can be taken per second and even a periodic movement of the vocal folds can also be picked up. The limitation of high-speed digital laryngoscopy is that the image size is reduced when frame rate increases because of technological limitation and it is solved by keeping the sampling frequency so that the image size will not be too small for analysis.

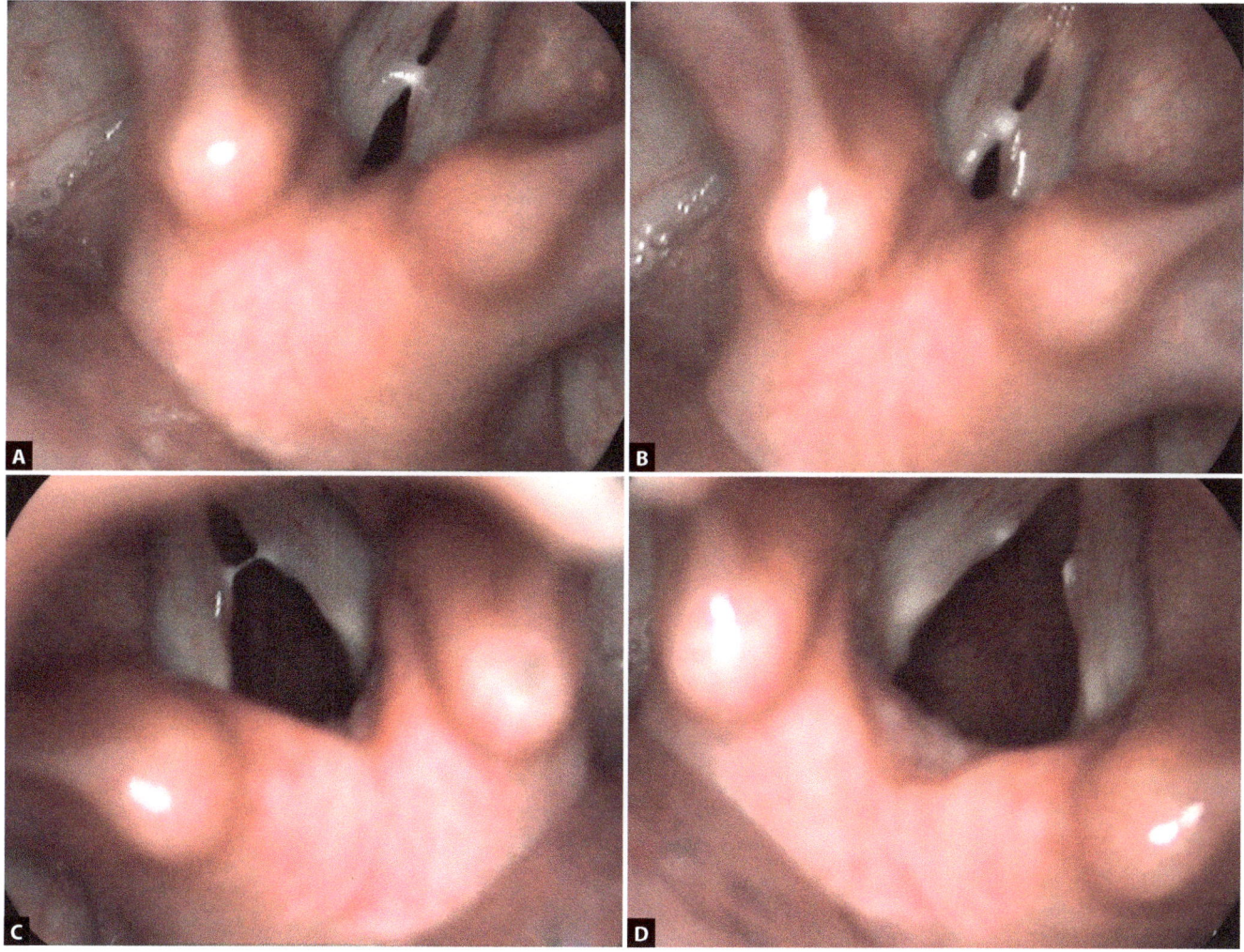

Figs 5A to D Vocal cord nodules seen with the strobe

It is mainly of advantage in two areas, i.e. variation of phonation with loudness and frequency changes and also in assessment of voice breaks and diplophonia.

Laryngeal Electromyography

It has been used as diagnostic tool since 1970. The first time report was in a thesis in 1958.[14] Standard laryngeal electromyography (EMG) tests thyroarytenoid and cricothyroid muscles of both sides.

Some clinical applications of laryngeal EMG are:

- Differentiate cricoarytenoid joint paralysis from vocal cord paralysis
- Assess whether paralyzed vocal cord function is going to return
- Botox injection in spasmodic dysphonia
- Differentiate myopathy from neuropathy
- Differentiate upper neuron lesions from lower motor neuron lesions in motor neuron disease

- Functional voice disorders.
  Interpretation of laryngeal EMG involves looking at:
- Denervation potentials
- Reinnervation potentials including polyphasic and giant potentials
- Irritability because of insertion.

Patient Scales

These are questionnaires completes by the patient or sometimes by the caregiver. These quantify patient satisfaction, life quality, general health, handicap or loss as result of the voice disorder.

- *Voice handicap index*: This scale assesses handicap, i.e. a social, economic or environmental disadvantage resulting from an impairment or a disability. It has 30 statements which patients rate at a 5-point equal appearing interval scale. The total possible score is 120 with higher scores depicting greater handicap.[15] It has been widely used to show voice handicap in specific groups of patients, comparisons between handicap and vocal function measures, and change with treatment.

- *Voice-related quality of life*:
  - It comprises of 10-points divided into physical functioning and social-emotional functioning subscales.
  - Each item is scored on a 5-point interval scale that depicts the severity of the disorder.
  - 100 is the highest possible score and reflects the best quality of life.[16]
- *Other scales include*:
  - Voice symptom scale (VoiSS)[17]
  - Voice activity and participation profile (VAPP)[18]
  - Reflux symptom index (RSI)[19]
  - Patient questionnaire of vocal performance (VPQ)[20]
  - Voice outcome survey (VOS).[21]

Perceptual Evaluation of Voice (Flow chart 1)

Auditory-perceptual Evaluation

Several scales have been used for auditory-perceptual evaluation. Two of the most commonly used have been described here:

1. *GRBAS*: It was developed by the Committee for Phonatory Function of the Japanese Society of Logopedics and Phoniatrics.[22,23] The "G" represents grade or overall quality, "R" for roughness, "B" for breathiness, "A" for asthenia, "S" for strain. Each parameter is rated on a 4-point scale:
   - 0: There is no deficit
   - 1: Mild deficit
   - 2: Moderate deficit
   - 3: Severe deficit.
2. *CAPE-V*: (Consensus Auditory-perceptual Evaluation of Voice Scale) was developed by the American Speech Language Hearing Association. Six core and other examiner selected parameters are evaluated on a visual analog scale. The clinician uses a tick mark to rate function on a 100 mm line and then measures distance from the left end of the line to establish a score; higher scores reveal a more deviation from the normal values. The CAPE-V is to be scored from two sustained vowels,

six standard sentences and at least 20 seconds of running speech.[24]

Some other aspects of speech production are:

- *Resonance*: It can either be hypernasal or hyponasal or cul-de sac.
- *Prosody*: This is the rate, repeated or prolonged syllables, rushes of speech, intonation and stress patterns.

Visual Perceptual Evaluation

It includes the following:
- General appearance factors
- Body posture and position, breathing and tension of muscles
- Any dysfunction of neurological system
- Any systemic disease.

Tactile Perceptual Evaluation

The manual examination of laryngeal musculoskeletal tension includes palpation of the suprahyoid group of muscles, hyoid bone, thyroid cartilage (cornu and lateral aspects), thyrohyoid space and the anterior border of the sternocleidomastoid muscle. It is useful to assess muscle tension both at rest and during phonation. Findings indicative of excessive musculoskeletal tension include:

- Excessive pain on palpation
- Decrease or absence of thyrohyoid space at rest or with phonation
- Muscle knots
- High carriage of the hyoid bone and thyroid cartilage
- Difficulty in rotating the larynx.

ACOUSTIC AND ELECTROLARYNGO-GRAPHIC VOICE EVALUATION

Fundamental Frequency (F_0)

Acoustic waveform produced by vocal fold vibrations can be considered as a series of sine waves. Fundamental frequency refers to lowest frequency of these sine waves.

The rate of change of the amplitude of the harmonic in accordance with the increase in frequency is known as spectral slope.

- *Microphones*: A good quality of microphone is must for correct measurements of the acoustic parameters. A quality microphone should have a minimum sensitivity of -60 dB. Reasonably flat frequency response across the range of human hearing frequency. The amplified signal is then recorded and analyzed by voice software.[25,26]

Flow chart 1 Auditory, visual and tactile perceptual evaluation

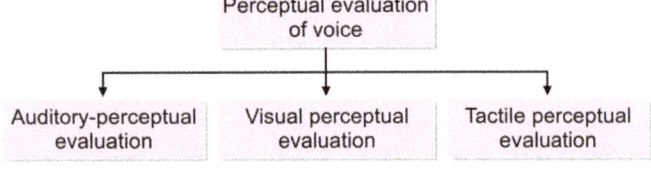

- *Electrolaryngograph*: Here two electrodes are placed on both sides of the thyroid cartilage. Current at a constant voltage is given and the changes in conductance when vocal folds vibrate are picked up. This signal is not affected by vocal cord resonance and is an accurate measure of fundamental frequency.[27]

AERODYNAMIC MEASURES

Measurements of airflow and pressure can provide precise and objective indicators of vocal function. The airflow exiting the mouth and nose can be directly and easily measured using a facemask, usually in terms of liters per second.

- *Mean phonatory flow rate*: It has been one of the easier, traditional measures to collect and is also the most common parameter to be reported in the literature. It is usually measured by a pneumotachograph, mounted on a full-face mask. Measurement is done during sustained phonation of a vowel. It is higher in cases of glottis incompetence and lower in cases of increased laryngeal resistance. The pneumotachograph measures airflow by calculating pressure decrease across a known resistance.[28] A yet another method of measuring airflow is by the use of hot-wire anemometry; it has a high-frequency response but does not measure actual volume.

- *Glottal airflow*: Airflow at the glottis can be measured by using a Rothenburg mask. This mask is circumferentially vented with multiple holes covered by fine wire mesh and uses a high frequency differential pressure transducer to measure airflow from the mouth and nose. The resultant waveform represents rapid airflow changes at the level of the glottis.[29]

- *Airflow open quotient*: Tells the time glottis aperture stays open as compared to full cycle of vocal fold vibration. It is useful in cases of incompetence or increases resistance.[30]

- *Maximum flow declination rate*: Its utility is in defining hyperfunctional and hypofunctional vocal states. It would be predictably low in cases of hypofunctional states because of the disability in completely closing the vocal folds and high in hyperfunctional states due to an increase in subglottal pressure and greater vibrational amplitudes.[31]

- *Peak glottal airflow*: It relates to the maximum glottal area during vocal fold vibration. Increase stiffness, decreased mucosal wave or any other pathological condition which restricts maximum displacement of the vocal folds, can alter this measurement.[32]

- *Alternating glottal airflow*: With increase stiffness of the vocal folds, this measurement typically decreases.

- *Minimal glottal airflow*: Indicator about the completeness of glottis closure by measuring airflow during the closed phase of vibratory cycle.[33]

- *Subglottal pressure*: It is difficult to measure directly as direct measurement would require a tracheal puncture. Thus, it is estimated by measuring intraoral pressure. It is assumed that subglottal and intraoral pressures are the same when the lips are sealed to form the consonant "P".[34]

- *Laryngeal resistance*: It is subglottal pressure divided by the mean phonatory flow rate. It reflects the actual physical function of the larynx. It is low in cases of glottal incompetence and high in cases of glottal strain.[35]

REFERENCES

1. Titze IR. Principles of voice production. Prentice Hall: Englewood Cliffs, New Jersey, 1994.
2. Mathieson L. Voice disorders: presentation and classification. In: Mathieson L (Ed). The voice and its disorders. London: Whurr Publishers; 2001. pp. 121-44.
3. Dejonckere PH, Bradley P, Clemente P, et al. A basic protocol for functional assessment of voice pathology, especially for investigating the efficacy of (phonosurgical) treatments and evaluating new assessment techniques. Guideline elaborated by the Committee on Phoniatrics of the European Laryngological Society (ELS). Eur Arch Otorhinolaryngol. 2001;258:77-82.
4. Dejonckere PH. Clinical implementation of a multidimensional basic protocol for assessing functional results of voice therapy. A preliminary study. Rev Laryngol Otol Rhinol. 2000;121:311-3.
5. Titze IR. Workshop on acoustic analysis: Summary statement. Iowa: National Centre for Voice and Speech, University of Iowa, 1995.
6. Scherer RC, Gould WJ, Titze IR, et al. Preliminary evaluation of selected acoustic and glottographic measures for phonatory analysis. J Voice. 1988;2:230-44.
7. Scherer RC, Vail VJ, Guo CG. Required number of tokens to determine representative voice perturbation values. J Speech Hearing Res. 1987;30:529-38.
8. Echternach M, Arndt S, Zander MF, et al. Voice diagnostics in professional sopranos: application of the protocol of the European Laryngological Society (ELS). HNO. 2009;57(3):266-72.
9. Schutte HK, Svec JG, Sram F. First results of clinical application of videokymography. Laryngoscope. 1998;108(1):1206-10.
10. Svec J, Schutte H. Videokymography: High-speed line scanning of vocal fold vibration. J Voice. 1996;10:201-5.
11. Kim DY, Kim LS, Kim KH, et al. Videostrobokymographic analysis of benign vocal fold lesions. Acta Otolaryngol. 2003;123(9):1102-9.
12. Wong, Nga-Kei. High speed digital imaging—the difference of vocal fold vibration between modal, falsetto, vocal fry registers and whisper. A dissertation submitted in partial fulfillment of the requirements for the Bachelor of Science (Speech and Hearing Sciences), The University of Hong Kong, 2004.
13. Hirose H. High speed digital imaging of vocal fold vibration. Acta Otolaryngol Suppl. 1988;458:151-3.
14. Anderson KF, Edfeldt AW. Electromyography of intrinsic and extrinsic laryngeal muscles during silent speech: correlation with reading activity. Acta Otolaryngol. 1958;49(6):478-2.

15. Jacobson GH, Johnson A, Grywalski C, et al. The voice handicap index (VHI): development and validation. Am J Speech Lang Pathol. 1997;6:66.

16. Hogikyan ND, Sethuraman G. Validation of an instrument to measure voice related quality of life (V-QOL). J Voice. 1999;13:557.

17. Deary IJ, Wilson JA, Carding PN, et al. VoiSS: a patient-derived voice symptom scale. J Psychosom Res. 2003;54(5):483-9.

18. Ma EP, Yiu EM. Voice activity and participation profile: Assessing the impact of voice disorders on daily activities. J Speech Lang Hear Res. 2001;44(3):511-24.

19. Belafsky PC, Postma GN, Koufman JA. Validity and reliability of the reflux symptom index (RSI). J Voice. 2002;16(2):274-7.

20. Deary IJ, Webb A, Mackenzie K, et al. Short, self-report voice symptom scales: psychometric characteristics of the voice handicap index-10 and the vocal performance questionnaire. Otolaryngol Head Neck Surg. 2004;131(3):232-5.

21. Gliklich RE, Glosky RM, Montgomery WW. Validation of a voice outcome survey for unilateral vocal cord paralysis. Otolaryngol Head Neck Surg. 1999;120(2):153-8.

22. Dejonckere PH, Remacle M, Fresnel-Elbaz E, et al. Differentiated perceptual evaluation of pathological voice quality: Reliability and correlations with acoustic measurements. Rev Laryngol Otol Rhinol. 1996;117:219-24.

23. De Bodt MS, Wuyts FL, Van de Heyning PH, et al. Test-retest study of the GRBAS scale: Influence of experience and professional background on perceptual rating of voice quality. J Voice. 1997;11:74-80.

24. Consensus Auditory-Perceptual Evaluation of Voice (CAPE-V) ASHA special interest division 3. Voice and its disorders (2003). Available from *www.asha.org/NR/rdonlyres/C6E5F616-972F-445A-AA40-7936BB49FCS3/0/ CAPEVprocedures.pdf.* Accessed May 2007.

25. Price DB, Sataloff RT. Technical note: A simple technique for consistent microphone placement in voice recording. J Voice. 1996;2:206-7.

26. Dejonckere PH, Bradley PJ, Clement P, et al. A basic protocol for functional assessment of voice pathology, especially for investigating the efficacy of (phonosurgical) treatment and evaluating new assessment techniques. Eur Arch Otorhinolaryngol. 2001;258:77-82.

27. Scherer RC, Drucker DG, Titze IR. Electroglottography and direct measurement of vocal fold contact area. In: Fujimura O (Ed). Vocal physiology: voice production, mechanisms and functions. New York: Raven Press, 1988.pp.279-91.

28. Prathanee B, Watthanathon J, Ruangjirachporn P. Phonation time, phonation volume and air flow rate in normal adults. J Med Assoc Thai. 1994;77(12):639-45.

29. Holmberg EB, Hillman RE, Perkell JS. Glottal airflow and transglottal air measurements for male and female speakers in soft, normal, and loud voice. J Acoust Soc Am. 1988;84(2):511-29.

30. Sapienza CM, Stathopoulos ET, Dromey C. Approximations of open-quotient and speed-quotient from glottal airflow and ECG waveforms: effects of measurement criteria and sound pressure level. J Voice. 1998;12(1):31-43.

31. Titze I. Theoretical analysis of maximum flow declination rate versus maximum area declination rate in phonation. J Speech Lang Hear Res. 2006;49(2):439-47.

32. Laukannen AM, Sundberg J. Peak-to-peak glottal airflow amplitude as a function of (F0). J Voice. 2008;22(6):614-21.

33. Jiang JJ, Tao C. The minimum glottal airflow to initiate vocal fold oscillation. J Acoust Soc Am. 2007;121(5):2873-81.

34. Herbst CT, Hess M, Muller F, et al. Glottal Adduction and Subgottal Pressure in Singing. J Voice. 2015;29(4):391-402.

35. Rieves AL, Hoffman MR, Jiang JJ. Indirect estimation of laryngeal resistance via airflow redirection. Ann Otol Rhinol Laryngol. 2009;118(2):124-30.

3

Imaging of Benign Laryngeal Pathology: Expanding Horizons

Smita Manchanda, Ashu Seith Bhalla

INTRODUCTION

Imaging plays a key supplementary role in the management of laryngeal pathology. It has a role primarily in determining the extent of disease and relation to the other anatomical structures. In addition, the distal airway may not be visualized in certain cases of complete obstruction due to tumors or stenosis. Multidetector computed tomography (MDCT) with its multiplanar reconstruction capabilities has a key role to play in these cases for anatomical delineation of the distal structures. The submucosal diseases are another subgroup where imaging, especially magnetic resonance imaging (MRI) is immensely useful.

IMAGING TECHNIQUES IN THE STUDY OF THE LARYNX

Plain Radiographs

Plain radiographs have a limited role, predominantly in the evaluation of pediatric airway. In young children presenting with stridor, frontal, and lateral radiographs of the soft tissues of neck are useful to look for foreign body. In addition, diagnosis such as epiglottitis and laryngotracheobronchitis[1] can be made, and immediate treatment initiated.

Ultrasonography

Ultrasonography (USG) is a complementary imaging technique for the evaluation of laryngeal pathology.[2] It can provide detailed information about laryngeal structures and the anatomical relationship of masses.

The false vocal folds are hyperechoic due to the presence of fibro-fatty tissues. The true vocal folds appear as bilateral triangular hypoechoic structures and their vibration during phonation can be easily visualized. The thyroid cartilage and the arytenoids are seen as hypoechoic structures, surrounded by an echogenic margin. The adduction–abduction movements of the arytenoids can be easily assessed during deep breathing.[3] The laryngeal landmarks have a key sonographic-appearance and can enable the radiologist to precisely diagnose the level of a lesion. Being a dynamic examination, ultrasound can be performed easily during respiration and phonation, showing the vocal folds in abduction as well as in adduction.

Cystic versus solid nature and internal characterization of any lesion can be easily assessed with USG. In addition, real-time dynamic evaluation can be easily performed. This requires minimal patient cooperation and involves no radiation exposure.[4] However, the inherent limitation of USG is nonavailability of an acoustic window in older patients with calcified cartilages.

Computed Tomography

Computed tomography imaging of the larynx was initially technically challenging. The motion artifacts of respiration, swallowing, and pulsation of the carotid arteries degrade the quality of images and require a high-speed of acquisition. The current MDCT scanners have overcome this problem.[5] These have from 16 to 320 detectors performing acquisition of high-resolution volumes of the neck in a single rotation (volume scanners). CT images can be reconstructed at subcentimeter thickness with soft tissue and bony filters.

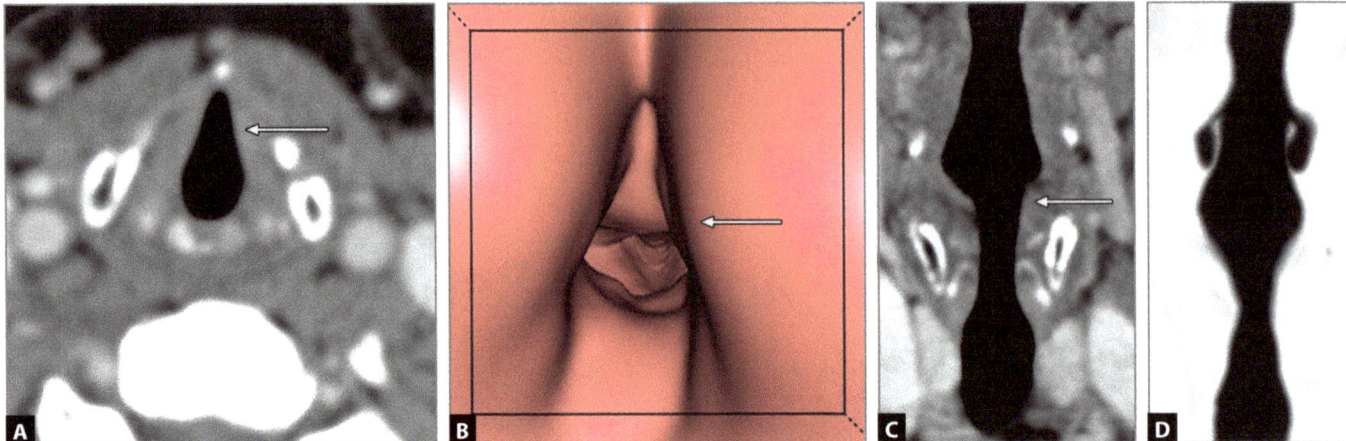

Figs 1A to D Multidetector CT images at the level of glottis. (A) Axial mediastinal window and (B) Virtual laryngoscopy image at the level of normal glottis (arrow); (C) The normal laryngeal air column is well depicted on coronal multiplanar reconstructed image (MPR), and (D) Coronal minimum intensity projection (minIP)

Axial images (Figs 1A to D) are evaluated in both soft tissue and bone window (required for the assessment of laryngeal cartilages and joints). Sagittal and coronal reformatted images and three-dimensional (3D) volume rendered reconstructions provide an excellent overview of the laryngeal anatomy and pathologies. Multiplanar reformatted (MPR) and minimum intensity projection (minIP) images can accurately demonstrate the site, degree and length in cases of stenosis. Virtual laryngoscopy is an exciting new technique, which allows viewing inside or beyond obstructed airways.

Magnetic Resonance Imaging

Magnetic resonance imaging of the larynx involves a multiparameter assessment in the form of T1-weighted, T2-weighted, diffusion-weighted and postcontrast acquisition. Imaging is performed with the neck in a hyperextended position and patients are instructed to breathe quietly and not to swallow. A number of flow compensation techniques like respiratory and cardiac gating and presaturation pulse techniques can be used to reduce motion artifacts.[6]

Acquisitions are obtained in coronal, axial, or sagittal planes and both T1- and T2-weighted sequences are performed, with a slice thickness of 3 mm with no or minimal interslice gap. Postgadolinium administration, 3D imaging is performed by acquisition of thin (1 mm) T1-weighted fat-suppressed images. The inherent superior contrast resolution of MRI provides excellent anatomical details and is useful in localization of pathologies and preoperative staging. However, there are certain limitations to MRI like cost, contraindications (cochlear implant, pacemaker) and poor compliance.

The imaging of benign conditions of larynx is discussed in the subsequent sections under the following headings:
- Laryngeal obstruction in the pediatric age group
- Stenosis (noncongenital)
- Cysts and laryngoceles
- Benign tumors of larynx
- Vocal cord paralysis
- Trauma

LARYNGEAL OBSTRUCTION IN THE PEDIATRIC AGE GROUP

Laryngomalacia

Laryngomalacia is a benign, self-limited condition characterized by abnormal redundancy of supraglottic tissue. It leads to a high-pitched and inspiratory stridor, which exacerbates in the supine position.

There is inferior and medial bowing of the arytenoids, aryepiglottic folds and epiglottis and dilatation of the laryngeal ventricle on fluoroscopy performed during inspiration.[1]

Laryngeal Clefts

Laryngo-tracheo-esophageal cleft (LC) is a rare congenital anomaly characterized by an abnormal, posterior communication between the laryngotracheal axis and the pharyngoesophageal axis. It presents with stridor and repeated aspirations.

Chest radiograph may reveal air space nodules and consolidation secondary to aspiration. Contrast esophagogram reveals tracking of contrast from the upper esophagus into the trachea. CT scan shows an abnormal communication or lack of soft tissue between trachea and esophagus. An abnormal anterior or intratracheal position of a nasogastric tube is also an indirect CT sign of presence of a laryngeal cleft.[1,7]

Congenital Subglottic Stenosis

Congenital subglottic stenosis is a cause of biphasic or inspiratory stridor in infants. The cricoid cartilage is small or malformed, with thickened submucosal layer.

Symmetric, circumferential subglottic narrowing with the typical hourglass-appearance is seen on plain radiograph. There is no phasic change with respiration in the narrowing on fluoroscopy.[1] CT scan is used to assess the location, degree and length of subglottic stenosis.

Multidetector CT has a key role to play in the evaluation of cases of subglottic stenosis (Figs 2A and B). Multiplanar reformats can be made in coronal, sagittal, and curved planes on a 3D workstation using both mediastinal and lung window settings. Thick-slab minIP images are reconstructed using a thickness range of 25–55 cm and viewed in various projections. The parameters assessed include degree, segment length and location of narrowing; distance from the vocal cord and status of the distal airway.[8]

Degree of narrowing is classified by the Myer-Cotton grading system, which divides it into four grades:
- *Grade I:* Luminal narrowing less than 50%
- *Grade II:* Luminal narrowing more than 50% but less than 70%
- *Grade III:* Luminal narrowing more than 70%
- *Grade IV:* No lumen detected.[9]

Segment length of narrowing is graded as:
- *Grade 0:* No narrowing
- *Grade I:* Less than one-third of the involved airway segment
- *Grade II:* One-third to two-thirds of the involved airway segment
- *Grade III:* More than two-thirds of the involved airway segment.

Laryngotracheobronchitis (Croup)

Croup is characterized by the inflammation of the subglottic larynx with occasional involvement of the trachea and bronchi. There is mucosal edema, which impinges upon the airway.

On the frontal radiograph, narrowing of the subglottic airway is seen for 1–2 cm, with loss of the subglottic arch ("wine-bottle" or "steeple-shaped" airway). Inspiratory films show ballooning of the hypopharynx with distension of the cervical trachea in expiration.[1]

Supraglottitis (Epiglottitis)

Epiglottitis or supraglottitis is a potentially fatal condition caused by *Haemophilus influenzae*. Fever, sore throat, drooling, dysphagia and inspiratory stridor are seen in young children (2–6 years) with rapid progression to complete airway obstruction.

Radiographs can be obtained where the clinical examination is equivocal. However, the child should not be restrained for this purpose and additional airway support should always be available. The lateral radiograph reveals thickened epiglottis with increased width of the aryepiglottic folds and arytenoids and ballooning of the hypopharynx.[1]

Ultrasonography can be easily performed at the bedside in suspicious cases.[10] The patient is placed in the sniffing position (head extended and neck flexed). The epiglottis is barely seen through thyrohyoid membrane in normal individuals. In longitudinal view, the swollen epiglottis is seen just by the side of hyoid bone with a hypoechoic halo around it as the "alphabet P-sign". The hyoid bone and its echogenic acoustic shadow form the straight line of the "P" whereas the pre-epiglottic space and the swollen epiglottis form the round of the "P".

STENOSIS (NONCONGENITAL)

Stenosis of the larynx or upper trachea can be iatrogenic or due to trauma. Iatrogenic stenosis occurs after prolonged cuffed tube intubation and starts in the anterior and lateral walls in the subglottic region and trachea. In later stages, the posterior wall is also involved and circumferential stenosis occurs. Structures of the posterior supraglottic larynx are seen characteristically in corrosive ingestion.

Axial CT demonstrates the extent of cross-sectional narrowing of the airway. Soft tissue scars and granulomas are seen as soft tissue thickening interposed between the

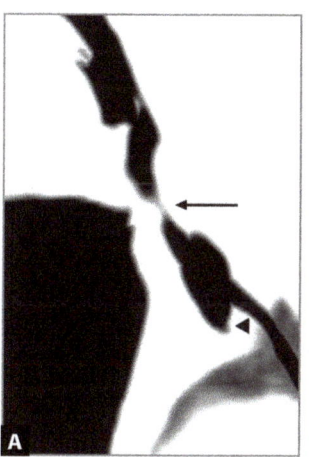 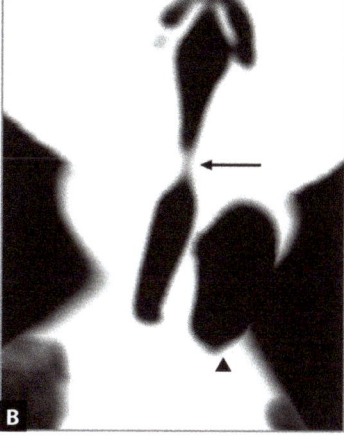

Figs 2A and B Congenital subglottic stenosis. (A) Sagittal; (B) Coronal minimal intensity projection images reveal short segment and circumferential narrowing of the subglottic region (arrow). Note the dilated proximal pouch (arrowhead) in case of associated esophageal atresia with distal tracheoesophageal fistula

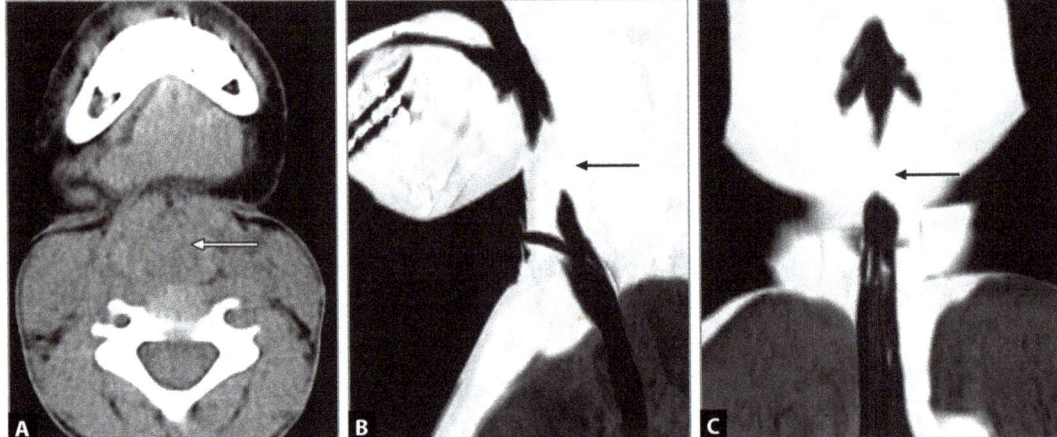

Figs 3A to C Postintubation subglottic stenosis. (A) Axial noncontrast-enhanced computed tomography image reveals complete occlusion of the subglottic airway; (B) Sagittal; (C) Coronal minimal intensity projection images demonstrate the vertical extent of the narrowing (arrow) and status of the distal airways

cartilage and air column. Traumatic displacement of the anterior cricoid causes narrowing of the subglottic area, which gets worsened by scarring.

Coronal and sagittal reformatted images (Figs 3A to C) provide an overview of the vertical extent of stenosis.[8,9] This has been discussed in detail above in the section on congenital subglottic stenosis.

CYSTS AND LARYNGOCELES

Saccule (also known as appendix of the laryngeal ventricle) extends from the ventricle superiorly into the paraglottic region of the supraglottic larynx. Enlargement of the saccule leads to formation of a submucosal mass which is known as saccular cyst. This lesion is also known as laryngocoele when it is air-filled and laryngeal mucocele or saccular cyst if it is fluid-filled.[1]

Etiology

These can result from inflammatory mucosal swelling or due to an obstructing lesion in the ventricle. Imaging and endoscopic evaluation is essential to rule out any underlying malignancy.

Imaging

On cross-sectional imaging (CT and MRI), fluid-filled or air-filled supraglottic lesion (Figs 4A and B) is seen extending through the paraglottic area of false cord to level of ventricle.[5] The margins are smooth and partially surrounded by the supraglottic fat. Thyrohyoid membrane is a key structure to evaluate for extralaryngeal extension in cases of external or mixed laryngoceles. Laryngocele should be differentiated from a normal air-filled ventricular appendix, which does not cause any submucosal deformity of the supraglottic margin.

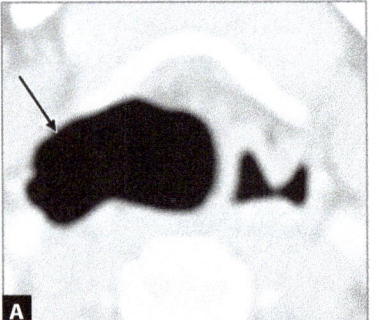
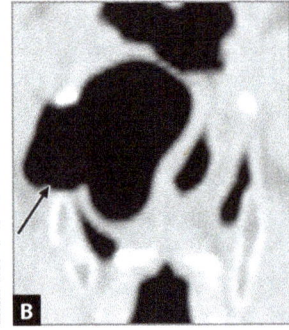

Figs 4A and B Laryngocele. (A) Axial and (B) coronal CT images reveal a large air-filled supraglottic lesion with extension through the thyrohyoid membrane (arrow) suggestive of mixed laryngocele

BENIGN TUMORS OR MASS LESIONS OF LARYNX

The following are the benign tumors of larynx.[1] Most of the lesions have nonspecific imaging appearances and are histopathological diagnosis.

Vocal Cord Nodule

These are soft tissue nodules seen between the anterior and middle third of the true cord usually in singers or teachers. On imaging, seen as small soft tissue projections along the margin of the cord bilaterally.

Vocal Cord Polyp

The most common benign neoplasm usually seen in males in the fourth decade. These are usually unilateral and larger than vocal cord nodules but difficult to differentiate from nodules on imaging.

Recurrent Respiratory Papillomatosis

A benign and self-limiting disease caused by recurrent growth of papillomas as a result of infection of the respiratory tract by human papilloma virus (HPV-6 and HPV-11). Usually limited to the larynx, multiple papillomas may also be seen in the nasopharynx and tracheobronchial tree.

Papillomas are seen on CT as multiple, small soft tissue density nodules in the true and false vocal cords, subglottis, and laryngeal surface of the epiglottis.[11]

Chest radiographs reveal multiple pulmonary nodules, few of which may show cavitation. CT chest shows the presence of multiple, well-defined nodules of varying sizes predominantly in the lung bases (Figs 5A to C). Cavitating nodules usually have thick walls and presence of air-fluid level. Nodules within the tracheobronchial tree are seen as polypoidal soft tissue masses with intraluminal projection. Complications include malignant degeneration and consolidation and bronchiectasis secondary to infection.[11,12]

Malignant degeneration is more common with tracheobronchial dissemination of the disease and has been reported in 1–10% of cases of laryngotracheobronchial papillomatosis.[12] The incidence is more common in smokers and patients treated with radiotherapy or chemotherapy with bleomycin. The imaging morphology is of squamous cell carcinoma of larynx (Fig. 5A) and lung as is seen in nonsyndromic cases.

Benign Nonepithelial or Mesenchymal Tumors

Benign nonepithelial or mesenchymal tumors include lipomas, hemangiomas, neural tumors, paragangliomas, leiomyomas, rhabdomyomas and chondromas.
- *Lipomas*: Well-defined lesions with characteristic fat attenuation [-50 to -100 Hounsfield units (HU) value on CT].

- *Hemangioma*: Hemangiomas are seen in the pediatric age group most commonly in the subglottis. There may be associated cutaneous hemangiomas. On plain radiographs (Fig. 6A), subglottic hemangiomas cause smooth and concentric narrowing of the airway, which is usually asymmetric. Lateral radiographs reveal a well-defined soft tissue bulge into the air column.
  On USG, the lesion is echogenic and shows internal color flow on color Doppler evaluation (Figs 6B and C).
  Computed tomography reveals intensely enhancing soft tissue density mass.[1,5] Similar morphology is seen on MRI with lesion appearing hypointense or isointense on T1-weighted image (T1WI) and hyperintense on T2-weighted image (T2WI) with occasional flow voids and intense postgadolinium enhancement.
- *Paragangliomas (glomus tumors)*: These are seen usually in the supraglottis as intensely enhancing submucosal masses on CT (Fig. 7). On MRI, they appear isointense on T1WI and hyperintense with flow voids ("salt and pepper appearance") on T2WI with intense postgadolinium enhancement.
- *Other lesions* like schwannomas (Figs 8A and B) and granular cell tumors are rare submucosal masses with nonspecific imaging findings.

Low-flow Vascular Malformations

Usually in the glottic or supraglottic location, low-flow vascular malformations are usually seen in the adult population. Phleboliths may be seen in *radiographs* of older patients. On *USG*, the lesion comprises of compressible, anechoic channels or spaces with no or minimal venous flow. Thrombosed areas may appear echogenic and give the appearance of a complex solid cystic mass. Mildly enhancing septated cystic lesion is seen on CT. MRI reveals a T1 hypointense and T2 hyperintense lesion with no flow voids and minimal delayed contrast enhancement (Figs 9A to C).

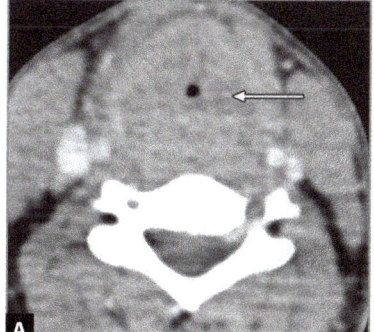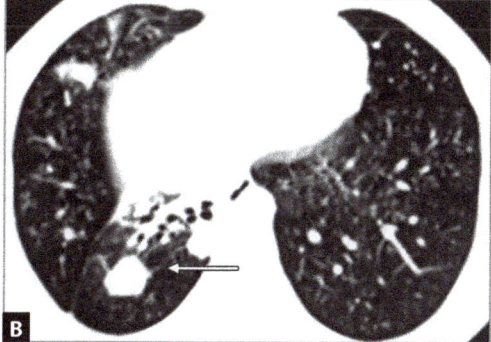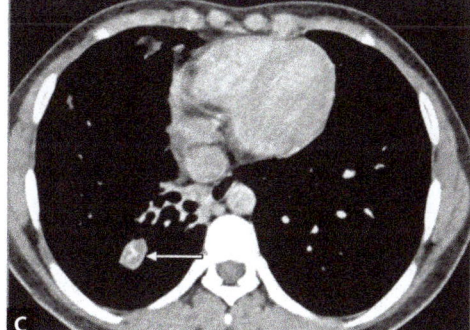

Figs 5A to C Recurrent respiratory papillomatosis (RRP). (A) Axial contrast-enhanced computed tomography (CT) image neck reveals hypoenhancing soft tissue transglottic mass with marked luminal narrowing suggestive of malignancy in a 17-year-old boy with RRP; (B) Axial CT chest lung, and (C) Mediastinal windows show multiple pulmonary nodules, few showing calcification (arrow)

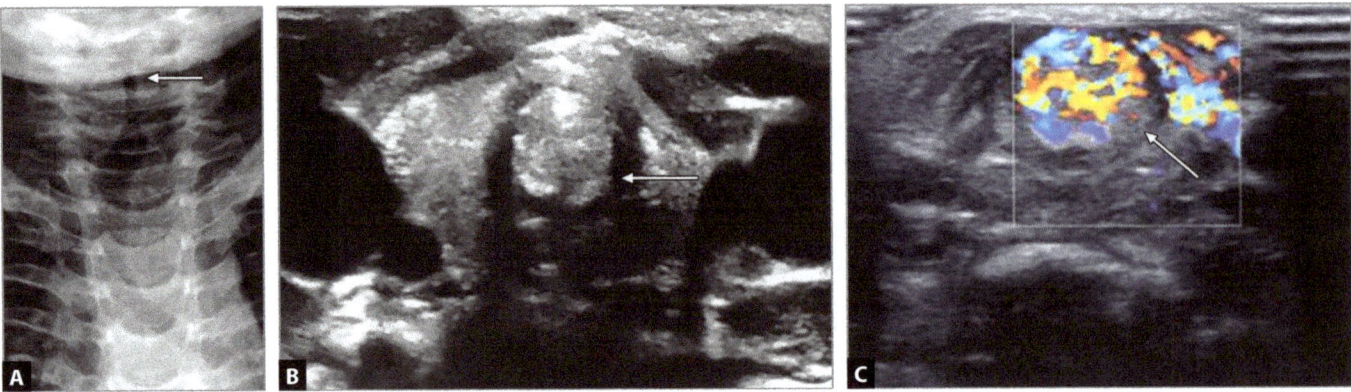

Figs. 6A to C Subglottic hemangioma. (A) Plain radiograph reveals concentric narrowing of the subglottic airway (arrow); (B) Ultrasonography shows an echogenic mass (arrow) causing near occlusion of the air column; (C) Intense vascularity is noted in the color Doppler image (arrow)

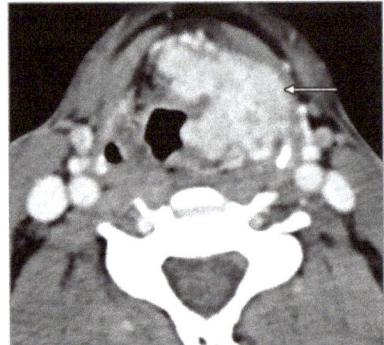

Fig. 7 Submucosal paraganglioma. Axial contrast-enhanced computed tomography image shows a markedly enhancing vascular mass in the pre-epiglottic and left paraglottic space

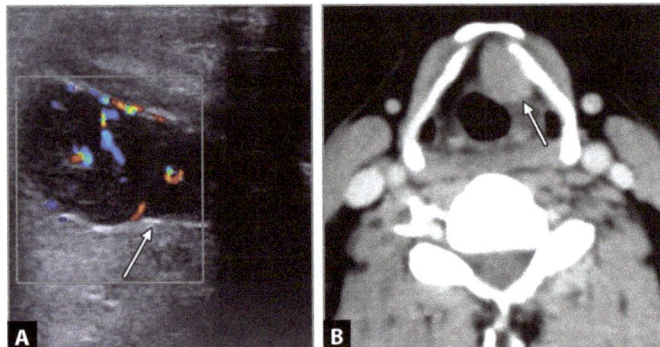

Figs 8A and B Submucosal schwannoma. (A) Axial color Doppler image reveals a well-defined hypoechoic solid mass with internal vascularity; (B) Axial contrast-enhanced computed tomography image shows a mildly enhancing well-defined mass in the left paraglottic space

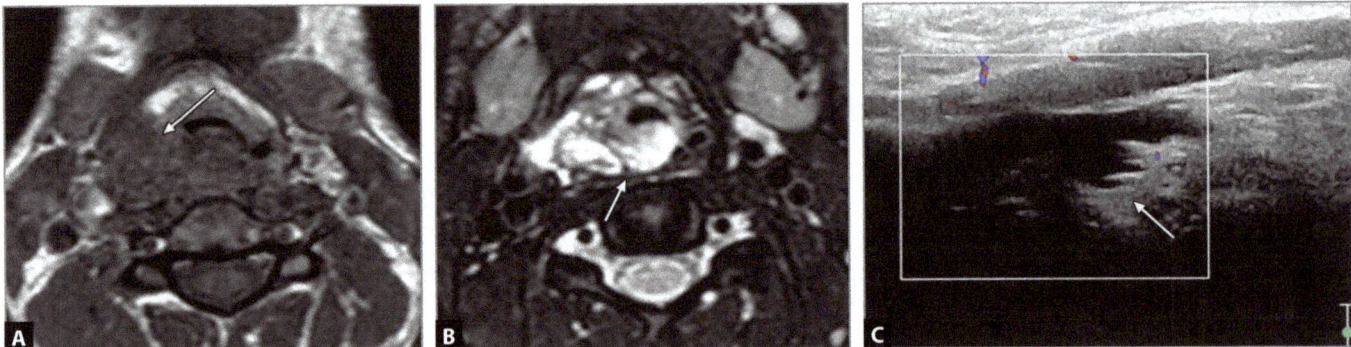

Figs 9A to C Low flow vascular malformation. (A) Axial MRI images T1-weighted image (T1WI) and (B) T2-weighted image (T2WI) reveal a multiloculated infiltrating lesion, predominantly hypointense on T1 and hyperintense on T2WI, involving the right supraglottis with extralaryngeal component; (C) Axial color Doppler image shows the lesion to be predominantly cystic with no internal color flow

VOCAL CORD PARALYSIS

Vocal cord paralysis[13] presents with hoarseness of voice and may be the first sign of pathology elsewhere. It can result from any lesion affecting the course of vagus nerve and its branches.

The recurrent laryngeal nerve (RLN) supplies the intrinsic muscles of larynx except the cricothyroid, which is supplied by the superior laryngeal branch of vagus.

Role of Cross-sectional Imaging (CT and MRI)

Because of the anatomical course of the RLN, the imaging of vocal cord palsy includes scanning from the skull base to below the aortopulmonary window. For evaluation of etiology of right cord palsy, the course of the right RLN from the vagal nerve-subclavian artery intersection to the tracheoesophageal groove should be carefully evaluated. Similarly on the left side, RLN after its origin in the mediastinum, crosses the vagus nerve and loops under the aortic arch to run between the aorta and the left pulmonary artery toward the tracheoesophageal groove. Hence, a careful evaluation of the superior mediastinum till the aortopulmonary window should be performed.

It is important to identify the signs of vocal cord palsy on cross-sectional imaging (CT/MRI). These include:[14,15]
- Dilatation of the ipsilateral laryngeal ventricle (Fig. 10A)
- Medial deviation and thickening of the ipsilateral aryepiglottic fold (Fig. 10B)
- Dilatation of the pyriform sinus
- Anteromedial deviation of the ipsilateral arytenoid cartilage
- Wide ipsilateral vallecula

- "Pointing" of the atrophied cord seen on coronal images as triangular shape and sharp medial margin of the cord in contrast to normal globular configuration (Fig. 10C)
- Flattening of the subglottic arch on coronal images.

The following signs indicate high vagal involvement as a cause of vocal cord palsy.
- Sternocleidomastoid and trapezius atrophy (accessory nerve involvement at the level of skull base)
- Atrophy and ballooning of the middle and inferior constrictors (pharyngeal plexus involvement at the skull base)
- Cricothyroid atrophy and subtle tilting of thyroid cartilage (superior laryngeal nerve involvement).

Etiology

In addition, an attempt should be made to search for the cause of palsy by tracing the course of vagal nerve and its branches.[15] The common etiologies include:
- *Iatrogenic (postoperative)*: Imaging usually not required as the cause is obvious
- *Tumors*: Scan along the course of vagus and RLNs (Figs 11A and B)
- *Vascular*: Aortic or carotid aneurysms, and dilated pulmonary artery (Ortner's cardiovocal syndrome)
- *Medical or inflammatory causes*: Diabetes, viral or infectious diseases (Figs 12A and B), multiple sclerosis, chemotherapy and radiotherapy to the neck
- *Central nervous system*: Infarct (dorsolateral aspect of the bulb), amyotrophic lateral sclerosis.

Role of Ultrasonography

Ultrasound has a key role to play in the evaluation of pediatric vocal cord palsy.[3] Being a safe and noninvasive technique, it

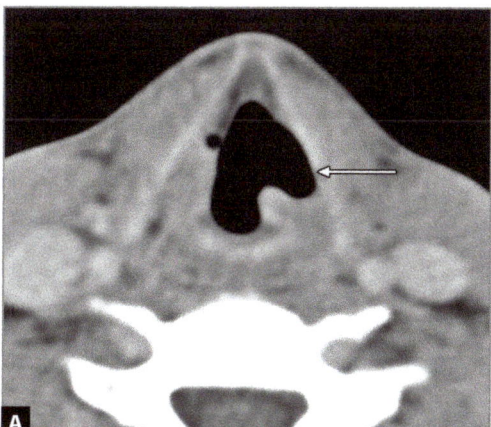 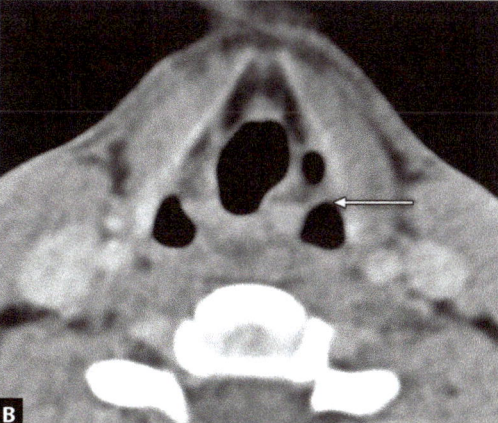 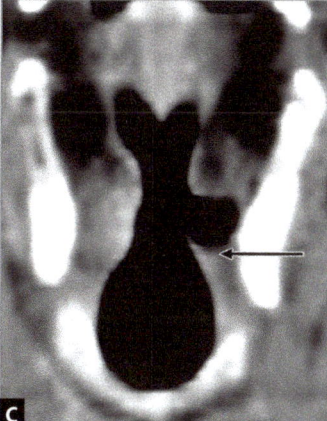

Figs 10A to C Vocal cord palsy (left). (A and B) Axial contrast-enhanced computed tomography image reveal dilatation of the left laryngeal ventricle (arrow in A) and medial deviation and thickening of the left aryepiglottic fold (arrow in B), and (C) "Pointing" of the atrophied cord is well seen on the coronal image as triangular shape and sharp medial margin of the left true cord (arrow)

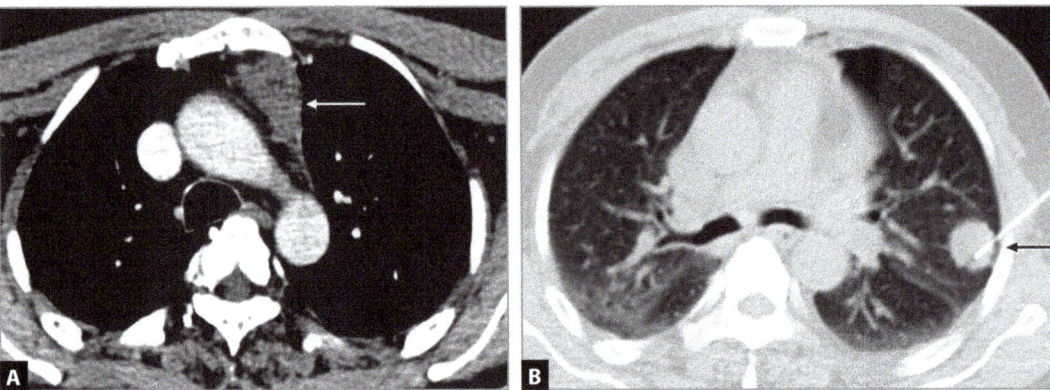

Figs 11A and B Metastatic lymphadenopathy from carcinoma lung causing left vocal cord palsy. (A) Axial contrast-enhanced computed tomography (CT) image mediastinal window reveals lymph nodal mass (arrow) in the prevascular location (the cause of left palsy); (B) CT-guided fine needle aspiration cytology (FNAC) from the lung nodule in left upper lobe revealed poorly differentiated carcinoma (arrow)

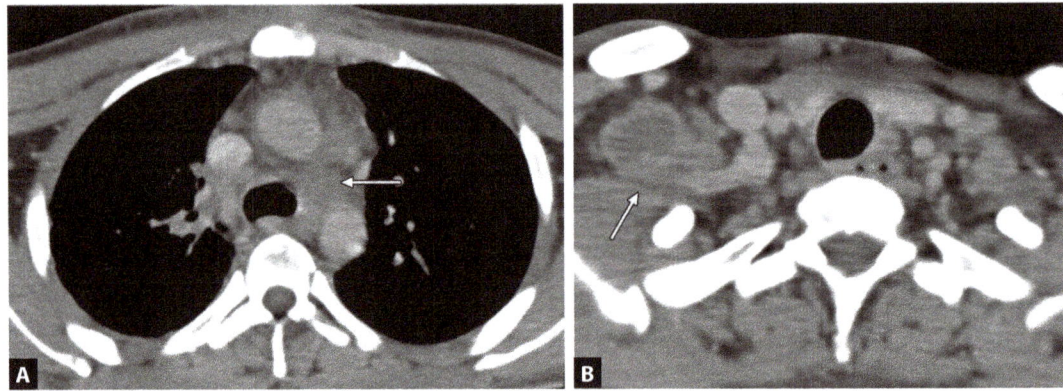

Figs 12A and B Tuberculous lymphadenopathy causing left vocal cord palsy. (A and B) Axial contrast-enhanced computed tomography images reveal necrotic lymph nodes (arrow in A) in the aortopulmonary window (the cause of left palsy) and right supraclavicular location (arrow in B)

is well-tolerated by children and can easily be performed at the bedside.

In vocal cord paralysis, abnormal mobility is the most important sign. On real-time evaluation by USG, different maneuvers (like phonation and valsalva) demonstrate absence of motion of the affected cord and normal motion of the contralateral side. This results in a gap at the level of the glottis, which is seen as a hyperechoic air-column band (Figs 13A and B). Any local pathology or cervical cause of the palsy can also be evaluated.[2,3]

TRAUMA

Injury to the larynx can occur in the form of mucosal tears, submucosal hematoma, cartilage fracture and joint dislocation. The mechanism is usually direct blow or penetrating trauma. The relatively lower position of the larynx with respect to mandible in adults makes it more susceptible to trauma especially dashboard or steering-wheel injury.

It is essential to secure airway before any radiological evaluation and the mucosal or submucosal injuries are better evaluated endoscopically. Trauma to the larynx in young patients with nonossified cartilages is difficult to identify. MDCT with its multiplanar reconstructions is beneficial for the evaluation of fractures and stability of the cartilages.[1,5]

Fractures of the Thyroid Cartilage

Fractures of the thyroid cartilage can be vertical (as a result of splaying of cartilage against the spine) and are well seen on axial CT. Horizontal fractures cross both thyroid alae with posterior displacement of the superior fragment and dislocation of epiglottis. These fractures are better appreciated on the coronal reformatted images. These can be associated with small hematomas which are seen as cystic or hypoechoic lesions on USG (Figs 14A and B).

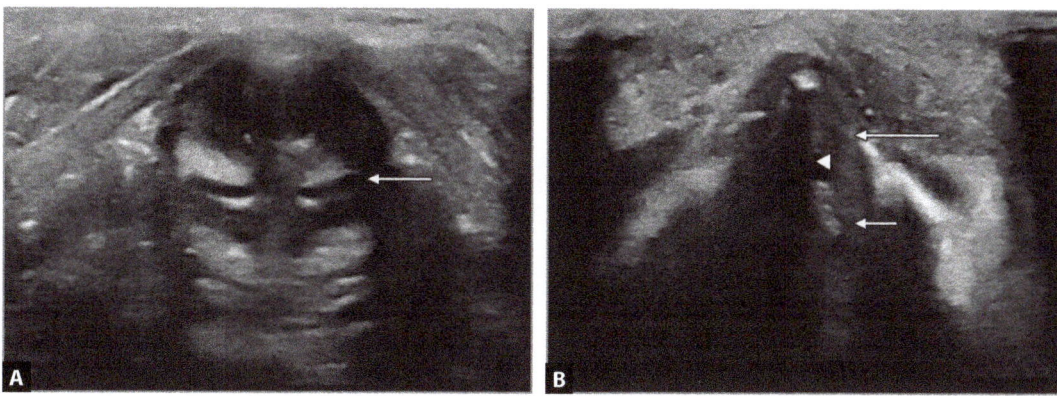

Figs 13A and B (A) Axial ultrasonography image during phonation of normal glottis and (B) left vocal cord paralysis. (A) The normal vocal folds are seen as paired hypoechoic structures and the arytenoid cartilages as symmetrical, paired hypoechoic structures with echogenic rim (arrow). (B) In case of vocal cord palsy, left vocal fold appears flaccid (long arrow) and the glottis is not closed tightly (arrowhead). Arytenoid cartilages are also asymmetrical (short arrows)

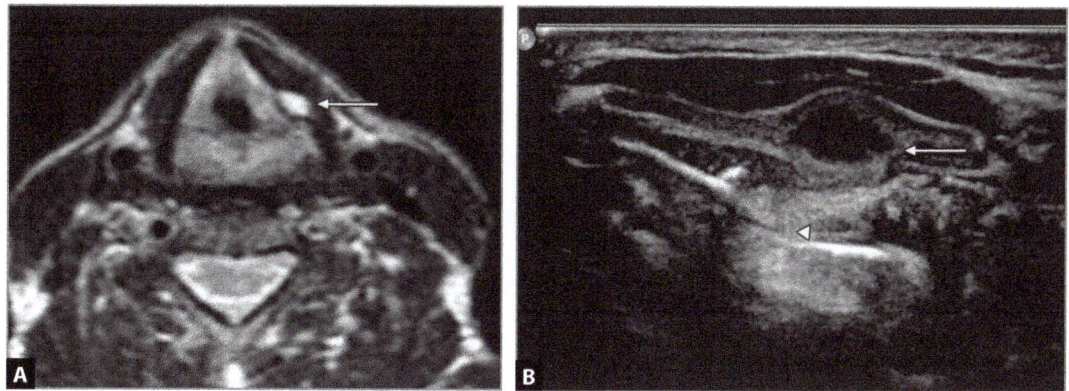

Figs 14A and B Post-traumatic hematoma and fracture. (A) Axial T2-weighted MRI reveals a small, well-defined hyperintense lesion (arrow) involving the left thyroid cartilage; (B) Ultrasonography image in longitudinal oblique plane shows the cystic lesion (arrow) and break in the continuity of the ossified thyroid cartilage (arrowhead)

Cricoid Fractures

Cricoid fractures occur on both sides of the cricoid ring with resultant anterior and posterior fragments. The anterior fragment can get posteriorly displaced and impinge on the airway. It is important to identify the shape of the subglottic airway—rounded contour is seen in case of fracture instead of normal oval shape. In addition, soft tissue may be seen between the cartilage and the air column due to mucosal edema.

Cricoarytenoid Joint Dislocation

Cricoarytenoid joint dislocation leads to hoarseness and may be associated with fracture of one of the laryngeal cartilages. On CT scan, the position of the arytenoid cartilage with respect to articular tubercle on upper margin of cricoid is altered (Fig. 15).

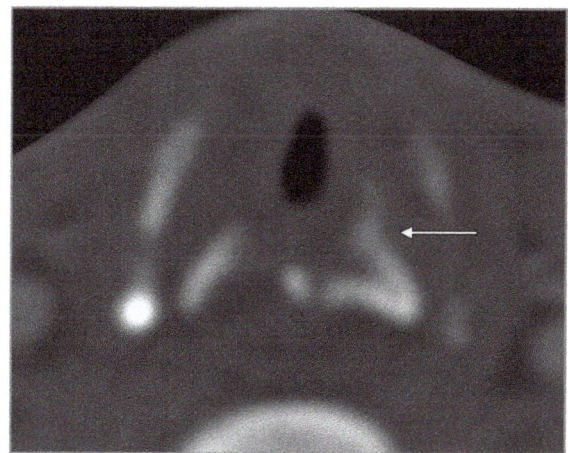

Fig. 15 Left cricoarytenoid joint dislocation. Axial CT bone window image reveals altered position of the arytenoid cartilage with respect to upper margin of cricoid (arrow)

Cricothyroid Joint Dislocation

Cricothyroid joint dislocation causes malalignment of the thyroid and cricoid cartilages. There is usually associated fracture of the inferior horn of thyroid cartilage causing an apparent separation of the cartilages.

Foreign Bodies

Foreign bodies are usually the result of ingestion or aspiration but can be seen occasionally in penetrating trauma. Foreign bodies can lodge in pyriform sinus and then enter laryngeal airway and the tracheobronchial tree. They may also penetrate into the paraglottic space. Plain radiographs can show a radiodense foreign body outlined against the air-filled laryngeal column.[1] *CT scan* is required in case of indeterminate radiographs or suspected complications like abscess formation.

REFERENCES

1. Curtin HD. The Larynx. In: Som PM, Curtin HD (Eds). Head and Neck imaging, 4th edition. St Louis: Mosby; 2003. pp. 1595-699.
2. Tsui PH, Wan YL, Chen CK. Ultrasound imaging of the larynx and vocal folds: recent applications and developments. Curr Opin Otolaryngol Head Neck Surg. 2012;20:437-42.
3. Wang LM, Zhu Q, Ma T, et al. Value of ultrasonography in diagnosis of pediatric vocal fold paralysis. Int J Pediatr Otorhinolaryngol. 2011;75(9):1186-90.
4. Bisetti MS, Segala F, Zappia F, et al. Non-invasive assessment of benign vocal folds lesions in children by means of ultrasonography. Int J Pediatr Otorhinolaryngol. 2009;73(8): 1160-2.
5. Storck C, Buitrago-Tellez C. Multidetector computed tomography in nonmalignant laryngeal disease. Curr Opin Otolaryngol Head Neck Surg. 2012;20:443-9.
6. Joshi VM, Wadhwa V, Mukherji SK. Imaging in laryngeal cancers. Indian J Radiol Imaging. 2012;22(3):209-26.
7. Leboulanger N, Garabédian EN. Laryngo-tracheo-oesophageal clefts. Orphanet J Rare Dis. 2011;6:81.
8. Sundarakumar DK, Bhalla AS, Sharma R, et al. Multidetector CT evaluation of central airways stenoses: Comparison of virtual bronchoscopy, minimal-intensity projection, and multiplanar reformatted images. Indian J Radiol Imaging. 2011;21(3): 191-4.
9. Myer CM, O'Connor DM, Cotton RT. Proposed grading system for subglottic stenosis based on endotracheal tube sizes. Ann Otol Rhinol Laryngol. 1994;103:319-23.
10. Hung TY, Li S, Chen PS, et al. Bedside ultrasonography as a safe and effective tool to diagnose acute epiglottitis. Am J Emerg Med. 2011;29(3):359.e1-3.
11. Marchiori E, Araujo Neto Cd, et al. Laryngotracheobronchial papillomatosis: findings on computed tomography scans of the chest. J Bras Pneumol. 2008;34(12):1084-9.
12. Katsenos S, Becker HD. Recurrent Respiratory Papillomatosis: A Rare Chronic Disease, Difficult to Treat, with Potential to Lung Cancer Transformation: Apropos of Two Cases and a Brief Literature Review. Case Rep Oncol. 2011;4:162-71.
13. Garcia DM, Magalhaes FP, Dadalto GB, et al. Imaging evaluation of vocal cord paralysis. Radiol Bras. 2009;42(5):321-6.
14. Kwong Y, Boddu S, Shah J. Radiology of vocal cord palsy. Clin Radiol. 2012;67:1108-14.
15. Dankbaar JW, Pameijer FA. Vocal cord paralysis: anatomy, imaging and pathology. Insights Imaging. 2014;5(6): 743-51.

Laryngopharyngeal Reflux

KK Handa, Aru Chhabra Handa, Ashutosh Hota

INTRODUCTION

Laryngopharyngeal reflux (LPR) is retrograde flow of gastric contents to the larynx and pharynx. In 1991, Koufman[1] first described LPR to be a distinct entity from the classic gastroesophageal reflux disease (GERD). Supraesophageal reflux, esophagopharyngeal reflux, extraesophageal reflux (EER), and posterior laryngitis are all synonyms to LPR. Poelmans et al.[2] estimated that 4–10% of patients presenting to ENT (ear, nose, and throat) clinics have symptoms or findings related to GERD. Chronic cough, chronic laryngitis, and asthma are significantly associated with GERD. Laryngotracheal stenosis, laryngeal papilloma, vocal cord granuloma, otitis media with effusion (OME) and even head and neck malignancy are some of the disorders for which LPR has been implicated. LPR symptoms may occur along with GERD symptoms or present alone. However, majority of patients of LPR may lack classic symptoms of GERD, i.e. heartburn so the term "silent reflux" was coined by Koufman.[1]

The diagnosis of LPR is not easy. The problem in diagnosis is because physiological reflux events in proximal as well as distal esophagus have been seen in healthy adults also.[3,4] Montreal definition by International Consensus Group defines GERD as a condition when reflux causes troublesome symptoms and/or complications.[5] Thus reflux without symptom is not a disease but physiological gastroesophageal reflux. Montreal classification further divides GERD into esophageal and extraesophageal considering laryngeal and pulmonary symptoms of cough, chronic laryngitis, and asthma in reflux as established extraesophageal features of reflux. In the same Global Evidence-based Consensus the association of sinusitis, pulmonary fibrosis, pharyngitis, or recurrent otitis media with reflux was proposed but with low evidence. The main objective of this chapter is to review the pathophysiology, clinical manifestations, diagnosis, and treatment of LPR.

PATHOPHYSIOLOGY

In LPR, the refluxate which has the potential to cause damage to the larynx and pharynx contains acid, pepsin, and sometimes bile juices and pancreatic enzymes. However, there are some natural defenses in place that prevent reflux. Upper esophageal sphincter (UES), lower esophageal sphincter (LES), esophageal acid clearance, and epithelial resistance are the four constituents of the barrier which prevent gastric reflux.

Lower Esophageal Sphincter

Lower esophageal sphincter is the first antireflux barrier. Gastroesophageal junction and diaphragmatic crura are the main constituents of LES. LES is not as well demarcated anatomically as the UES but functionally it acts as a stronger barrier than UES. The sphincter relaxes in response to swallowing to allow the ingested particles to pass into the stomach. At all other times the pressure in the LES must be more than the intra-abdominal pressure to prevent gastric reflux. Lax LES (relaxed sphincter) and increase in stomach pressure allows reverse movement of stomach contents into esophagus. The length of the esophagus that presents below the crura is detrimental for LES. Large hiatus hernia also disrupts the sphincteric action of the LES. The LES pressure is also controlled by many hormones secreted in the gastric tract.

Chronic hypotonicity of LES is seen in diseases like CREST syndrome (*calcinosis, Raynaud's phenomenon, esophageal dysmotility, sclerodactyly, and telangiectasia*), scleroderma, and isolated Reynaud's phenomenon. In pregnancy LES tone decreases due to progesterone[6] and also, due to the growing fetus, the intra-abdominal pressure increases and exceeds the sphincteric pressure of the LES causing LPR.

Esophageal Acid Clearance

Esophageal acid clearance protects the esophageal mucosa from damage caused by reflux. It is achieved by esophageal motor motility pushing reflux back to stomach and neutralization by bicarbonate in swallowed saliva. If the acid clearance capacity of esophagus is compromised due to esophageal motility disorder, the chance of LPR is increased. Xerostomia, which can be caused by Sjögren's disease, certain medications, and previous radiotherapy, may also abolish this important antireflux barrier by reducing the amount of saliva produced. A study by Postma et al.[7] showed that LPR patients have reflux in upright position and the esophageal acid clearance is reduced to some extent compared to control. Same study also showed that esophageal motility is more severely affected in GERD compared to LPR patients. So the exposure of the esophagus to reflux is less in LPR compared to GERD. This can explain lack of heartburn in LPR patients.

Upper Esophageal Sphincter

Upper esophageal sphincter is the final gatekeeper in preventing the entry of gastric contents into the upper aerodigestive tract. It is made up of the cricopharyngeus, the thyropharyngeus, and the proximal cervical esophagus. The innervation is by the pharyngeal plexus and the motor innervation is mainly by the vagus nerve. The sphincteric action of the UES is compromised by general anesthetics, sleep state, cigarette smoking, and peppermint consumption. Main mechanism causing LPR is nonswallow-related transient relaxation of UES.[8]

Epithelial Resistance

Epithelial resistance is achieved by esophageal secretions and swallowed saliva which protect the esophagus from the damaging effect of the refluxate. But laryngeal epithelium is more sensitive to gastric juice compared to the esophageal epithelium. In the larynx acidified pepsin causes breach in mucosal barrier by causing loss in function of E-cadherin complex which has an important role in the maintenance of epithelial integrity.[9] Ultrastructural study with electron microscopy of oropharyngeal biopsy in LPR patients with sore throat have shown dilatation of intercellular spaces at squamous basal and suprabasal level suggesting reflux caused damage.[10]

Another defense mechanism is through carbonic anhydrase III (CA III) which regulates pH by converting carbon dioxide and water into carbonic acid, protons, and bicarbonate ions. Bicarbonates protect tissues from damage by neutralizing acid. In the esophagus, bicarbonate production in the extracellular space plays critical role in pH buffering after acid reflux.[11] However in larynx CA III protein which is normally found in non LPR patients was not detectable in 64% (47/75) of biopsy specimens from vocal fold and ventricle in the larynx of LPR patients. Lack of CA III could be a major factor in making larynx susceptible to injury by refluxate. In contrast posterior larynx is protected from reflux damage by the presence of CA III despite the presence of pepsin.[9,12]

Role of Pepsin and Nonacid Reflux

In the study by Parkkila et al.[11] pepsin was found in all the laryngeal samples from LPR patients thus implicating pepsin for the absence of key protective proteins like CA III and E-cadherin. Pepsin in the reflux gets adhered to epithelium in extraesophageal sites. There it gets reactivated when exposed to acid and this acidified pepsin causes tissue damage. Even without acid the pepsin can get activated after it enters the cell by endocytosis thus damaging the cell. This suggests that nonacidic components of the reflux are capable of bigger damage to the extraesophageal tissues.

MECHANISM OF SYMPTOMS

According to Hogan and Shaker[13] injury to larynx in LPR involves two pathways:
1. Direct reflux
2. Vagal reflux.

Direct Reflux

Irritation due to direct reflux can cause coughing and choking (laryngospasm) as local inflammation leads to upregulation in laryngeal sensitivity. Combination of factors then leads to vocal fold edema, contact ulcers, and granulomas that cause other LPR-associated symptoms: hoarseness, globus pharyngeus, and sore throat.[1]

Though physiological refluxes into the esophagus are common but as few as three LPR episodes per week can produce ciliary dysfunction due to severe damage to the ciliary respiratory epithelial lining the larynx especially the posterior larynx. This results in mucus stasis as damaged cilia are unable to clear the mucus. This causes foreign body sensation or postnasal drip feeling leading to frequent throat clearing.

Vagal Reflux

Both esophagus and airway have common innervations by vagus. So irritation of the esophagus by reflux can cause bronchoconstriction of larynx and cough by esophagobronchial reflux.

SIGNS AND SYMPTOMS

Symptoms

Patients with LPR may present with chronic cough, frequent throat clearing, throat irritation not associated with cold, change in voice, choking episodes, foreign body sensation, difficulty in swallowing, or a feeling of lump in the throat. Other common symptoms are postnasal drip, mucus stuck in the throat or feeling of fullness in the throat even on empty stomach leading to loss of appetite.

Common regions involved and related disease complications associated with LPR have been shown in Table 1.

Signs

Physical findings frequently observed in patients of LPR include laryngeal pseudosulcus,[14] diffuse laryngeal edema, erythema, and posterior commissure hypertrophy[15] commonly referred to as pachydermia. Classically, posterior laryngeal changes, such as pachydermia, have been linked to LPR but recent studies have demonstrated that the entire larynx can undergo significant changes when exposed to gastric contents.

Posterior commissure hypertrophy is a common finding in patients of LPR; a scheme of grading[15] has been postulated based on endoscopic findings.
- *Grade 1*: Mild posterior commissure hypertrophy.
- *Grade 2*: Posterior commissure hypertrophy characterized by a mustache-like appearance, but the posterior commissure has a convex configuration.
- *Grade 3*: Posterior commissure hypertrophy; the epithelium creates a straight-line across the back of the larynx.
- *Grade 4*: Posterior commissure hypertrophy; begins to encroach on to the airway.

Differential Diagnosis

Symptoms in LPR are nonspecific. Patients with postnasal drip due to rhinopharyngitis, sinusitis, and allergy may have similar clinical presentation. Some of the laryngeal symptoms of LPR are difficult to differentiate from those seen in mild throat infection, vocal abuse hypothyroidism, and some autoimmune disorders. Problems such as cough, asthma,

Table 1 Common symptoms and related disease complications associated with laryngopharyngeal reflux

Region	Manifestation
Chest	• Bronchial asthma • Pulmonary fibrosis • Pulmonary collapse • Chronic bronchitis • Bronchiectasis • Chronic obstructive pulmonary disease • Pneumonia • Croup/stridor
Laryngeal	• Laryngitis • Hoarseness • Chronic cough • Throat clearing • Chronic laryngitis • Globus sensation • Vocal cord ulcers • Granulomas • Laryngeal spasm • Laryngeal stenosis • Laryngeal cancer • Subglottic stenosis • Torticollis (Sandifer syndrome)
Oral cavity and pharynx	• Loss of dental/gingival strictures • Buccal burning • Mouth ulcers • Loss of taste • Otalgia • Otitis • Chronic sinusitis • Postnasal drip

and laryngitis are multifactorial with LPR as one of the factors causing it. Older patients with vocal cord atrophy and glottic insufficiency also suffer from mucus sensation and throat clearing seen in LPR and get unnecessarily treated with proton pump inhibitors.[16]

Majority of LPR patients have globus sensation which is also seen in patients having abnormal UES, esophageal motor diseases, upper aerodigestive tract malignancy, cervical hypertropic gastric mucosa, and psychological factors.[16] Pharyngeal irritation due to smoking and environmental pollution can be misdiagnosed as LPR. To avoid over diagnosis a detailed history taking is must to rule out other diseases having similar complaints or findings thus avoiding unnecessary expense on treating a disease which is not.[17]

LPR versus GERD

It is not clear why some patients have reflux limited to esophagus causing GERD and some have reflux reaching all the way to pharynx as in LPR. Different studies[7,18] have shown that the pathophysiology, symptoms, signs, and treatment in

LPR are different from GERD. Primary defect in LPR seems to be in the UES, whereas GERD patients have problem in LES and esophageal motility thus causing prolonged acid clearance in the esophagus. The pathophysiology in both may be entirely different as it has been seen that LPR patients have day time reflux in upright position while GERD patients have nocturnal reflux in supine position. Symptoms in LPR patients are throat and upper airway related; on the other hand GERD patients complain more of epigastric pain and heartburn. On endoscopic examination LPR patients have laryngeal changes but no esophagitis. Because of the severity of tissue damage, the proton pump inhibitor (PPI) therapy in LPR is double the dose and duration compared to GERD. All these differences could be because acid reflux is the main cause of damage in GERD, and nonacid reflux by pepsin or acidified pepsin mediates LPR disease (LPRD).

EFFECTS OF REFLUX IN AERODIGESTIVE TRACT

Effect of Reflux on Larynx

Kambic and Radsel[19] postulated that LPR causes histological transformation of tissue confined to the interarytenoid area. Epithelial hyperplasia with some degree of keratinization occurs in the prickle and basal cell layers due to chronic exposure of the gastric contents. In larynx the damage due to refluxate is more to subglottis compared to posterior commissure. This alteration is quite irreversible even with appropriate medical therapy. So physical finding simply signify that the patient had been exposed to the LPR in the past, but it does not essentially indicate an active disease. Acidified pepsin can damage the larynx even at pH 6. Johnston et al. in a study on porcine larynx model found that the damage to the larynx is more with pepsin containing acidified buffer than with acidified buffer of same pH alone.[20]

Chronic Cough and Laryngopharyngeal Reflux

Chronic cough sometimes is the only manifestation of LPR. Forty percent of patients of LPR are reported to have a cough-related problem in the course of the disease. LPR should be suspected, if cough is associated with intake of food, heartburn, reflux-related irritation of the larynx, and choking feeling. Later is more common when the patient is sleeping. The origin of cough can be peripherally mediated by proximal acid exposure of larynx causing laryngeal inflammation and hypersensitization.[1]

Cough can also be due to microaspiration of refluxate directly stimulating tracheobronchial receptors.[21] Indirectly cough can be induced by vagus nerve-mediated esophagobronchial reflux after distal esophageal acid exposure.[22,23]

Reflux and Otitis Media with Effusion

Both OME and reflux are common in first 3–4 years in children. Various studies have found presence of pepsin or antipepsin antibody from middle ear fluids of children.[24,25] Eustachian tube in children being more horizontal and shorter helps in passage of infection and probably refluxate to go from nasopharynx to middle ear. So there may be a potential role of gastric reflux in causing inflammation and edema of the Eustachian tube and thus the development of OME in children. Tasker et al.[23] investigated the potential role of gastric reflux in the development of OME (glue ear) in children who had undergone myringotomy. Of 65 tested effusion samples, measured in enzyme-linked immunosorbent assay (ELISA) using antipepsin antibody, 59 (91%) effusions gave a positive result. However, a cause-effect relationship between pepsin or pepsinogen in middle ear and otitis media is unclear. Reflux being common in children, its high prevalence in pediatric age group could be related to physiologic reflux. The results of empirical treatment for reflux in otitis media are not very encouraging. So keeping in view the side effects of antireflux therapy it cannot be advised in children with OME on the basis of literature available.[26]

Pediatric Laryngopharyngeal Reflux

Pediatric laryngopharyngeal reflux (PLPR) deserves special mention as infants are predisposed to reflux due to a shorter intra-abdominal esophagus and an immature LES. Fifty percent of normal infants have regurgitation, which in the majority of cases spontaneously resolves by the age of 2 years. Symptomatology in children is different than adults. For the evaluation of reflux different questionnaires need to be developed in infants and children. Children with LPR can present with chronic cough, hoarseness, or even failure to thrive. Frequent awakening at night, regurgitation of food, and frequent lower respiratory tract infections can also be caused by reflux. Apnea recurrent croup, anorexia, or dysphagia may be more common in infants, while school going children demonstrate globus sensation, sore throat, dyspnea, and dysphonia.[27,28] There need to be a high degree of clinical suspicion in children presenting with varied nonspecific laryngeal and pharyngeal symptoms. Complications associated with LPR in pediatric populations are refractory asthma, aspiration, recurrent bronchitis, laryngomalacia, subglottic stenosis[29] and middle ear effusion. PLPR is also considered as a predisposing factor for recurrent respiratory papillomatosis. LPR has been shown to complicate conditions such as croup, vocal fold nodules[30] and possibly sudden infant death syndrome.[31,32]

Reflux and Malignancy

Chronic hypertrophic laryngitis is seen in patients who suffer from frequent LPR. Chronic hypertrophic laryngitis is a precursor lesion of laryngeal carcinoma as described by Glanz and Kleinsasser in 1976.[33] Ward and Hanson[34] described that reflux is an important factor in patients of laryngeal carcinoma who are nonsmokers. Koufman[1] also described LPR as a causative factor of laryngeal carcinoma in 58% of cases. In a recent study higher levels of total pepsin and bile acid were detected in the saliva of laryngeal cancer patients compared to healthy volunteers. It has been demonstrated that nonacid reflux plays a significant role in the carcinogenesis.[35]

Chronic Rhinosinusitis and Reflux

The mechanism of how LPR may contribute to chronic rhinosinusitis (CRS) is a controversial topic, direct peptic-acid injury and vagus nerve-mediated neurophysiologic changes are the most frequently suspected mechanisms.[36] The possibility that *Helicobacter pylori* may facilitate the disease was only proposed recently.[37] Patients with LPR were reported to have intermittent acid reflux that sometimes reached up into the airway to the nasopharynx[38,39] Also, in some other studies, gastric pepsin was detected in laryngeal and sinus tissue, pulmonary secretions, sputum, and middle ear effusions.[40]

Bola F Olusola et al.[41] in their study demonstrated a high prevalence of GERD in patients with CRS, many of whom experienced sinus symptom improvement after using twice daily omeprazole for 3 months, thus providing a strong basis for LPR as an etiology of CRS. The prevalence of LPR in patients of CRS is not precisely known, however, it is estimated that 5–48% of patients of sinusitis have symptoms of LPR.[41,42]

INVESTIGATIONS

History

A good case history is very critical to both the diagnosis and the treatment of patients with EER. The clinician must not only identify symptoms but also behavioral and medical risk factors. Many symptom and sign scores have been used in literature for evaluation, pre- and post-treatment response. In a series of patients with LPR hoarseness or dysphonia (71%) was found to be the most common symptom. Other symptoms were cough (51%), globus pharyngeus (41%), throat clearing (42%), and dysphagia (35%). Some surveys have found all these symptoms in the range of 95–98%.[43]

Belafsky, Postma, and Koufman[44] developed the reflux symptom index (RSI), a self-administered survey of nine questions used to assess patients with EER with a maximal score of 45 points. A score greater than 13 is considered suggesting LPR. They demonstrated that the instrument is reliable and that it provides reproducible and valid findings. Normative data gathered by these authors support that RSI of more than 10 is associated with a high likelihood of positive dual-channel pH probe study.

Reflux Symptom Index

The use of the RSI has been validated in pH test proven patients with LPR and has been used in different centers all over the world. However, the scale does not include throat pain, one of the most common symptoms of LPR. Also, one of the items incorporates heartburn, which might induce a bias in favor of the nonplacebo limb,[45] because some authorities now define heartburn as "that which responds to PPI therapy".[46]

Laryngoscopy or the Reflux Finding Score

Laryngoscopic findings are used by otorhinolaryngologists to diagnose LPR. However, laryngoscopic changes are very nonspecific and have subjective variability. Beleskey et al.[15] introduced "the reflux finding score" as an eight-item grading scale that was developed to standardize the laryngoscopic findings of LPR so that laryngologists may better diagnose, evaluate clinical improvement, and assess therapeutic efficacy of patients with LPR (Figs 1A to C).

Based on their analysis, they concluded that one can be 95% certain that a patient with a reflux finding score of 7 or more will have LPR.

In the laryngeal findings presence of pseudosulcus of the vocal fold is a good predictor of LPR and has been found in 90% of LPR cases.[14] It is actually infraglottic edema caused by either refluxate or repeated throat clearance and cough in patients with LPR. It needs to be differentiated from sulcus vocalis which is caused by adhesion of the vocal fold epithelium to the vocal ligament. In sulcus vocalis the linear indentation is present at the free edge of the cord and ends at the vocal process whereas in pseudosulcus edema ventral to the cords extends all the way to posterior commissure.

Next important laryngoscopic finding is ventricular obliteration. In this the ventricle, a trough between the vestibular fold and vocal fold, gets obliterated due to edema of the false cords and true cords. Depending on the severity and time duration of reflux, the edema of the larynx may be limited to one particular area like arytenoids, vocal folds or can be diffuse involving the whole larynx.

Laryngoscopic changes in LPR can be categorized into three types, namely, (1) alterations in epithelium, (2) erythema, and (3) edema. The main regions of larynx evaluated are arytenoids, interarytenoid notch, vestibular folds, and vocal cords. Of these posterior larynx

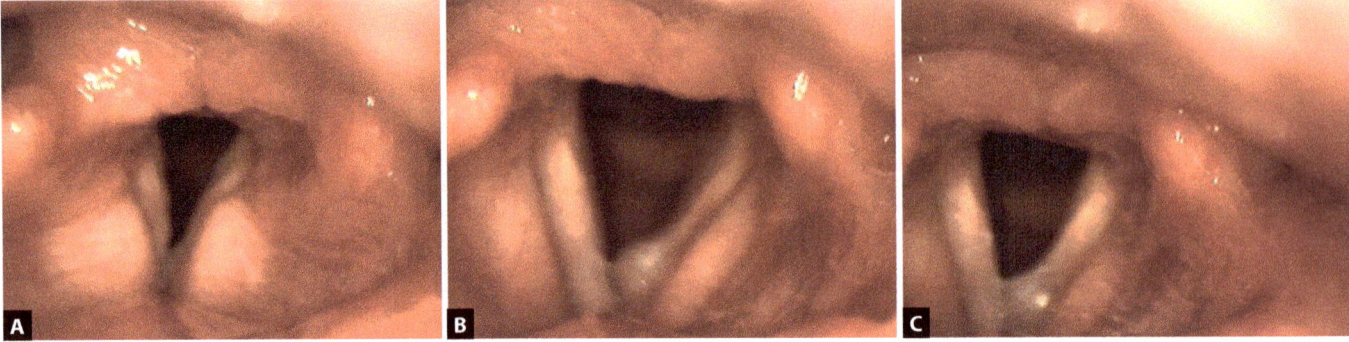

Figs 1A to C Laryngoscope findings in a patient with severe laryngopharyngeal reflux including: (A) Posterior commissure hypertrophy, (B) mucus and (C) an unrelated anterior small mucus retention cyst on its true cord

(interarytenoid notch) and arytenoids are more commonly found to be involved. Laryngeal examination is superior to endoscopy for diagnosing LPR.[47]

Videostroboscopy

Laryngovideostroboscopy (LVS) is currently recommended for use in the dynamic evaluation of laryngeal disorders.[48,49] Digital LVS further improves resolution and image extraction and is particularly useful in the detection of subtle findings of chronic inflammation caused by LPRD.

Voice Analysis

Dysphonia is common in LPR. Voice analysis is sometimes done pre- and post-treatment to know the efficacy of LPR treatment. On GRABSI (grade, roughness, asthenia, breathiness, strain, instability) scale in perceptual voice assessment, roughness is found to be the most common characteristic of voice to be affected in LP. Hanson and colleagues[50,51] reviewed the voice quality and measures of jitter, shimmer, and signal-to-noise ratios in 16 patients undergoing treatment for chronic posterior laryngitis. Perceptual analysis did not show correlation with acoustic measures, and it did not show significant change with treatment. The authors demonstrated that measures of jitter, shimmer, and signal-to-noise ratio improve significantly with anti-secretory and antireflux treatment of chronic posterior laryngitis. The acoustic parameters are improved with the treatment of PPI as it reduces the inflammation and swelling in the vocal cord mucosa. But some studies in literature also state no significant response in voice parameters after treatment, thus making voice analysis a controversial diagnostic entity.[52]

Barium Studies

Barium esophagram is often negative in LPR as there is no associated esophagitis. It is a traditional test for GERD and not routinely advised in all suspected cases of LPR. It is a convenient, inexpensive, and noninvasive diagnostic test. It is a useful method to diagnose structural and functional abnormalities of the esophagus, including hiatal hernia, erosive esophagitis, strictures, Barrett's esophagus, esophageal rings, extrinsic compression, motility disorders, diverticula, possible malignancy, cricopharyngeal spasm, aspiration, and esophageal shortening. Fluoroscopic evaluation is often used to look for the presence of reflux, and it is often combined with provocative maneuvers, such as Valsalva's maneuver, cough, rolling from the supine to the right lateral position, and the water siphon test (the patient drinks 60 mL of water through a straw while supine). The sensitivity of barium esophagram to detect gastroesophageal reflux is between 20% and 60%, with a specificity of 64–90% and accuracy of 6%.[53]

Flexible Endoscopy

Aviv and colleagues[54] have noted that LPR can be observed during flexible endoscopic evaluation of swallowing and sensory testing (FEESST) examinations. In a prospective pilot study, the authors evaluated 20 dysphagic patients (without neurologic etiology) and 20 controls with FEESST. Eighteen out of twenty of the dysphagic patients were noted to have reflux, i.e. passage of material from the esophageal inlet retrograde into the laryngopharynx before, during, or after the swallow during FEESST, whereas no reflux was noted in any of control subjects. Apart from laryngoscopic findings and reflux, laryngopharyngeal sensory changes can also be tested with FEESST.

Esophagoscopy

Esophagogastroduodenoscopy is useful for the direct visualization of the esophagus, along with biopsies and cultures in patients with esophagitis and gastritis. In patients with GERD, it may be valuable in esophagitis. McMurray and colleagues found a weak correlation between laryngoscopic findings of EER and postcricoid biopsy findings.[55] The necessity of esophageal endoscopy in patients with EER without GERD is unclear, and the procedure may be unnecessary.

Manometry Studies

Although manometry is valuable in a certain subset of patients with EER, it may not be useful as a diagnostic test for EER. Esophageal manometry measures the tone of the sphincter at one point in time. Reflux occurs due to transient relaxations of LES so manometry may not accurately assess patients for the events of relaxations of the LES and, therefore, EER.[53]

Radionuclide Studies

Radionuclide scanning involves the oral administration of saline with technetium followed by a gamma scan that looks for reflux. The reflux scan can also be used to quantify delayed gastric emptyig.[53] The sensitivity of this test has been found to be between 14% and 90%, and it is considered to have low sensitivity in patients with EER.

Acidification Tests

Acidification tests, such as the Tuttle test and the Bernstein test, are rarely used today in clinical practice. The sensitivity of this test for the detection of GERD has been reported to be 32–95%[3,56] It is not as useful for the diagnosis of EER, because only a fraction of these patients have concurrent symptoms of GERD.

Bronchoalveolar Lavage

Bronchoalveolar lavage sampled tracheal aspirates are used to look for lipid-laden macrophages, and is a test for aspiration into the lower respiratory tract. It has been shown to be 85% sensitive, and it becomes positive within 6 hours of the reflux event and stays positive for up to 3 days.[53] Lipid-laden macrophages have been shown to be increased in children with pulmonary complications of EER. The advantage of this test is that it provides the ability to track EER days after the event; the disadvantage is that it requires bronchoscopy to acquire the sample.

pH Monitoring

Continuous pH monitoring studies are considered to be the gold standard study for GRD[53] but less reliable in LR.[57] Probes that sense pH changes can be placed in different locations in the esophagus, pharynx, or hypopharynx. Probe placement can be verified using manometry, endoscopy, or fluoroscopy. Manometric localization of pH probe location is the most commonly used technique. Fiber-optic laryngoscopy is also used sometimes to make sure that proximal sensor is surrounded by the mucosa of the esophagus.

Dual probe pH monitoring was started to detect reflux in the proximal esophagus. One sensor is placed 5 cm above the LES and second near the UES. However, it is difficult to achieve uniform positioning of proximal probe relative to UES. Some investigators even tried placing the proximal sensor in the pharynx to detect pharyngeal reflux. The limitation is that it is an invasive test also if the probes are kept in the pharynx, they dry out, get covered with food or mucus or the reference electrode loses control with the mucosa breaking the electrical continuity and give unreliable readings.[58] A 24-hour pH monitoring by this method is not helpful in nonacid reflux and does not permit relief of LPR symptoms by acid suppression therapy or surgery.

Restech pH Probe or Dx-pH Measurement

Restech pH measurement system (Respiratory Technology Corporation, San Diego, CA, USA) is a small catheter put through the nose into the pharynx. Its teardrop design overcomes the shortcomings of dual pH probe, and light-emitting diode (LED) at the tip guides the placement in the pharynx to monitor pH in the pharynx. It can detect liquid as well as aerosolized acid. The investigators established discriminating pH thresholds and defined normal values during upright and supine period.[59] Desjardin M et al. in their study found that all pharyngeal pH drops found with this probe were not associated with reflux. So this technique alone is not very reliable in detecting reflux events.[60]

Multichannel Intraluminal Impedance Monitoring

Multichannel intraluminal impedance (MII) using a pH sensor (MII-pH) equipment is a flexible catheter placed transnasally and has impedance measuring sites at distal and proximal esophagus. The pH sensor on this is positioned so that it can be located 5 cm above the proximal border of LES.[61]

Multichannel intraluminal impedance-pH is used for diagnosis and characterization of LPR. MII testing allows one to detect the direction, composition (gas, liquid, or mixed), and height of material flow. Furthermore, adding pH monitoring to the impedance analysis can detect both acid and nonacid reflux events. The test can be performed in ambulatory conditions. This is an expensive and invasive test.

Pharyngoesophageal Scintigraphy

Pharyngoesophageal scintigraphy is a noninvasive technique used for qualitative and quantitative analysis of swallowing and has also been used to diagnose and quantify reflux. It can differentiate between GERD and LPR. Radiolabeled water is given to the patient to swallow. High resolution, low energy collimator gamma camera is used to evaluate transit through upper and lower esophageal sphincter. This is followed by no radiolabeled water to wash out remaining radiation dose. Persistence of radioactivity is indicative of inflammation. Dynamic images of pharynx, esophagus, and stomach are taken in upright and supine position with or without Valsalva to look for reflux. Galli et al.[62] propose this test to be used as a screening tool and when done along with barium swallow it can differentiate GERD from LPR. However, this test involves some radiation exposure and cannot be done in pregnant women.

Salivary Pepsin

Pepsin is proteolytic enzyme of stomach which when present in saliva is considered a good marker for reflux. Pepsin in saliva or exhaled breath in patients of LPR can be detected by simple, rapid, noninvasive, inexpensive immunoassay test using two monoclonal antibodies to human pepsin.[63]

DIAGNOSIS

It is not very easy to make diagnosis of LPR. All the tests available till date suffer from poor sensitivity and specificity or do not have enough data to support their use for making definitive diagnosis of LPR. Failure to recognize the problem of LPR can be frustrating and sometimes even dangerous for the patient. At the same time over diagnosis can cause financial burden and side effects due to unnecessary use of PPIs.

As most of the tests available are invasive initial diagnosis are made on the basis of symptoms and laryngoscopic findings by subjecting the patient to RSI (Box 1) and reflux finding score (Table 2). Patients are then put on therapeutic trial of twice daily dose of PPI for 2–3 months. Response to the therapeutic trial, in cases suspected to be having LPR, is also considered diagnostic of LPR. Patients who do not show good response are then subjected to one of the diagnostic tests elaborated in the list of investigations. Of all the investigations MII-pH has shown promising results in not only diagnosing but also in characterizing reflux.

TREATMENT

The treatment is divided into three phases as described by Silva:[64]

1. *Phase 1*: Lifestyle modifications
2. *Phase 2:* Medical management
3. *Phase 3*: Surgery.

Box 1 Reflux symptom index

Within the past month, how did the following problems affect you? Rank them from 0 (no problem) to 5 (severe problem).
- Hoarseness or a problem with your voice
- Clearing your throat
- Excess throat mucus or postnasal drip
- Difficulty swallowing food, liquids, or pills
- Coughing after you have eaten or after lying down
- Breathing difficulties or choking episodes
- Troublesome or annoying cough
- Sensations of something sticking in your throat or a lump in your throat
- Heartburn, chest pain, indigestion, or stomach acid coming up

Table 2 Reflux finding score

Pseudosulcus	0, absent; 2, present
Ventricular obliteration	0, none; 2, partial; 4, complete
Erythema/hyperemia	0, none; 2, arytenoids only; 4, diffuse
Vocal fold edema	0, none; 1, mild; 2, moderate; 3, severe; 4, polypoid
Diffuse laryngeal edema	0, none; 1, mild; 2, moderate; 3, severe; 4, obstructing
Posterior commissure hypertrophy	0, none; 1, mild; 2, moderate; 3, severe; 4, obstructing
Granuloma/granulation	0, absent; 2, present
Thick endolaryngeal mucus	0, absent; 2, present

Lifestyle Modification

Dietary and behavioral changes aimed at reducing episodes of reflux may be critical to the successful management of EER. Fatty food and certain other food items increase the frequency of reflux by reducing LES pressure or by prolonging gastric emptying. Increased intake of spicy food irritates already inflamed mucosa and causes burning feeling. High calorie food (1,000 Kcal vs 500 Kcal) is also seen to increase the esophageal acid exposure.[65,66]

Hanson, Kamel, and Kahrilas[51] have shown that nocturnal reflux precautions alone will result in symptomatic improvement in approximately 50% of patients with posterior laryngitis and chronic dysphonia. Common modifications recommended in patients with reflux include the following:

Dietary Modifications

Dietary modification includes:
- Avoidance of eating or drinking 2 hours before sleeping
- Having small frequent meals
- Avoidance of tobacco products, alcohol, carbonated drinks, chocolate, milk, tea, caffeine, hot pepper, and peppermint.

- Avoidance of fried, fatty, spicy, or sour (tomatoes, citrus, and other acidic foods) foods
- Increasing bread and fiber[67] in the diet
- Eliminating all foods and drinks at pH less than 5 in LPR patients and more so in PPI resistant cases have shown to improve symptoms and signs of LPR. Tissue-bound pepsin in larynx and pharynx is thought to be the culprit in these patients as it gets reactivated when exposed to acidic environment and causes tissue damage.[68]

Physical Activity

Physical exercise has a protective role against reflux. Nocon and colleagues in a study reported that subjects having GERD symptoms exercised less compared to those without symptoms.[69] While exercising following precautions need to be taken:
- Avoid bending forward
- No exercise for 2 hours after eating
- Regular physical activity on empty stomach.

General

- Avoidance of tight-fitting clothing
- Sleeping in left lateral recumbent position[70]
- Elevation of the head of the bed by 6–8 inches[71]
- Reduction of weight in overweight people helps in reflux.
- Overweight [Body Mass Index (BMI) 25–30 kg/m²] and obese (BMI>30 kg/m²) persons are more prone to GRD.[72] However, similar correlation has not been seen in LPR patients. Halum et al.[73] found that patients with isolated LPR are not obese.

Medical Treatment

There is lack of high quality evidence supporting efficacy of PPI in EER still the mainstay of treatment in LPR is acid inhibition with PPI. As larynx is more sensitive to acid reflux, patients with LPR require longer and double the dose treatment to get symptomatic relief compared to patients having GERD.[74] Empirically most patients are given twice daily dose of PPI, about half an hour before morning and evening meals. A double standard dose of PPIs was recommended for at least 3 months and if possible for 6 months for LPR was proposed in the first multidisciplinary international symposium on supraesophageal complications of GERD.[75] PPI is also recommended in asthma patient with a history of LPR. It reduces the severity of the asthmatic episode. PPI for at least 2–3 months can also be used empirically in the treatment of idiopathic chronic cough.[76] Younger patients show a better response to PPI therapy than older patients.[77] Symptoms of LPR recover over 2 months of therapy but laryngeal signs take longer to improve.[78] Response to the empiric trial of therapy also helps to confirm the diagnosis of LPR. Nonresponders are subjected to further tests. Failure to therapy can be either due to nonacid reflux or wrong diagnosis.

Management of Nonresponders

Patients who do not respond to PPI therapy need to be further evaluated to look for other factors contributing in reflux or investigated further for correcting the diagnosis.

In a study significant number (57%) of patients of LPRD were found to have *Helicobacter pylori* stomach infection. These patients showed higher incidence of symptom relief and cure with triple therapy, consisting of PPI, amoxicillin sodium and clarithromycin, compared to monotherapy with PPI alone.[79]

Since pepsin plays an important role in cause LPR-related symptoms, many patients do not show good response to PPI therapy. Alginate, a dietary fiber derived from sea weed, has shown some encouraging results in reducing nonacid reflux in LPR patients.[80] But more studies are needed to validate their effect.

Baclofen is gamma-aminobutyric acid (GABA) receptor agonist which helps to reduce transient LES relaxations and therefore reflux. It has been shown to significantly reduce upright reflux and belching. However, more long-term studies are requied.[81] It shows response in both acid and nonacid reflux.

Antacids are effective as a result of their acid-neutralizing properties. Antacids may be used as first-line therapy in patients with minor LPR or as an adjunct to other treatment modalities.[82] Antacids work best when taken half an hour after meals.

Several H_2-receptor blockers are currently available by prescription and over the counter. These act at the histamine type 2 receptor by competitive binding, and they reduce gastric acid secretion along with pepsin production, compared to PPI H_2-receptor antagonists.

Metoclopramide is a dopamine antagonist, and it is effective against GER. It increases LES pressure, improves gastric emptying, and may increase esophageal clearnce.[83] Another salt sucralfate has been shown to enhance mucosal resistance to trauma, is effective for promoting the healing of duodenal ulcers, and has been shown in animal studies to protect esophageal mucosa against injury from acid.

Surgical Treatment

Surgical treatment is reserved for patients who fail aggressive medical management and continue to have life-threatening complications of reflux. Antireflux surgery involves replacing the LES into the abdomen and then augmenting the LES as an antireflux barrier. The Nissen fundoplication involves the use of a 360° wrap of the gastric fundus around the intra-abdominal esophagus.[84] Ten-year success rates for the treatment of GERD are quoted to be around 90%, with a mortality rate of 1%.

REFERENCES

1. Koufman JA. The otolaryngologic manifestations of gastroesophageal reflux disease (GERD): a clinical investigation of 225 patients using ambulatory 24-hour pH monitoring and an experimental investigation of the role of acid and pepsin in the development of laryngeal injury. Laryngoscope. 1991;101(53):1-78.
2. Poelmans J, Feenstra L, Demedts I, et al. Yield of upper GI endoscopy in patients with suspected reflux related chronic ENT symptoms. Am J Gastroenterol. 2004;99(8):1419-26.
3. Shay S, Tutuian R, Sifrim D, et al. Twenty-four-hour ambulatory simultaneous impedance and pH monitoring: a multicenter report of normal values from 60 healthy volunteers. Am J Gastroenterol. 2004;99:1037-43.
4. Zerbib F, Des Varannes SB, Roman S, et al. Normal values and day-to-day variability of 24-h ambulatory oesophageal impedance-pH monitoring in a Belgian–French cohort of healthy subjects. Aliment Pharmacol Ther. 2005;22:1011-21.
5. Vakil N, van Zanten SV, Kahrilas P, et al. The Montreal definition and classification of gastroesophageal reflux disease: a global evidence-based consensus. Am J Gastroenterol. 2006;101(8):1900-20.
6. Castell DO, Harris LD. Hormonal control of gastroesophageal-sphincter strength. N Engl J Med. 1970;282(16):886-9.
7. Postma GN, Tomek MS, Belafsky PC, et al. Esophageal motor function in laryngopharyngeal reflux is superior to that in classic gastroesophageal reflux disease. Ann Otol Rhinol Laryngol. 2001;110:1114-6.
8. Szczesniak MM, Williams RB, Cook IJ. Mechanisms of esophago-pharyngeal acid regurgitation in human subjects. PLoS One. 2011;6(7):e22630.
9. Gill GA, Johnston N, Buda A, et al. Laryngeal epithelial defenses against laryngopharyngeal reflux: investigations of E-cadherin, carbonic anhydrase isoenzyme III, and pepsin. Ann Otol Rhinol Laryngol. 2005;114(12):913-21.
10. Amin SM, Abdel Mated KH, Naser AY, et al. Laryngopharyngeal reflux with sore throat: an ultrastructural study of oropharyngeal epithelium. Ann Otol Rhinol Laryngol. 2009;118(5):362-7.
11. Parkkila S, Parkkila AK. Carbonic anhydrase in the alimentary tract. Roles of the different isozymes and salivary factors in the maintenance of optimal conditions in the gastrointestinal canal. Scand J Gastroenterol. 1996;31:305-17.
12. Afford SE, Sharp N, Ross PE, et al. Cell biology of laryngeal epithelial defenses in health and disease: preliminary studies. Ann Otol Rhinol Laryngol. 2001;110:1099-108.
13. Hogan WJ, Shaker R. Supraesophageal complications of gastroesophageal reflux. Dis Mon. 2000;46(3):193-232.
14. Hickson CA, Simpson CB, Falcon R. Laryngeal pseudosulcus as a predictor of laryngopharyngeal reflux. Laryngoscope. 2001;111:1742-5.
15. Belafsky PC, Postma GN, Koufman JA. The validity and reliability of the Reflux Finding Score (RFS). Laryngoscope. 2001;111:1313-7.
16. Patel AK, Mildenhall NR, Kim W, et al. Symptom overlap between laryngopharyngeal reflux and glottic insufficiency in vocal fold atrophy patients. Ann Otol Rhinol Laryngol. 2014;123(4):265-70.
17. Bong Eun Lee, Gwang Ha Kim. Globus pharyngeus: A review of its etiology, diagnosis and treatment. World J Gastroenterol. 2012;18(20):2462-71.
18. Koufman JA. Laryngopharyngeal reflux is different from classic gastroesophageal reflux disease. Ear Nose Throat J. 2002;81:7
19. Kambic V, Radsel Z. Acid posterior laryngitis. Aetiology, histology, diagnosis, and treatment. J Laryngol Otol. 1984;98:1237-40.
20. Johnston N, Bulmer D, Gill GA, et al. Cell biology of laryngeal epithelial defences in health and disease: further studies. Ann Otol Rhinol Laryngol. 2003;112:481-91.
21. Irwin RS, Zawacki JK, Curley FJ, et al. Chronic cough as the sole presenting manifestation of gastroesophageal reflux. Am Rev Respir Dis. 1989;140(5):1294-300.
22. Altman KW, Simpson CB, Amin MR, et al. Cough and paradoxical vocal fold motion. Otolaryngol Head Neck Surg. 2002;127:501-11.
23. Harding SM, Richter JE. The role of gastroesophageal reflux in chronic cough and asthma. Chest. 1997;111:1389-402.
24. Tasker A, Dettmar PW, Panetti M, et al. Is gastric reflux a cause of otitis media with effusion in children? Laryngoscope. 2002;112:1930-4.
25. He Z, O'Reilly RC, Bolling L, et al. Detection of gastric pepsin in middle ear fluid of children with otitis media. Otolaryngol Head Neck Surg. 2007;137(1):59-64.
26. Miura MS, Mascaro M, Rosenfeld RM. Association between otitis media and gastroesophageal reflux: a systematic review. Otolaryngol Head Neck Surg. 2012;146(3):345-52.
27. Deal L, Gold BD, Gremse DA, et al. Age specific questionnaires distinguish GERD symptom frequency and severity in infants and young children: development and initial validation. J Pediatr Gastroenterol Nutr. 2005;41(2):178-85.
28. Venkatesan NN, Pine HS, Underbrink M. Laryngopharyngeal reflux disease in children. Pediatr Clin North Am. 2013;60(4):865-78.
29. Halstead LA. Gastroesophageal reflux: a critical factor in pediatric subglottic stenosis. Otolaryngol Head Neck Surg. 1999;120:683-8.
30. Halstead LA. Role of gastroesophageal reflux in pediatric upper airway disorders. Otolaryngol Head Neck Surg. 1999;120:208-14.
31. Loughlin CJ, Koufman JA, Averill DB, et al. Acid-induced laryngospasm in a canine model. Laryngoscope. 1996;106:1506-9.
32. Duke SA, Postma GN, McGuirt WF, et al. Laryngospasm and diaphragmatic arrest in immature dogs after laryngeal acid exposure: a possible model for sudden infant death syndrome. Ann Otol Rhinol Laryngol. 2001;110:729-33.
33. Glanz H, Kleinsasser O. Chronic laryngitis and carcinoma. Arch Otorhinolaryngol. 1976;212:57-75.

34. Ward PH, Hanson DG. Reflux as an etiological factor of carcinoma of the laryngopharynx. Laryngoscope. 1988;98:1195-9.

35. Sereg-Bahar M, Jerin A, Hocevar-Boltezar I. Higher levels of total pepsin and bile acids in the saliva as a possible risk factor for early laryngeal cancer. Radiol Oncol. 2015;49(1):59-64.

36. Loehrl TA, Smith TL, Darling RJ. Autonomic dysfunction, vasomotor rhinitis and extraesophageal manifestations of gastroesophageal reflux. Otolaryngol Head Neck Surg. 2002;126:382-7.

37. Dinis PB, Subtil J. Helicobacter pylori and laryngopharyngeal reflux in chronic rhinosinusitis. Otolaryngol Head Neck Surg. 2006;134:67-72.

38. Contencin P, Narcy P. Nasopharyngeal pH monitoring in infants and children with chronic rhinopharyngitis. Int J Ped Otorhinolaryngol. 1991;22:249-56.

39. Del Gaudio JM. Direct Nasopharyngeal reflux of gastric acid is a contributing factor in refractory chronic rhinosinusitis. Laryngoscope. 2005;115:946-57.

40. Krishnan U, Mitchell JD, Messina I, et al. Assay of tracheal pepsin as a marker of reflux aspiration. J Pediatr Gastroenterol Nutr. 2002;35:303-8.

41. Olusola BF, Dibaise JK, Huerter JV, et al. Role of GERG in Chronic Resistant Sinusitis (CRS): Results of a prospective, open-label pilot trial and chronic resistant sinusitis. Am J Gastroenterol. 2002;97:843-50.

42. Barbero GJ. Gastroesophageal reflux and upper airway disease. Otolaryngol Clin North Am. 1996;29:27-38.

43. Book DT, Rhee JS, Toohill RJ, et al. Perspectives in laryngopharyngeal reflux: an international survey. Laryngoscope. 2002;112:1399-406.

44. Belafsky PC, Postma GN, Koufman JA. Validity and reliability of the Reflux Symptom Index (RSI). J Voice. 2002;16(2):274-7.

45. Karkos D, Wilson JA. Empiric treatment of laryngopharyngeal reflux with proton pump inhibitors: A systematic review. Laryngoscope. 2006;116:144-8.

46. Carlsson R, Dent J, Bolling-Sternevald E, et al. The usefulness of a structured questionnaire in the assessment of symptomatic gastroesophageal reflux disease. Scand J Gastroenterol. 2003;33:1023-9.

47. Jonaitis L, Pribuisiene R, Kupcinskas L, et al. Laryngeal examination is superior to endoscopy in the diagnosis of the laryngopharyngeal form of gastroesophageal reflux disease. Scand J Gastroenterol. 2006;41:131-7.

48. Casiano RR, Zaveri V, Lundy DS. Efficacy of videostroboscopy in the diagnosis of voice disorders. Otolaryngol Head Neck Surg. 1992;107:95-100.

49. Remacle M. The contribution of videostroboscopy in daily ENT practice. Acta Otorhinolaryngol Belg. 1996;50:265-81.

50. Lechien JR, Finck C, Costa de Araujo P, et al. Voice outcomes of laryngopharyngeal reflux treatment: a systematic review of 1483 patients. Eur Arch Otorhinolaryngol. 2016;23.

51. Hanson DG, Jiang JJ, Chen J, et al. Acoustic measurement of change in voice quality with treatment for chronic posterior laryngitis. Ann Otol Rhinol Laryngol. 2007;106:279.

52. Jin BJ, Lee YS, Jeong SW, et al. Change of acoustic parameters before and after treatment in laryngopharyngeal reflux patients. Laryngoscope. 2008;118:938-41.

53. Zalzal GH, Tran LP. Paediatric gastroesophageal reflux & laryngopharyngeal reflux. Otolaryngol Clin North Am. 2000;33(1):151-61.

54. Aviv JE, Parides M, Fellowes J, et al. Endoscopic evaluation of swallowing as an alternative to 24 hr pH monitoring for diagnosis of extraesophageal reflux. Ann Otol Rhinol Laryngol. 2000;184:25-7.

55. McMurray JS, Gerber M, Stern Y, et al. Role of laryngoscopy, dual pH probe monitoring and laryngeal mucosal biopsy in the diagnosis of pharyngoesophageal reflux. Ann Otol Rhinol Laryngol. 2001;110:299-304.

56. Rival R, Wong R, Mendelsohn M, et al. Role of gastroesophageal reflux disease in patients with cervical symptoms. Otolaryngol Head Neck Surg. 1995;113(4):364-9.

57. Postma GN. Ambulatory pH monitoring methodology. Ann Otol Rhinol Laryngol Suppl. 2000;184:10-4.

58. Mathus-Vliegen EM, Smit CF, Devriese PP. Artifacts in 24-h pharyngeal and oesopharyngeal pH monitoring: is simplification of pH data analysis feasible? Scand J Gastroenterol. 2004;39(1):14-9.

59. Ayazi S, Lipham JC, Hagen JA, et al. A new technique for measurement of pharyngeal pH: normal values and discriminating pH threshold. J Gastrointest Surg. 2009;13:1422-9.

60. Desjardin M, Roman S, Varannes SB, et al. Pharyngeal pH alone is not reliable for the detection of pharyngeal reflux events: A study with oesophageal and pharyngeal pH-impedance monitoring. United European Gastroenterol J. 2013;1(6):438-44.

61. Tutuian R, Vela MF, Shay SS, et al. Multichannel intraluminal impedance in esophageal function testing and gastroesophageal reflux monitoring. J Clin Gastroenterol. 2003;37(3):206-15.

62. Galli J, Volante M, Parrilla C, et al. Oropharyngoesophageal scintigraphy in the diagnostic algorithm of laryngopharyngeal reflux disease: A useful exam? Otolaryngol Head Neck Surg. 2005;132:717-21.

63. Vaez MF. New tests for the evaluation of laryngopharyngeal reflux. Gastroenterol Hepatol (NY). 2013;9(2):115-7.

64. Silva AB, Hotaling AA. Pediatric gastroesophageal reflux disease. Curr Opin Otolaryngol Head Neck Surg. 1994;2:508.

65. Hanson DG, Kamel PL, Kahrilas PJ. Outcomes of antireflux therapy for treatment of chronic laryngitis. Ann Otol Rhinol Laryngol. 1995;104-7:550-5.

66. Fox M, Barr C, Nolan S, et al. The effects of dietary fat and calorie density on esophageal acid exposure and reflux symptoms. Clin Gastroenterol Hepatol. 2007;5(4):439-44.

67. El-Serag HB, Satia JA, Rabeneck L. Dietary intake and the risk of gastro-oesophageal reflux disease: a cross sectional study in volunteers. Gut. 2005;54(1):11-7.

68. Koufman JA. Low-acid diet for recalcitrant laryngopharyngeal reflux: therapeutic benefits and their implications. Ann Otol Rhinol Laryngol. 2011;120(5):281-7.

69. Nocon M, Labenz J, Willich SN. Lifestyle factors and symptoms of gastro-oesophageal reflux—a population-based study. Aliment Pharmacol Ther. 2006;23(1):169-74.

70. Khoury RM, Camacho-Lobato L, Katz PO, et al. Influence of spontaneous sleep positions on night time recumbent

reflux in patients with gastroesophageal reflux disease. Am J Gastroenterol. 1999;94(8):2069-73.

71. Shaw GY, Searl JP. Laryngeal manifestations of gastroesophageal reflux before and after treatment with omeprazole. South Med J. 1997;90:115.

72. Dore MP, Maragkoudakis E, Fraley K, et al. Diet, lifestyle and gender in gastro-esophageal reflux disease. Dig Dis Sci. 2008;53(8):2027-32.

73. Halum SL, Postma GN, Johnston C, et al. Patients with isolated laryngopharyngeal reflux are not obese. Laryngoscope. 2005;115(6):1042-5.

74. Ford CN. Evaluation and management of laryngopharyngeal reflux. JAMA. 2005;294(12):1534-40.

75. First multidisciplinary international symposium on supra-esophageal reflux disease. Workshop consensus reports. Am J Med. 1997;103:149S-50S.

76. Ford GA, Oliver PS, Prior JS, et al. Omeprazole in the treatment of asthmatics with nocturnal symptoms and gastro-oesophageal reflux: a placebo-controlled cross-over study. Postgrad Med J. 1994;70:350-4.

77. Lee YC, Lee JS, Kim SW, et al. Influence of age on treatment with proton pump inhibitors in patients with laryngopharyngeal reflux disease: a prospective multicenter study. JAMA Otolaryngol Head Neck Surg. 2013;139(12):1291-5.

78. Belafsky PC, Postma GN, Koufman JA. Laryngopharyngeal reflux symptoms improve before changes in physical findings. Laryngoscope. 2001;111(6):979-81.

79. Youssef TF, Ahmed MR. Treatment of clinically diagnosed laryngopharyngeal reflux disease. Arch Otolaryngol Head Neck Surg. 2010;136(11);1089-92.

80. Bardhan KD, Strugala V, Dettmar PW. Reflux revisited: advancing the role of pepsin. Int J Otolaryngol. 2012;2012:646901.

81. Cossentino MJ, Mann K, Armbruster SP, et al. Randomised Clinical Trial: The effect of baclofen in patients with gastro-oesophageal reflux a randomised prospective study. Aliment Pharmacol Ther. 2012;35(9):1036-44.

82. Postma GN, Johnson LF, Koufman JA. Treatment of laryngopharyngeal reflux. Ear Nose Throat J. 2002;81(9): 24-6.

83. Orihata M, Sarna SK. Contractile mechanism of action of gastroprokinetic agents: cisapride, metoclopramide, and domperidone. Am J Physiol. 1994;266:G665-76.

84. Hinder RA, Perdikis G, Klinger PJ, et al. The surgical option for gastroesophageal reflux. Am J Med. 1997;103(5A):144S-8S.

Spasmodic Dysphonia

KK Handa

INTRODUCTION

Dystonia patients have sustained, uncontrolled muscle contractions causing actions which are not normal and involuntary.[1] They can be characterized as focal affecting only a group of muscles or generalized which affect the full body. The credit for describing condition of spasmodic dysphonia (SD) goes to Aronson.[2] It consists of an adductor, abductor and mixed type. It is a focal laryngeal dystonia which affects intrinsic muscles of the larynx. The hallmark of the condition is intermittent or continuous hyperadduction (coming together) of the vocal cords.[3] The overclosure of the cords causes phonatory breaks and choked strangulated voice. These spasms often interrupt the sound, squeezing the voice to nothing in the middle of a sentence. However, voice is normal during other activities, such as breathing, swallowing, and laughing. This condition has lot of effect on productivity and patient's quality of life.[4] It is most common in ideal age females. The diagnosis is made on listening to the patient as she enters the doctor's chamber.[5] On the other hand, patients with abductor SD patients have a breathy voice which takes a lot of effort to produce and interspersed with sudden voice stopping. In some patients, there are features of both and this variety is termed as mixed type. In fact, Connito et al.[5] believe that abductor and adductor elements are there in all patients and preponderance of one variety leads to more of that type of symptoms.

Stress and anxiety cause deterioration of symptoms of SD patients. On the other hand, alcohol and some sedatives cause some improvement in the symptoms.

Initially it was considered as a psychogenic disorder; however, the concept changed after Dedo[6] found that section of the recurrent laryngeal nerve (RLN) in his patients caused good improvement in the symptoms. Block of RLN has been used to diagnose adductor SD and to select suitable patients for surgery.[7] Adductor variety is very often confused with muscle tension dysphonia and here recurrent nerve block may be of help in correct diagnosis.

ETIOPATHOGENESIS

Exact etiology is not known. There is evidence of genetic component including familial involvement. There was a 12% familial history in one series.[8]

There is evidence of neurogenic origin in a number of studies. Basal ganglia[9] involvement was seen in a series while another study showed involvement of primary somatosensory cortex.[10]

Three mechanisms involved in SD are: (1) reduced inhibition, (2) more plasticity, and (3) sensory inputs which are not normal. Reduction or absent inhibition is known in SD.[11] Many spinal and brainstem reflexes are not normal along with the central motor cortex which has a inhibition loss.[12,13] These measures have been found to have deficits in patients with SD.[14] This concept is used in treating SD where emphasis is on increasing inhibition or making excitability less.[15] Fine motor movements, which are affected by center surround inhibition, may be reduced in SD and other dystonias.[14] In patients with writer's cramp motor training of specific finger movements greatly makes patients' writing skills better.[16]

Patients with writer's cramp have greater plasticity. This is shown by paired associative stimulation showing more excitability.[17] In dystonia the cause of abnormal response to repetitive activity or increased use is increased plasticity.[18]

There is reduced amount of temporal and spatial discrimination. Sensory abnormalities in hand dystonia include less than normal temporal and spatial discrimination.[19,20] There is also decrease in cerebral response to vibrotactile stimulation of the hand in sensorimotor and other motor areas.[21] Disordered motor output is likely to be because of disordered sensory input.

MANAGEMENT

Medical Therapy

The symptoms may show partial and temporary improvement with sedatives and some anticholinergics, and dopamine drugs. However, they can only be used sparingly because of central nervous system side effects.

Voice Therapy

There is very limited or no role of voice therapy. However, it may be used by patients to understand their own voice and hence reduce associated muscle tension and other compensatory behavior. The limited role of voice therapy is applicable to:

- Psychogenic dysphonia
- Mild, intermittent symptoms of adductor SD
- In abductor SD patients who have not received benefit from botox injections
- Patients who while trying to compensate for muscle spasms develop significant muscle tension dysphonia.

The gold standard of treatment is intracordal botulinum toxin injection (Fig. 1). It works if injected in the correct place; however, effect lasts for a limited time.

Botulinum Toxin in Spasmodic Dysphonia

This is the gold standard and accepted treatment for SD. The toxin is produced by a bacteria called *Clostridium botulinum*. This toxin has widespread uses in medical field. Toxin

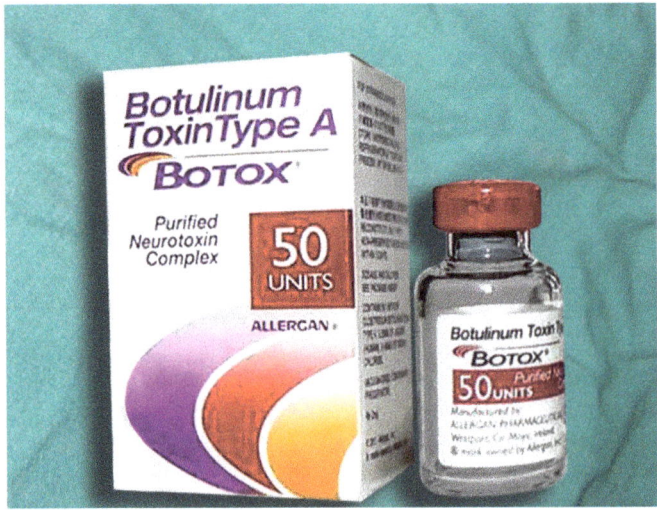

Fig. 1 Botulinum toxin

types A and B are used for medicinal purposes. The drug works by blocking release of acetylcholine at nerve muscle endings.

The most common brand is Botox which is marketed by company Allergan. Other known brands are:

- Dysport (Company: Ipsen)
- Xeomin (Company: Merz Pharma)
- Myoblock (Company: Solstice)
- Neuronox (Company: Medy-Tox Inc.).

The patient is informed that Botox only improves the symptoms and is not the cure. Botox comes in lyophilized form in 50 or 100 unit vials.

Adductor Spasmodic Dysphonia

The injection can be given by either of the following methods:

- External approach through:
  - The cricothyroid membrane
  - Thyroid membrane with an endoscopic visualization
- Injection channel of fiberoptic laryngoscope.

Botulinum injection is given with patient being in a supine or seating position with the neck extended. It is better to give it without gloves to increase the tactile feel. The thyroid and cricoid cartilages are palpated and cricothyroid membrane is identified. The injection is carried out about 2–3 mm from center with needle facing 30° up and lateral. It is preferred to do injection under electromyography (EMG) control with a 27 number Teflon-coated needle and asking the patient to see "ee". Once correct placement is confirmed, aspiration is done through the syringe. The injection is done into thyroarytenoid (TA) muscle and can be done unilaterally or bilaterally. The Botox vial comes as 50 Mu or 100 Mu. Adding 4 cc of preservative-free normal saline to 50 Mu vial will have 1.25 units per 0.1 cc. However, now there are study reports of doing injection directly without EMG control.

About 90–95% patients improve after Botulinum toxin injection in adductor SD. Nonresponders may be because of incorrect diagnosis of the condition and the needle is not going into TA muscle. However, it is seen that with repeat injections the effect goes down which may be due to formation of an antibody.[22]

The patients injected with Botox may have a "Mickey mouse" breathy voice for a week.

Abductor Spasmodic Dysphonia

Here injection of the Botox is done into the posterior cricoarytenoid. It is technically more demanding. It is best done through the lateral approach by holding the thyroid cartilage between thumb and index finger and rotating towards the side to be injected. Needle is injected into the posterior cricoarytenoid by pushing it behind the posterior edge of the thyroid cartilage and the patient is asked to sniff and injection is done on getting the maximum response on EMG.

Normally about 3–4 Mu is injected unilaterally. Normally one-sided injection is done as injecting both sides can lead to breathing problem. The results are slightly unpredictable in abductor SD and about 70% patients improve.

The response starts in 2–3 days. Initially, the jerks go away but the voice is breathy and some patients may experience cough on taking liquids. This is temporary; however, some patients may need some swallow exercises.

A recent study[23] has shown efficacy and side effects to be similar between fresh reconstituted Botulinum toxin and stored (frozen for 4–8 weeks) reconstituted Botulinum toxin.

SURGERY FOR SPASMODIC DYSPHONIA

The aim of any surgery for SD is to replicate action of Botulinum toxin for a longer or permanent period. Most described surgeries try to reduce the action of intrinsic muscles of larynx going into spasms.

Recurrent Laryngeal Nerve Sectioning

First nerve-related operation for SD was done by Dedo HH[6] from San Francisco in USA in the year 1976. His surgical technique consisted of doing section of one side RLN and removing a portion of the cut nerve. He removed 1 cm of the nerve near the inferior thyroid pole. Some patients reported good improvement in symptoms but some postoperatively developed significant hoarseness. There was also coming back of spasms in some operated patients. To improve results and minimize the side effects there have been several modifications in this surgery since then.

However, subsequent studies found that about 64% of patients had return of spasms within 3 years[24,25] and 48% had a voice worst than before surgery. Most likely cause of postsurgical recurrences was reinnervation as demonstrated by further studies.[26] However, Dedo claimed that he achieved better results because of surgical step of turning back each stump after removing section of nerve and ligating it and also by postoperative voice therapy. Later he also advised doing laser thinning of vocal folds to prevent overpressure.[27] The disadvantage is that patient will have vocal cord paralysis for long even after reinnervation.

Avulsion of Recurrent Laryngeal Nerve

A more extensive surgery was developed by Netterville called recurrent nerve avulsion.[28] He attempted this to avoid problems of reinnervation as seen with RLN section. He traced all branches of RLN and avulsed them from their insertion into muscles. The proximal end of the nerve is dissected for 3–4 cm below the clavicle and ligated. Total length of 9 cm of the nerve is removed as compared to 2 cm with RLN section. This procedure had a recurrence rate of 22% which was much lower than with nerve section.

Selective Denervation with Reinnervation (Berke)

This surgery was done by Berke[29] and it attempted to achieve a permanent bilateral adductor weakness so as to mimic the action of Botulinum toxin. The surgery consisted of bilateral section of the adductor RLN branch to the TA muscle and lateral cricoarytenoid (LCA) muscle with anastomosis of the distal stump to ansa cervicalis nerve. Most of the patients had the symptoms improving from severe to mild. However, there is only limited experience with this procedure. The reasoning was that cutting the branch to the TA muscle and then trying to make sure that the nerve did not regrow could be accomplished with a nerve transfer graft. Cutting the nerve supply to TA weakens the vocal cords and if done alone gives a breathy voice with air escape. However, when a new nerve grows into the vocal cord muscle (TA), the bulk of the muscle is restored, though it may not move completely normally. This is enough to allow the other muscles within the larynx to work. This however does not cure vocal cord tremor.

Type II Thyroplasty

First description of type II thyroplasty was by Professor Ishikki in the year 2000.[30] This procedure entails separating the vocal folds. It was originally described for cord lateralization. In type II thyroplasty, previously also described as lateralization thyroplasty, the surgeon separates the vocal folds to limit their ability to come in contact with one another. The operation is performed under local anesthesia with monitored anesthesia so that voice can be tested and adjusted while the surgeon adjusts the distance between the separated thyroid and amyotrophic lateral sclerosis (ALS). The result is a slightly weaker voice with little or no spasms. It is a safe operation with no side effects although the results are slightly variable.

After doing 6 patients in the first year,[31] the number of cases done by Professor Ishikki had increased to 26 by the year 2004.[32]

Sanuki and Isshiki[33] reported satisfactory results by doing type II thyroplasty with a bridge made of titanium (to maintain correct distance between separated thyroid cartilage) in a larger group of patients. Significant improvement was seen in operated patient's perceptual voice parameters.

Surgical Steps

It is preferably done under local anesthesia under monitoring. Subplatysmal flaps are elevated and strap muscles are also split in the midline. Thyroid cartilage is split in the midline. Caution is exercised so as not to enter the anterior commissure as anteriorly there is no muscle and only Broyle's ligament is present. Silastic shims 2–3 mm wide are used to keep split thyroid ala apart (Figs 2A and B). Usually 2–3 silastic shims suffix. Alternatively 4 mm titanium miniplates can also be used. The surgery has the effect of getting both the ala apart and reducing the hyperadduction of the vocal cords and in turn reducing the spasms. The voice is tested on the table and appropriate modification done in distance between the separated thyroid ala to achieve the best voice results. A small drain is kept in the wound before closure (Figs 3A to D).

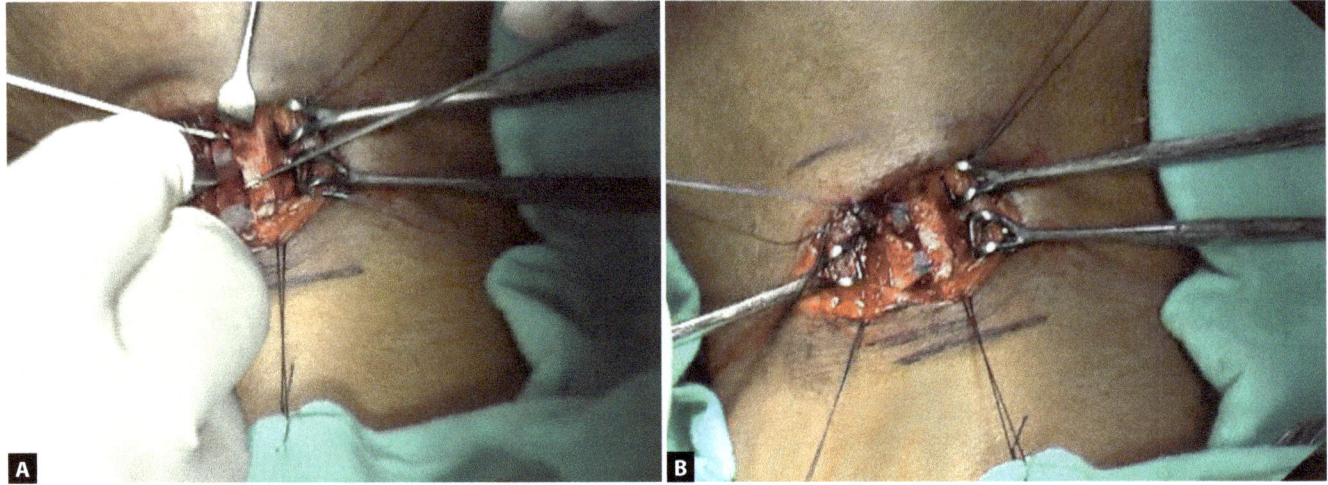

Figs 2A and B (A) Type II thyroplasty splitting of thyroid cartilage in midline and (B) Insertion of 3 mm × 2 mm silastic shims

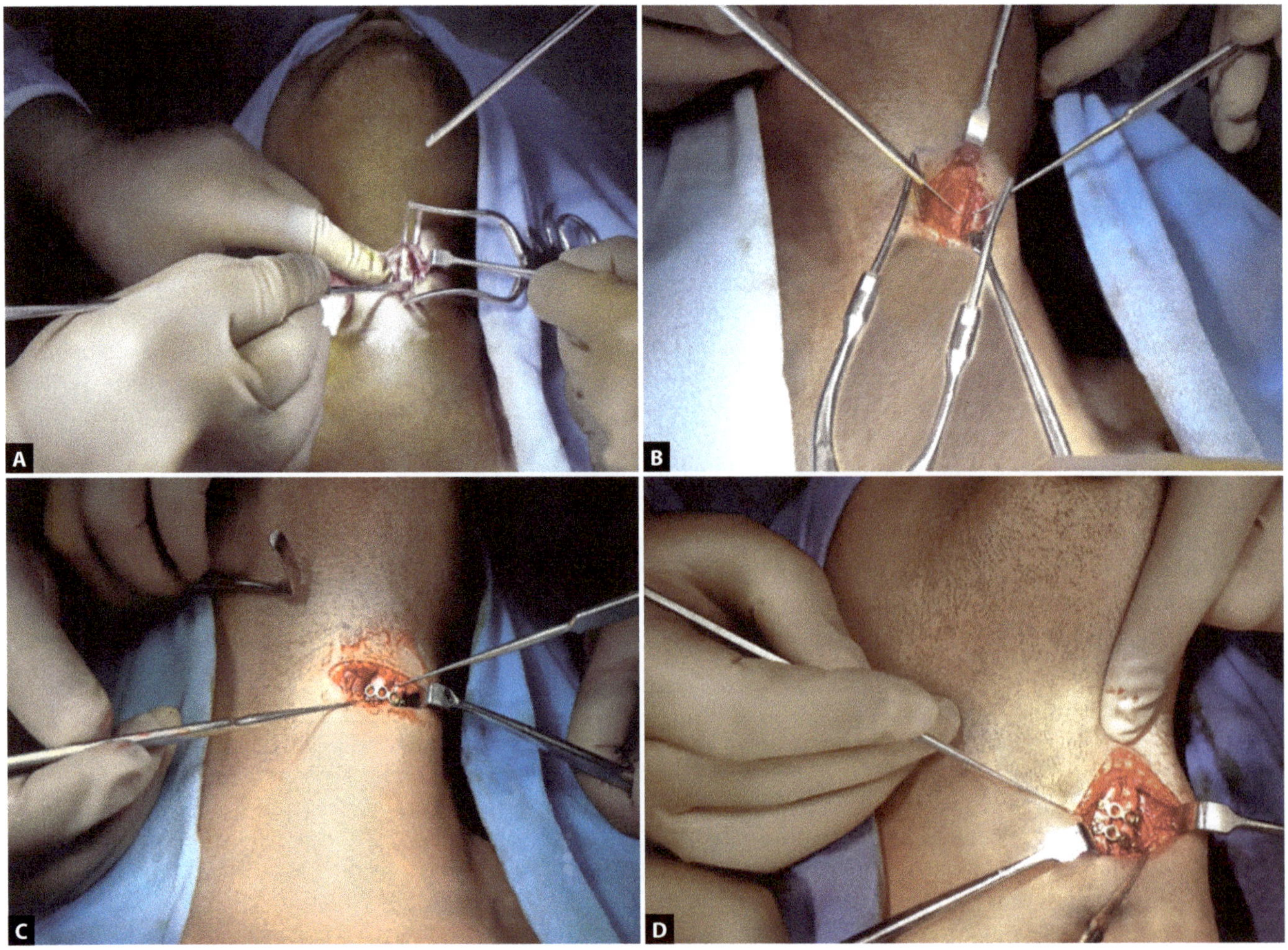

Figs 3A to D Type II thyroplasty; use of titanium miniplates to stabilize the separated thyroid ala

Endoscopic Laser Thyroarytenoid Myoneurectomy

This surgery consists of ablating the selective branch of RLN to TA muscle along with reduction of the TA muscle. Either CO_2 laser through rod delivery or a fiber laser can be used.

Tsuji et al.[34] reported 15 patients operated by this technique. Surgery was performed in 11 females and 4 males, aged between 29 years and 73 years, diagnosed with adductor SD. Voice Handicap Index (VHI) was obtained before and after surgery. A significant improvement in VHI was observed after surgery. 80% of operated patients showed subjective improvement.

Thyroarytenoid Myomectomy

Thyroarytenoid myomectomy (TAM) is an external approach via a thyroid window and in this procedure TA muscle is coagulated using bipolar cautery along with that the branch of RLN to TA muscle is also cut.

Nomoto et al.[35] did a comparison of type II thyroplasty and TAM procedure in a series of 35 and 30 patients, respectively. Compared with type II thyroplasty, TAM improves choking, interruption and tremor of voice. However, voice tends to be more breathy postoperatively. Postoperative VHI 10 scores did not differ significantly between the two procedures. Hence both surgical procedures can be used as per requirement of the situation.

Treatment has also been tried recently with a neuromodulating electrical implant. An electrode is placed into the TA muscle with a postauricular stimulator.[36] This is based on hypothesis that the benefit of Botulinum toxin injections is because of modulation of gamma loop of the muscle spindle via inhibition of motor neuron and not just because of weakness.[37] The initial results indicated that SD symptoms improved after electrical stimulation of the thyroarytenoid at levels below alpha motor neuron afferent. However, a bigger series with a longer follow-up is required for further validation.

REFERENCES

1. Fahn S. The varied clinical expressions of dystonia. Neurol Clin. 1984;2:541-54.
2. Aronson AE. Clinical voice disorders. New York: Thieme Medical Publishers; 1985.
3. Brin MF, Fahn S, Blitzer A, et al. Movement disorders of the larynx. In: Blitzer A, Brin MF, Sasaki CT, Fahn S, Harris KS (Eds). Neurological Disorders of the Larynx. New York: Thieme Medical Publishers; 1992. pp. 248-72.
4. Meyer TK, HU A, Hillel AD. Voice disorders in the workplace: productivity in spasmodic dysphonia and the impact of Botulinium toxin. Laryngoscope. 2013;123:S1-4.
5. Cannito MP, Woodson G. The spasmodic dysphonias. In: Kent RD, Ball M (Eds). Voice Quality Measurement. San Diego, CA: Singular; 2000. pp. 411-30.
6. Dedo HH. Recurrent laryngeal nerve section for Spastic dysphonia. Ann Otol Rhinol Laryngol. 1976;85(4):451-9.
7. Smith ME, Roy N, Wilson C. Lidocaine block of the recurrent laryngeal nerve in adductor spasmodic dysphonia: A multidimensional assessment. Laryngoscope. 2006;116:591-5.
8. Blitzer A, Brin MF. Laryngeal dystonia: a series with Botulinum toxin therapy. Ann Otol Rhinol Laryngol. 1991;100(2):85-9.
9. Marsden CD, Obeso JA, Zarrang JJ, et al. The anatomical basis of symptomatic hemidystonia. Brain. 1985;108(2):463-83.
10. Simonyan K, Ludlow CL. Abnormal activation of the primary somatosensory cortex in spasmodic dysphonia: an MRI study. Cereb Cortex. 2010;20(11):2749-59.
11. Cohen LG, Ludlow CL, Warden M, et al. Blink reflex curves in patients with spasmodic dysphonia. Neurolog. 1989;39:572-7.
12. Ibanez V, Sadato N, Karp B, et al. Deficient activation of the motor cortical network in patients with writer's cramp. Neurology. 1999;53:96-105.
13. Butefisch CM, Boroojerdi B, Chen R, et al. Task-dependent intracortical inhibition is impaired in focal hand dystonia. Mov Disord. 2005;20:545-51.
14. Sohn YH, Hallett M. Surround inhibition in human motor system. Exp Brain Res. 2004;158:397-404.
15. Boroojerdi B, Cohen LG, Hallett M. Effects of botulinum toxin on motor system excitability in patients with writer's cramp. Neurology. 2003;61:1546-50.
16. Zeuner KE, Shill HA, Sohn YH, et al. Motor training as treatment in focal hand dystonia. Mov Disord. 2005;20:335-41.
17. Quartarone A, Bagnato S, Rizzo V, et al. Abnormal associative plasticity of the human motor cortex in writer's cramp. Brain. 2003;126:2586-96.
18. Quartarone A, Siebner HR, Rothwell JC. Task-specific hand dystonia: can too much plasticity be bad for you? Trends Neurosci. 2006;29:192-9.
19. Bara-Jimenez W, Shelton P, Sanger TD, et al. Sensory discrimination capabilities in patients with focal hand dystonia. Ann Neurol. 2000;47:377-80.
20. Bara-Jimenez W, Catalan MJ, Hallett M, et al. Abnormal somatosensory homunculus in dystonia of the hand. Ann Neurol. 1998;44:828-31.
21. Tempel LW, Perlmutter JS. Abnormal vibration-induced cerebral blood flow responses in idiopathic dystonia. Brain. 1990;113:691-707.
22. Dezfulian M, Hatheway CI, Yolken RH, et al. Enzyme linked immunosorbent assay for detection of *Clostridium botulinum* type A and type B toxins in stool samples of infants with botulism. J Clin Microbiol. 1984;20(3):379-83.
23. Thomas JP, Siupsinskiene N. Frozen versus fresh reconstituted botox for laryngeal dystonia. Otolaryngol Head Neck Surg. 2006;135(2):204-8.
24. Aronson AE, Desanto LW. Adductor spasmodic dysphonia: 1.5 years after recurrent laryngeal nerve section. Laryngoscope. 1983;93:1-8.
25. Fritzell B, Feuer E, Haglund S, et al. Experiences with recurrent laryngeal nerve section for spastic dysphonia. Folia Phoniatr. 1982;34:160-7.

26. Dedo HH, Izdebski K. Intermediate results of 306 recurrent laryngeal nerve sections for spastic dysphonia. Laryngoscope. 1983;93:9-16.

27. Dedo HH, Izdebski K. Problems with surgical (RLN section) treatment of spasmodic dysphonia. Laryngoscope. 1983;93(3):268-71.

28. Netterville JL, Stone RE, Rainey C, et al. Recurrent laryngeal nerve avulsion for treatment of spastic dysphonia. Ann Otol Rhinol. 1991;100(1):10-4.

29. Berke GS, Blackwell KE, Gerratt BR, et al. Selective laryngeal adductor denervation—reinnervation; a new surgical treatment for adductor spasmodic dysphonia. Ann Otol Rhinol Laryngol. 1999;108(3):227-31.

30. Isshiki N, Tsuji DH, Yamamoto Y, et al. Midline lateralization thyroplasty for adductor spasmodic dysphonia. Ann Otol Rhinol Laryngol. 2000;109(2):187-93.

31. Isshiki N, Haji T, Yamamoto Y, et al. Thyroplasty for adductor spasmodic dysphonia: further experiences. Laryngoscope. 2001;111(4 Pt 1):615-21.

32. Isshiki N, Yamamoto I, Fukagai S. Type 2 thyroplasty for spasmodic dysphonia; fixation using a titanium bridge. Acta Otolaryngol. 2004;124(3):309-12.

33. Sanuki T, Isshiki N. Overall evaluation of effectiveness of type II thyroplasty for adductor spasmodic dysphonia. Laryngoscope. 2007;117(12):2255-9.

34. Tsuji DH, Takahashi MT, Imamura R, et al. Endoscopic laser thyroarytenoid myoneurectomy in patients with adductor spasmodic dysphonia: a pilot study on long-term outcome on voice quality. J Voice. 2012;26(5):666.e7-12.

35. Nomoto M, Tokashiki R, Hiramatsu H, et al. The comparison of thyroarytenoid muscle myectomy and type II thyroplasty for spasmodic dysphonia. J Voice. 2015;29(4):501-6.

36. Pitman MJ. Treatment of spasmodic dysphonia with a neuromodulating electrical implant. Laryngoscope. 2014;124: 2537-43.

37. Rosales RL, Dressler D. On muscle spindles, dystonia and botulinum toxin. Eur J Neurol. 2010;17:71-80.

6

Care of Singing Voice

Jaya Kumar Menon

INTRODUCTION

Singing voice is unique and complex. The singers need to realize the full potential of their voice not only in its pitch range and loudness, but also in the resonance. All this needs to be done without undue strain on the vocal apparatus. If a faulty technique creeps in, the voice starts losing its smoothness and flexibility, thereby leading to inability to express the finer nuances of musical notes. There can be nothing more heartbreaking for a singer than losing the ability to express the subtle variations in the pitch and resonance, which is very much in his or her mind. In almost all disease status, prevention is better than cure. It is especially true in case of singing voice. To learn a healthy singing voice, production technique is to prevent the chance of developing voice strain later.

VOICE PRODUCTION

Voice production includes three major levels. The vibrating force is the exhaled air, the vibrators are the vocal folds and the resonance is imparted by the supraglottic air column or the vocal tract up to the lips. For a vocalist rendering as well as diction is equally important. Hence these two factors also need to be taken into consideration. Then there is something called vocal hygiene, which is essentially about what is good for the voice and what is not so good. In the ensuing section, we will look into these areas which encompass the true singing voice care.

Vibrating Force

Exhaled air is the vibrating force.[1] Even though most of us can produce voice on inhaled air, it is rarely being resorted to. Usually in respiratory cycle, inspiration is more prolonged

than expiration. However, in vocalization, especially during singing, the exhalation phase has to be more prolonged in a controlled fashion. So, in order to have a good exhalation, one needs a good inhalation technique. During inhalation, the chest cage expands and let the air fill the lungs. This expansion of the chest cage is done by various methods. Some of these techniques are quietly efficient, while some others may be very inefficient.

Good Breathing Techniques

Chest breathing and abdominal breathing both are efficient inhalation techniques. In chest breathing or thoracic breathing, the chest cage expands in more of a horizontal plane, while in abdominal or diaphragmatic breathing the expansion happens in the vertical plane. The former expansion method is brought about by the intercostal muscles, while the latter is the result of diaphragmatic contraction.[2] To identify the breathing technique, ask the singer to place one palm over the central chest and the other one over the anterior abdominal wall just below the xiphisternum. Watch the singer from the side and note which hand is being displaced anteriorly. If the hand over the anterior chest wall is moving predominantly, then it is chest breathing. Conversely, if it is the lower hand which is moving then the person is having abdominal breathing. It is not uncommon to find in certain persons both the hands moving equally well. It simply suggests that the person has both chest and abdominal breathing, which is all the more good.

Bad Breathing Techniques

Many children and ladies use what is known as the neck breathing or clavicular breathing. This is said to occur, when the clavicles are pulled up by the sternomastoid muscles on both sides during inspiration. As a result, only the apical parts of the lungs get filled with air, which is much less than the full capacity. Here the effort is more, but the result is poor. Another relatively inefficient breathing technique is the shoulder breathing, wherein the shoulders are lifted during each inspiratory effort. This is also known as the upper chest breathing or pectoral breathing. Though not as inefficient as the neck breathing, shoulder breathing also causes suboptimal volume of the inhaled air and consequently having a detrimental effect on the exhalation. A third type of undesirable inhalation is the paradoxical breathing. In this type of breathing, the person uses chest breathing causing expansion of the chest cage in a horizontal plane. But this is undermined by the upward movement of the diaphragm, which happens at the same time as the chest expansion. While the chest will be seen expanding, the anterior abdominal wall will be moving inwards, secondary to the upward movement of the dome of the diaphragm.

Exhalation

To have a good voice technique, one should have not just a great breathing in technique, but also an efficient breathing out technique. While breathing out for vocalization, three key points are there. First of all, it is very important not to waste any air. Many nervous singers will take a good inhalation, but will surrender all its benefits by wasting significant amounts of air before starting phonation. Second abnormal exhalation behavior is leaking of air while phonating. This happens because the vocal folds are not snugly meeting each other. Instead they have a phonatory gap through which significant amount of exhaled air is wasted. This usually happens in muscle tension dysphonia, especially in those with vocal nodules. Even more common is the third abnormal exhalation technique, in which the singer forces the air through. This amounts to colossal waste of energy, both in the form of air as well as in the form of muscle contraction.

ASSESSING THE BREATH SUPPORT

This is best done by the simple test of maximum phonation duration (MPD). The singer is asked to take a deep breath and without wasting any air asked to produce an "ee" sound in the habitual pitch and loudness for as long as he or she can. Minimum three trials are needed and the best value is taken. It is advisable to have an MPD of 15 seconds or more. MPD is best assessed on empty stomach, though taking water prior to the test is advisable.

Phonation

The vocal folds vibrate in various frequencies during singing. This happens after both of them meet in the midline.

Depending upon the way in which they adduct, the modes of vocal fold vibrations can be divided into three groups known as vocal registers. The lower most of the pitch range is produced, with vocal folds medial margin thick and round,[3] while at the other extreme, vocal folds do not completely meet each other during the falsetto register. During this register, the vibratory margin of the vocal folds is extremely thin. The middle register is the one most commonly used by the singers. Three-fourths of the pitch range is produced in this register. There is a fourth register called whistle register for producing the extreme high pitches. This is not used by the singers in India.

The registers can be compared to the gears of a motor vehicle. The lowest register or the vocal fry is comparable to the first gear of the motor vehicle. It can only produce very low frequencies like first gear capable of lower speeds only. The middle register produces the biggest chunk of the pitch range and the upper one-fourths of the pitch spectrum is produced by the falsetto register. Just like in case of a motor vehicle, where smooth transition from one gear to the next is of great importance to produce a smooth ride, transition from one register to the next should be flowing. This smooth transition from one register to another is known as passaggio.[4] Instead of being smooth, if the register to register transmission is jerky, then the voice suffers from pitch breaks and can result in unpleasant auditory effect.

While most singers will be quite comfortable in the middle range of pitch, many will struggle at the extremes, especially at the high-pitch range. Increased pitch is produced by making the vocal cord thin and taught. Many singers will have the wrong technique of increasing the subglottic pressure to produce high pitch. Nothing can be more counterproductive. When a singer pushes at the voice, the flexibility and the sweetness of the voice are lost and consequently the ability to bring in subtle variations will be lost.

Resonance

Resonance is the key to the individuality of the voice as well as the voice projection.[5] By voice projection, what is meant is the ability to make the voice louder without straining. There are many resonating chambers in the human vocal tract. Pharynx is the most important among them. Oral cavity and nasal passages are the second and third important resonating chambers. A key area in singers is the epilaryngeal zone, which is bounded by the epiglottis in front, aryepiglottic folds on both sides and arytenoids posteriorly. The volume of this chamber is very small compared to the previously mentioned resonating chambers. Because of that the resonance imparted by the epilaryngeal zone is on the higher pitches, usually around 3,000 Hz. Each of these resonating chambers helps to amplify one or more of the overtones produced by the vocal folds. These frequencies are then known as formants.

The formant produced by the epilaryngeal zone is called the singers formant.[6]

The major organs responsible for altering the resonance are tongue, lips, and palate. The base tongue is responsible for changing the volume of the retrolingual space and consequently decides the "openness" or "closeness" of the voice. The anterior two-thirds of the tongue can alter the volume of the oral cavity and thus alter the resonance as well as the voice projection. Soft palate also can alter the oral cavity resonance by moving down and up. Oral cavity can be considered as a room with tongue its floor and palate its roof. Both of these walls can move in various directions and consequently can change the size and shape of the oral resonating chamber. In addition to this, the soft palate also plays a critical role in determining the nasal resonance. It can completely or partially cut-off the nasal cavity from the oral cavity and adjust the nasality. Lips are very important in vowel production as well as labial sounds. They also impart resonance by opening laterally and rounding the oral aperture.

Diction and Rendering

The correct pronunciation with suitable expression is called diction. To many it comes naturally. If not, it is not impossible to train them. Rendering denotes the emphasis while producing the consonants. In soft rendering the emphasis is minimal, while in hard rendering it is more. Rendering and diction varies according to the mood of the songs.

ASSESSMENT OF SINGING VOICE

A thorough history taking is of paramount importance. Specific complaints regarding the singing voice has to be recorded in the history chart.[7] Ask whether the speaking voice is normal or not. If the speaking voice also is affected, chances are that the person is suffering from a structural lesion of the vocal fold. More commonly the complaint will be that singing voice is abnormal, but the speaking voice is normal. This is sometimes referred to as dysodia and almost certainly suggests that the vocal folds are structurally normal, but there is some problem with the way they are functioning. Specific complaints, like loss of pitch range, shift of pitch range, easy vocal fatigability, inability to raise the volume, frequent clearing of the throat and irritation of the throat, should be noted.

A detailed history of the vocal demands is of great importance in reaching the diagnosis as well as charting out treatment options. Ask for any medication the singer is on. Drugs, like aspirin and clopidogrel, significantly increase the risk of submucosal hemorrhage of the vocal folds. Antihistamines and vitamin C can produce significant drying effect and can adversely affect the smooth phonation.[8] Long-term steroid inhalers are known to produce bowing of the vocal folds. History of use of tobacco and alcohol is specifically asked as is the food habits. In case of females, menstrual history needs to be asked.

Check the MPD and the confortable pitch range. Usually, most singers will be comfortable singing two octaves. Look for the breathing technique. Watch the mouth opening, lip movements, tongue position, palate lifting, and lower jaw thrust. Measure the pitch range and formants if facilities are available.

Flexible endoscopic evaluation of the singing voice is the next step. This is done in the sitting position with minimal or no local anesthesia. First of all, the singer is asked to sing ascending and descending notes and then a relatively easy song and finally a song which he or she finds difficult. Look for abnormal muscle tension dysphonia patterns like phonatory gap with or without nodules, ventricular band adduction, anteroposterior compression, persistent falsetto mode and pharyngeal squeeze.[9] Of these it is not uncommon to find unilateral muscle tension dysphonia pattern with ventricular band adduction and pharyngeal squeeze. Also look for any structural lesions, submucosal hemorrhage or features of laryngopharyngeal reflux disorder. Gradually withdraw the scope and fix it just above the tongue base. Look for the tongue base position to decide whether the person is singing with an open throat resonance or a closed throat resonance. Withdraw the scope further and locate the tip just above the soft palate so as to see the movement of the velopharyngeal sphincter so as to assess the control of nasality.

In certain cases, videofluoroscopy will be a good tool to assess the resonance, especially the oral resonance. But this is not routinely needed. A dynamic magnetic resonance imaging (MRI) also will give excellent assessment of the resonating chambers. But it is more expensive than the fluoroscopy.

MANAGEMENT

Acute Dysphonia in Singers

The common two causes of acute dysphonia in singers are laryngitis and submucosal hemorrhage. The former may occur as an isolated entity or as part of the upper airway tract infection. Most of them are viral. Hence, there is no need of antibiotics. But if the singer has a program which cannot be cancelled, then one is justified in prescribing steroids like prednisolone 30 mg daily in divided doses along with proton pump inhibitors.[10] The steroids can be rapidly tapered off once the performance is over. Antihistamines are better avoided as they are known to produce significant drying of the mucosa. If there is an associated nasal obstruction secondary to rhinosinusitis local decongestants like xylometazoline should be prescribed. It is important to warn the singer that the highest pitch ranges are better avoided. They should also be instructed to take frequent sips of warm water.

Submucosal hemorrhage is a more severe form of acute dysphonia. It is better to avoid performing till the hemorrhage has completely resolved. This may take up to 2 weeks. Performing in presence of submucosal hemorrhage increases the risk of opening up the submucosal capillaries and thus causing even bigger hemorrhage.

Chronic Dysphonia in Singers

Systematic assessment of the singing voice described earlier will give valuable clues regarding the management of chronic dysphonia in singers. If it is secondary to a bad breathing technique like neck, shoulder or paradoxical breathing, then the correction of dysphonia should be attempted by teaching the chest and/or abdominal breathing. Making the patient sit in front of a mirror and watching the breathing technique while singing will help in a big way. Some singers will have wrong exhalation technique while singing, despite having a good inhalation technique. They will be found using more than necessary force during singing. This is forcing out or squeezing out the voice and is not at all desirable. During singing their neck, chest, and abdominal muscle will be seen contracting vigorously. Lax vox technique will be a very useful method to correct this fault.[11] In this method, singer is asked to produce a note through a wide bore straw, which has its other end immersed in water filled up to a quarter of a glass. Next, ascending and descending notes are produced and finally various songs' tunes are played. If the singer uses too much of force, the bubbling will increase. Using this as a feedback, the singer can adjust and avoid any excessive force during voice production.

Many singers will complain about the difficulty in reaching the higher pitches. More often than not, this is due to technical faults. If not properly counseled these singers will try wrong forcing techniques and end up having even lesser range of pitch. It is important to understand that for extreme high pitch the vocal folds need to be stretched fully.[12] This is best brought about by not just cricothyroid and suprahyoid strap muscles, but also by protruding the lower jaw, slightly elevating the face and imparting more nasality. Bringing the chin down and turning it to one side or the other will be counterproductive.

Another not so rare problem faced by the singers is the inability to smoothly transit from one register to another. The smooth transition from one register to the next is known as passaggio. Its absence will cause unpleasant pitch breaks. Passaggio training can be done with a simple technique. The singer is asked to keep his right index finger just above the thyroid notch and then to produce notes in the ascending order. If the transition from the modal voice to falsetto is smooth, the larynx will lift the finger in a gradual fashion to the uppermost part of the neck. On the contrary, if passaggio is conspicuously absent, the larynx will abruptly slip under the finger, when the singer switches on to the falsetto register. Practicing yodeling, which involves deliberate abrupt register transfer, though difficult, is an efficient way of learning passaggio.

Resonance is the key to having very impressive singing voice. If the singer is using a clenched teeth technique, that should be corrected by teaching the open mouth technique. Similarly pronounced movement of upper lip should be taught, if the singer does not move the lip that too well. The position of the tongue in the oral cavity is denoted by the term "tongue carriage". Ideally the tongue tip should be just behind the lower central incisor teeth. If the tongue is held in a posterior position, it is called "posterior tongue carriage" and when held high up in the oral cavity, it is called "superior tongue carriage". Both of these positions are not conductive for good voice projection. So if these behaviors are noted they should be corrected with visual and auditory feedbacks. Lifting the soft palate gives an excellent voice quality and power. If the singer is unable to do it intentionally, it can be taught by the semiyawning technique. In this technique, the singer is asked to do a yawning and at the height of yawning asked to produce a note. The voice produced will be really powerful. The role of lower jaw protrusion has already been discussed.

VOCAL HYGIENE

There are things which are good for the voice and things which are bad for the voice. Practicing the former and avoiding the latter essentially constitutes vocal hygiene. Adequately hydrating the vocal folds by taking enough water is probably the most important must do thing for voice.[13] Bathroom singing is a very good technique for hydrating the vocal folds, because you are breathing in air which is coming through the water particles and thus moist. By the same token, "jalasadhakam" practiced in India in the years gone by imparts humidification of the breathing air. It also has the added advantage of strengthening the breath power. In this method, the singer stands neck deep in water and sings. Because the chest is underneath the water level, each time the singer takes in breath, the lungs have to expand against the resistance of water, which is more than the resistance offered by the air. Thus, somebody who has practiced this technique regularly finds it easy to breathe in during singing, because the resistance offered by atmospheric pressure is much less.

Dryness obviously will be harmful to the vocal function. Gastroesophageal reflux will cause the acid to fall on the laryngeal mucosa and thus nullify the effect of moisture on the vocal folds. So, it is imperative for the singers to have regular food habits. Eating too much and too little is best avoided. Avoiding fatty spicy foods, especially for the dinner, is preferable. There should be a minimum of 2 hours between dinner and going to bed. Excessive coffee and tea cause drying of the vocal folds and hence to be limited. Alcohol also has drying effect as well as stimulation of acid secretion in the stomach. Smoking obviously is a greater hazard and can even cause malignancy of the larynx.

Almost everybody knows that speaking very loud is not a good thing for the vocal health. But, what many do not understand is the fact that speaking faster is as bad or even worse. Speaking in noisy surrounding is another bad habit. Singers also should know that it is very important not to engage in other vocal activities like mimicry, dubbing and ventriloquy. Improper valving can occur while lifting weights and playing power games. This can cause microtrauma to the medial margin of the vocal folds, more so if the person happens to take any blood thinning agents like aspirin or clopidogrel.

Female singers in the reproductive age group should understand the effects of the female sex hormones on the voice. Estrogen is the voice beautifying hormone, while progesterone makes the voice low pitched and coarse. Hence during the premenstrual period, the highest pitch range may not be possible.[14] Without knowing this, if the singer tries to hit the higher pitches, she may damage her vocal folds. Even submucosal hemorrhages of the vocal folds are likely to occur during this period.

Finally, the importance of voice rest needs to be understood by all singers. Vocal folds, being very fragile structures, need lots of rest period for recuperating the energy and for repair of the microtrauma that can happen with sustained singing. A general rule will be about 16 hours of voice rest and 8 hours of vocal activity in a day. Like in any other art or sport, practice makes perfect singing voice. Every singer should understand the basic functioning of the vocal apparatus and nurture it properly to have a long and successful career.

REFERENCES

1. van den Bergh J. Myoelastic-aerodynamic theory of voice production. J Speech Hear Res. 1958;1(3):227-44.
2. LoVetri JL. Treatment of injured singers and professional speakers: The singer/actor, singer/dancer, and singer/musician. In: Benninger MS, Murry T (Eds). The Singer's Voice. California, CA, USA: Plural Publishing; 2006. pp. 209-18.
3. Titze IR, Luschei ES, Hirano M. Role of the thyroarytenoid muscle in the regulation of fundamental frequency. J Voice. 1989;3:213-24.
4. Titze IR. Principles of voice production. Englewood Cliffs, NJ, USA: Prentice Hall Incorporation; 1994.
5. American Standards Association. American Standard Acoustical Terminology (Including Mechanical Shock and Vibration). New York, NY, USA: American Standards Association; 1960.
6. Sundberg J. Perceptual aspects of singing. J Voice. 1994;8(2):106-22.
7. Sataloff RT. Efficient history taking in professional singers. Laryngoscope. 1984. pp. 1111-4.
8. Lawrence VL. Medical care for professional voice. In: Lawrence VL (Ed). Transcripts from the annual symposium: care of the professional voice (Volume 3). New York, NY, USA: The Voice Foundation; 1978. pp. 17-8.
9. Belafsky PC, Postma GN, Reulbach TR, et al. Muscle tension dysphonia as a sign of underlying glottal insufficiency. Otolaryngol Head Neck Surg. 2002;127(5):448-51.
10. Thompson AR. Pharmacological agents with effects on voice. Am J Otolaryngol. 1995;16(1):12-8.
11. Sihvo M, Denizoglu I. Lax vox: voice therapy technique. Turkey: Ad Izir; 2007.
12. Sundberg J. The science of the singing voice. DeKalb, IL, USA: Northern Illinois University Press; 1987.
13. Verdolini K, Titze IR, Fennell A. Dependence of phonatory effort on hydration level. J Speech Hear Res. 1994;37(5):1001-7.
14. Abitbol J, Abitbol P, Abitbol B. Sex hormones and the female voice. J Voice. 1999;13(3):424-46.

The Aging Voice

Joseph P Bradley, Michael M Johns

INTRODUCTION

The world population has continued to grow significantly in the past century. Not only is our population growing, but it is also aging. The number of individuals over age of 60 years is expected to more than double by 2050 (from 841 million in 2013 to over 2 billion by 2050).[1] The incidence of vocal disorders is estimated to be between 12 and 35% in the older population.[2-4] As a result, we can expect that the number of older Indians seeking medical care for assorted vocal complains will also increase.

Vocal complains in the older population have an impact on patient's quality of life, particularly in patients who are already struggling with communication issues. 13% of these patients note a marked reduction in their quality of life because of their dysphonia.[5] There are changes in the acoustic properties of the voice—increased breathiness, decreased loudness, increased jitter and shimmer, and increased fundamental frequency (F_0) in men and decreased F_0 in women.[6] These patients complain of voice instability and generally avoid more social situations as a result.[6]

Geriatric voice dysfunction may be caused by a number of factors—vocal fold atrophy, neurologic conditions, decreased lung capacity, lesions of the larynx, inflammatory or infectious disorders, vocal fold paralysis.[2] The goal of this chapter is to discuss the physiology behind the aging voice and to learn how to identify and treat the major causes of vocal distress in the aging population.

GERIATRIC DYSPHONIA

Presbyphonia

Presbyphonia, or age-related dysphonia, is a diagnosis given to patients after a thorough examination and workup excludes other pathology. Some might argue that presbyphonia is not a true pathology, but rather a pattern of symptoms involving several organ systems that result from the normal aging process.

While not part of the larynx, the actuator of the voice is the lungs. The normal aging process leads to a significant decrease in the compliance of the chest wall, in elastic recoil of the lungs, and in respiratory muscle strength. Compared with a 20-year-old person, compliance of the respiratory system is approximately 20% less in a 60-year-old person, leading to an increase in the work to be just to maintain tidal volumes.[7] Together with increased functional reserve capacity (FRC), it becomes more difficult to overcome subglottal pressure and to power the voice.[8]

The neuromuscular anatomy and function of the larynx are also prone to the effects of aging. Human cadaveric studies of the recurrent laryngeal nerve have indicated a loss of large axons with a slenderization of the remaining axons with loss of myelin in older patients.[9] Connor and colleagues demonstrated a reduction in axon terminal area and an increased number of unoccupied postsynaptic acetylcholine receptors similar to that of denervated muscle in the neuromuscular junction (NMJ) of the thyroarytenoid (TA) muscle.[10] Direct muscle changes also occur within the aging larynx—a loss of type I (slow-twitch fibers), compensatory hypertrophy of the remaining type I fibers, and an age-related increase in type 1 and type 2 myosin heavy-chain isoforms.[11] This is indicative of motor-unit remodeling similar to denervation-reinnervation. There is also demonstrable evidence that the TA muscle becomes weaker, slower, and more fatigable with age.[12]

The epithelial and lamina propria also exhibit age-related changes. Collagen normally forms a "wicker-basket" type of appearance within the lamina propria, providing tension and elasticity. In older adults, this organization becomes much more disarrayed throughout all the layers of the lamina propria and becomes more abundant, along with a loss of hyaluronic acid (HA) and elastin.[13,14] These changes lead to loss of the viscoelastic properties and a thinning of the vocal fold. Combined with TA muscle atrophy, this leads to the classic bowed membranous vocal fold.

The larynx descends into the neck, while the laryngeal cartilages start to ossify, which has an impact on vocal resonance.[8] As with other joints in the body, the articular surfaces breakdown and decreased range of motion of the cricoarytenoid joints.[15,16] In aging adults, there is less laryngeal mucous with a higher viscosity and, therefore, less overall lubrication.[17]

Central Nervous System Pathology

There are a number of central nervous system (CNS) pathologies seen in older adults that may also have an impact on the voice. These include stroke, tremor, amyotrophic lateral sclerosis (ALS), and Parkinson's disease. Broadly speaking, the laryngologic manifestations of neurologic disease can be categorized as motor neuron disease, extrapyramidal disease, cerebrovascular event, or multiple sclerosis (MS).

Lesions involving motor neurons can exclusively affect the upper motor neurons, the lower motor neurons, or a combination of both. Upper motor neuron disease presents with spasticity of laryngeal and orofacial muscles, leading to laryngospasm, myoclonus, and a tense dysphonia.[18] Lower motor neuron disease presents with a flaccid paralysis and muscle atrophy, manifesting as vocal fold bowing. This leads to a greater amount of glottal insufficiency along with hypernasal speech secondary to poor palate elevation.[18] ALS is the classic example of mixed motor neuron disease with symptoms of both upper and lower pathology, including a weak, breathy voice, weak cough, and dysarthria.[18]

Multiple sclerosis is a neurodegenerative disease of the myelin sheaths of the CNS. A variety of laryngopharyngeal complaints can be seen in these patients. Scanning speech is very frequently found in patients with MS, in which syllables of words are separated by pauses.[19] They may also suffer from dysphagia, vocal tremor, and vocal spasm. Acoustic analysis demonstrates that women with MS have a higher fundamental frequency, while men tend to have more jitter.[19]

Neurolaryngology diseases involving the extrapyramidal system include Parkinson's disease, spasmodic dysphonia, and essential tremor. Parkinson's disease results from degeneration of dopamine-producing cells of the *substantia nigra* in the brainstem. Because of the systemic weaknesses associated with Parkinson's disease, over 70% of patients may experience glottal insufficiency, poor respiratory support, laryngeal tremor, dysarthria and dysphagia.[18]

Essential tremor is an action tremor of the upper limbs, and, less commonly, the head and neck that presents without other neurologic signs. While there are several types, Marsden type 2 tremor includes the lips, tongue, head and voice, and shows abnormal motor unit entrainment at frequencies of 4–12 Hz.[20] The oscillating nature of the tremor creates an unstable voice with frequent breaks.[18]

HISTORY AND EXAMINATION

As with any patient encounter, a complete patient history is necessary. It is important to ascertain the level of vocal use, both historically and currently. This can help to gauge the amount of trauma endured and to identify the level of voice necessary for functional daily activities. Diet, use of tobacco and alcohol are also key pieces of information in putting the puzzle together. The most important part of the clinic visit, however, comes from imaging of the larynx, especially via the videostroboscopic examination. Figure 1A of the glottis in the open phase demonstrates increased ventricular visibility, atrophy of structures, and prominence of the vocal processes. Figure 1B of the glottis in the closed phase demonstrates vocal fold bowing, and the spindle-shaped glottic chink. These important examination findings are characteristic for presbylarynx.[8,21,22] The increased glottal gap seen in these patients does not necessarily correlate with the severity of the dysphonia. This is likely due to the compensatory mechanisms of the larynx. On stroboscopy, the vocal folds will demonstrate irregular or aperiodic vibration, asymmetric mucosal wave, and increased amplitude.[8] As a diagnosis of exclusion, the practitioner must rule out other causes of dysphonia, including lesions of the vocal folds, neurologic disorders, and reduced lung function.

REJUVENATION OF THE AGING VOICE

A multidisciplinary approach by the laryngologist and speech pathologist is a key to treating the aging voice, much as with other vocal complaints. Key to determining the optimal approach, one must examine factors such as the severity of the patient's problem, the patient's desires, comorbidities, and the ability to undergo an intervention. One of the most important, but often more forgotten, things that the practitioner can do is to provide reassurance to the patient. These patients are often referred because of vocal changes that give worry for malignancy. Many of these patients still have a very serviceable voice and not need any further intervention.

The most conservative therapy is voice therapy. Therapy that focuses on phonatory and respiratory strengthening exercises would seem ideal for increasing neuromuscular coordination needed to overcome age changes. The therapy focuses on educating the patient about the etiology of the problem, producing a resonant tone for optimal vocal postures, and standard vocal function exercises (VFEs). Therapy requires multiple sessions, but, more importantly, requires patients to work on the exercises outside of formal therapy sessions. Voice therapy alone has been demonstrated to be highly efficacious in improving voice quality of life measures, with a mean improvement in voice-related quality of life (VRQOL) score of 19.21 after roughly four sessions in a 5-month period.[23] Sauder et al. demonstrated that VFEs serve to improve functional and perceptual voice parameters, voice problem severity, breathiness, and strain with demonstrable reductions in Voice Handicap Index (VHI).[24] These exercises strengthen and rebalance the laryngeal musculature and improve vocal fold adduction. Phonation resistance training exercise (PhoRTE) is another novel therapy that aims to treat presbylarynx. It is modeled after Lee Silverman Voice Therapy (LSVT) and consists of four exercises: (1) loud maximum sustained phonation on /a/; (2) ascending and descending pitch glides on /a/; (3) shouting specific word lists/phrases using a loud and high voice, and (4) shouting those same phrases using a low and authoritative voice. The goal of these exercises is to target the degenerative and age-related changes to the respiratory system and larynx. While both VFE and PhoRTE demonstrate improvement on VRQOL scores, only the PhoRTE group demonstrates an improvement in perceived phonatory effort.[25] For patient with a more severe dysphonia or for elderly patient who cannot travel distances or with frequency, then voice therapy may not work as well.

The next least invasive intervention is vocal fold augmentation via injection. Injection laryngoplasty was initially developed for treating glottic insufficiency for unilateral vocal fold paralysis by augmenting the paraglottic space and medializing the true vocal fold. Postma and colleagues demonstrated that this intervention was also successful for treating glottal insufficiency for bilateral vocal fold atrophy.[26] There are a number of substances in the market, most being some form of dermal or collagen matrix—Cymetra, Restylane, Radiesse Voice Gel, etc. All of these substances are temporary, with variable times for resorption. The utility in a temporary material is to give the patient and practitioner an idea of how much benefit can be achieved by augmentation. Classically, injection laryngoplasty has been performed in the operating room under general anesthesia, which provides the most precision and control of augmenting the paraglottic space. The disadvantage to injecting under general anesthesia is that the provider cannot titrate the patient's voice. In recent years, percutaneous and per oral techniques in the awake setting have grown increasingly at common place. This avoids the need for the time and expense required with going to the operating room and allows for titration of the patient's voice. There is less precision with the awake technique and multiple injections may be required to achieve the desired result.

Just as injection laryngoplasty was transferred from treating first unilateral vocal fold palsy to treating bilateral vocal fold atrophy, laryngeal framework surgery as a more permanent solution has developed similarly. With the patient sedated in the operating room, the neck is opened centrally and small thyroid cartilage windows are fashioned bilaterally to expose the paraglottic space. Silastic or Gore-Tex implants are fashioned to fit in the paraglottic space and provide medialization bilaterally while the patient phonates.[27] While this technique is useful because of its permanence, limitations include a dynamic glottal closure and the risk of implant extrusion or inflammatory reaction.

PROFESSIONAL VOCALIST

Increased awareness by the practitioner is paramount when treating those individuals whose livelihood depends on their voice. Attention to healthy mechanics is a key to continued use of that instrument, despite aging effects. Voice coaching by the speech-language pathologist will help to correct and maintain the appropriate mechanics to overcome age-related effects.

FUTURE DIRECTIONS

While both speech therapy and surgical techniques successfully improve presbyphonia, neither addresses the underlying structural changes. Basic fibroblast growth factor (bFGF) has demonstrated the ability to reduce collagen production while increasing the presence of HA, which may be an ideal way to rejuvenate aged vocal folds.[28] The increased production of matrix metalloproteinase and HA synthase by injection of hepatic growth factor (HGF) has been demonstrated by Ohno and colleagues, thereby increasing HA.[29] Hydrogels serving as delivery systems for HGF demonstrated improvement in mucosal wave amplitude, vocal fold bowing, and glottal incompetence. The use of HGF has been limited in human studies because of the need to clarify safety concerns.[30] Injection of a synthetic derivative of HA to improve viscoelasticity of the superficial lamina propria (SLP) has also been described.[31] Much work remains to be done to translate what we know on the cellular level into clinical treatments.

CASE STUDIES

Case Study 1

Patient number 1 is a 65-year-old male with a several year history of increasing high-pitched voice. He reports that he is often confused as a woman on the phone or an intercom system. When he has tried to speak in a more normal pitch for a male, his voice becomes soft, breathy, and he becomes quickly fatigued. His speaking fundamental frequency was 138 Hz. He was intermittently seen for voice therapy over a 2-year period, but was inconsistent and subsequently developed a larger magnitude of glottal insufficiency. His

videostroboscopic examination demonstrated prominent vocal processes, concave bowing of the bilateral true vocal folds, patulous ventricles, and a spindle-shaped glottis closure (Figs 1A and B). The patient was taken to the endoscopic suite for an awake endoscopic bilateral injection laryngoplasty using Restylane-L. Two weeks after his injections, his breathy dysphonia was no longer present, he had increased vocal endurance, and a lower-pitch to his voice. Videostroboscopic examination demonstrated a loss of bowing with complete glottal closure (Fig. 1C).

Case Study 2

Patient number 2 is an 87-year-old male with a several year history of progressive dysphonia characterized by breathy dysphonia, increased pitch of the voice, decreased vocal endurance, increased vocal fatigue, decreased projection with difficulty being heard in noisy environments and some

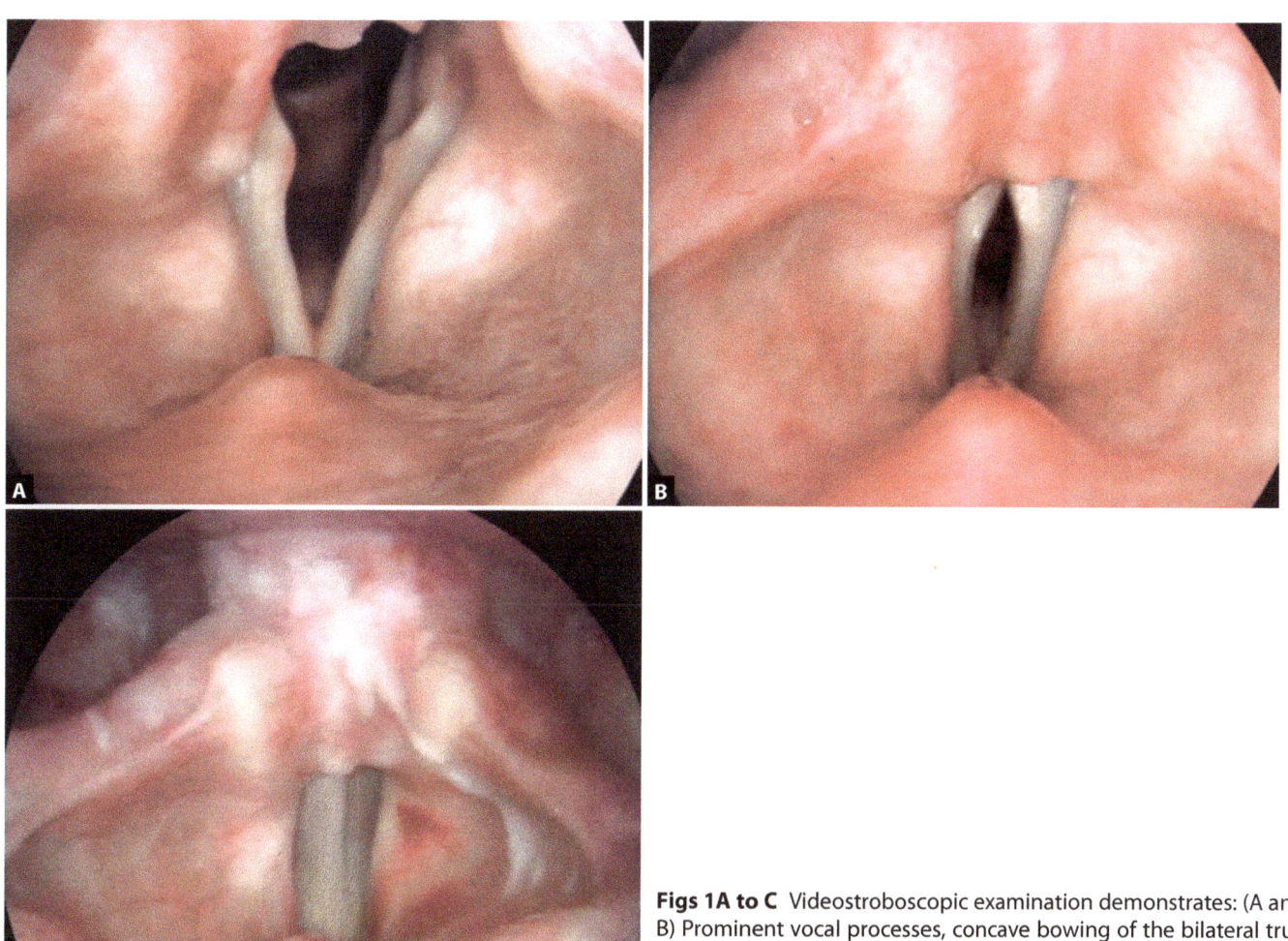

Figs 1A to C Videostroboscopic examination demonstrates: (A and B) Prominent vocal processes, concave bowing of the bilateral true vocal folds, patulous ventricles and a spindle-shaped glottis closure; (C) A loss of bowing with complete glottal closure

complaints of dysphagia. He underwent voice therapy with some improvement in his voice. However, he still noted problems with decreased projection, making it difficult for him to teach. He chose to undergo awake endoscopic bilateral injection laryngoplasty using Cymetra. He had a very good response with increased projection and vocal endurance. For the next 2 years, he chose not to proceed with any further interventions for his voice; although he began to experience his original symptoms as the Cymetra was resorbed. He was given the option of repeat injection laryngoplasty with long-acting material (calcium hydroxyapatite) versus bilateral type I thyroplasties with Gore-Tex. He chose to undergo bilateral thyroplasties, which were performed in the standard fashion. Figures 2A and B show his preoperative videostroboscopic findings, while Figures 2C and D show his postoperative videostroboscopic results.

CONCLUSION

Care of the aging voice is a unique treatment opportunity for voice practitioners, given the challenge to diagnose true presbyphonia exists versus an underlying neurologic disorder. Treatment modalities are not so complex that most practitioners cannot easily perform them. Moreover, the multidisciplinary approach undertaken for these patients offers a significantly improved quality of life. Given the increased number of patients over age of 60 years expected in the next few decades, having a fundamental understanding

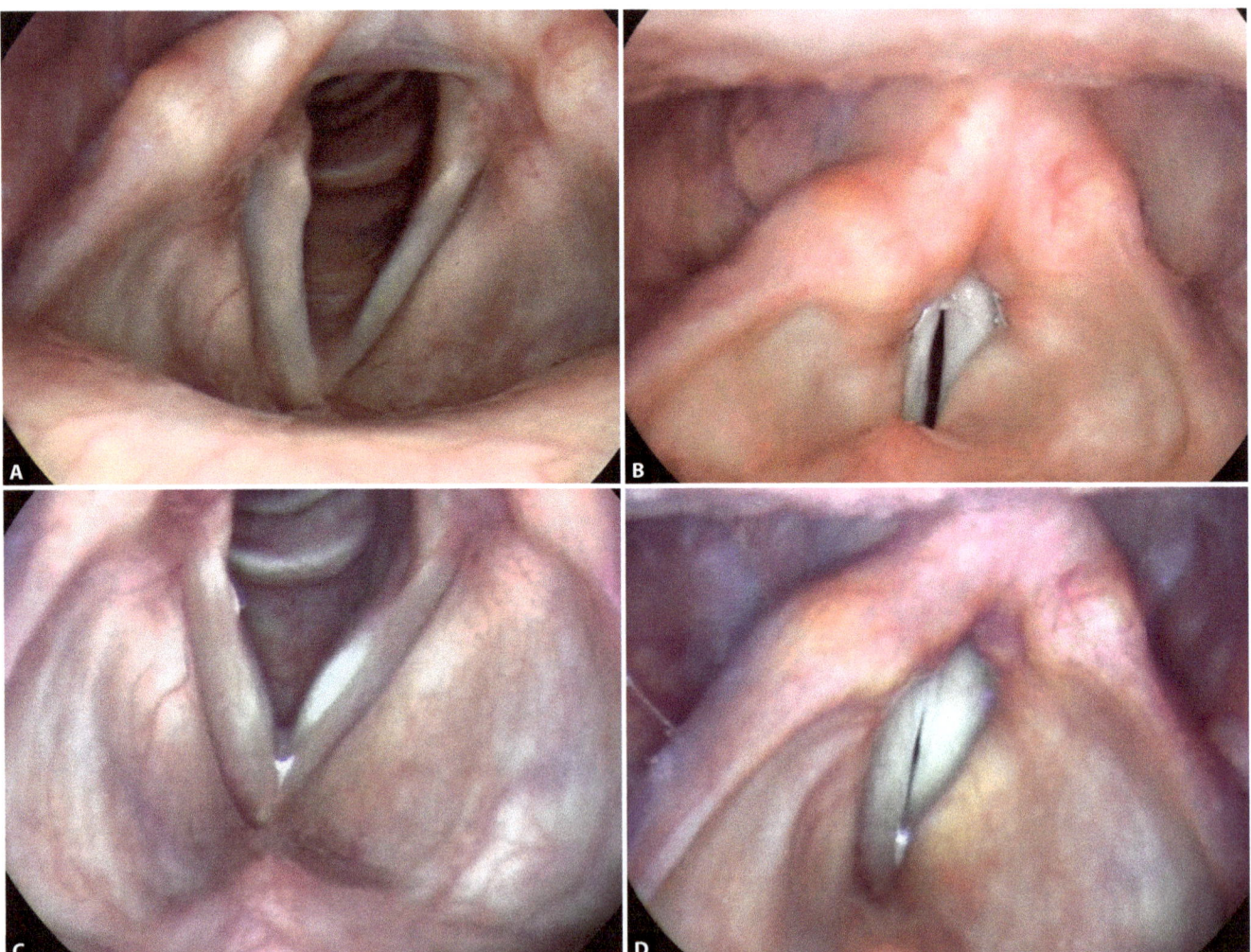

Figs 2A to D (A and B) Preoperative videostroboscopic findings; (C and D) Postoperative videostroboscopic results

of the diagnosis, treatment, and societal impact of the aging voice is crucial to the practice of otolaryngologists.

REFERENCES

1. United Nations, Department of Economic and Social Affairs, Population Division. (2013). World Population Ageing 2013.pp.1-11. [online] Available from *www.un.org/en/development/desa/population/publications/pdf/ageing/WorldPopulationAgeing2013.pdf*. [Accessed November, 2016].
2. Davids T, Klein AM, Johns MM 3rd. Current dysphonia trends in patients over the age of 65: is vocal atrophy becoming more prevalent? Laryngoscope. 2012;122(2):332-5.
3. Roy N, Stemple J, Merrill RM, et al. Epidemiology of voice disorders in the elderly: preliminary findings. Laryngoscope. 2007;117(4):628-33.
4. Turley R, Cohen S. Impact of voice and swallowing problems in the elderly. Otolaryngol Head Neck Surg. 2009;140(1):33-6.
5. Golub JS, Chen PH, Otto KJ, et al. Prevalence of perceived dysphonia in a geriatric population. J Am Geriatr Soc. 2006;54(11):1736-9.
6. Verdonck-de Leeuw IM, Mahieu HF. Vocal aging and the impact on daily life: a longitudinal study. J Voice. 2004;18(2):193-202.
7. Janssens JP. Aging of the respiratory system: impact on pulmonary function tests and adaptation to exertion. Clin Chest Med. 2005;26(3):469-84.
8. Johns MM, Arviso LC, Ramadan F. Challenges and opportunities in the management of the aging voice. Otolaryngol Head Neck Surg. 2011;145(1):1-6.
9. Nakai T, Goto N, Moriyama H, et al. The human recurrent laryngeal nerve during the aging process. Okajimas Folia Anat Jpn. 2000;76(6):363-7.
10. Connor NP, Suzuki T, Lee K, et al. Neuromuscular junction changes in aged rat thyroarytenoid muscle. Ann Otol Rhinol Laryngol. 2002;111(7 Pt 1):579-86.
11. Malmgren LT, Fisher PJ, Bookman LM, et al. Age-related changes in muscle fiber types in the human thyroarytenoid muscle: an immunohistochemical and stereological study using confocal laser scanning microscopy. Otolaryngol Head Neck Surg. 1999;121(4):441-51.
12. McMullen CA, Andrade FH. Contractile dysfunction and altered metabolic profile of the aging rat thyroarytenoid muscle. J Appl Physiol. 2006;100(2):602-8.
13. Madruga de Melo EC, Lemos M, Aragão Ximenes Filho J, et al. Distribution of collagen in the lamina propria of the human vocal fold. Laryngoscope. 2003;113(12):2187-91.
14. Sato K, Hirano M, Nakashima T. Age-related changes of collagenous fibers in the human vocal fold mucosa. Ann Otol Rhinol Laryngol. 2002;111(1):15-20.
15. Dedivitis RA, Abrahão M, de Jesus Simões M, et al. Cricoarytenoid joint: histological changes during aging. Sao Paulo Med J. 2001;119(2):89-90.
16. Paulsen F, Kimpel M, Lockemann U, et al. Effects of ageing on the insertion zones of the human vocal fold. J Anat. 2000;196(Pt 1):41-54.
17. Sato K, Hirano M. Age-related changes in the human laryngeal glands. Ann Otol Rhinol Laryngol. 1998;107(6):525-9.
18. Núñez-Batalla F, Díaz-Molina JP, Costales-Marcos M, et al. [Neurolaryngology]. Acta Otorrinolaringol Esp. 2012;63(2):132-40.
19. Feijó AV, Parente MA, Behlau M, et al. Acoustic analysis of voice in multiple sclerosis patients. J Voice. 2004;18(3):341-7.
20. Elble RJ. What is essential tremor? Curr Neurol Neurosci Rep. 2013;13(6):353.
21. Honjo I, Isshiki N. Laryngoscopic and voice characteristics of aged persons. Arch Otolaryngol. 1980;106(3):149-50.
22. Pontes P, Brasolotto A, Behlau M. Glottic characteristics and voice complaint in the elderly. J Voice. 2005;19(1):84-94.
23. Berg EE, Hapner E, Klein A, et al. Voice therapy improves quality of life in age-related dysphonia: a case-control study. J Voice. 2008;22(1):70-4.
24. Sauder C, Roy N, Tanner K, et al. Vocal function exercises for presbylaryngis: a multidimensional assessment of treatment outcomes. Ann Otol Rhinol Laryngol. 2010;119(7):460-7.
25. Ziegler A, Verdolini Abbott K, Johns M, et al. Preliminary data on two voice therapy interventions in the treatment of presbyphonia. Laryngoscope. 2014;124(8):1869-76.
26. Postma GN, Blalock PD, Koufman JA. Bilateral medialization laryngoplasty. Laryngoscope. 1998;108(10):1429-34.
27. Zeitels SM, Mauri M, Dailey SH. Medialization laryngoplasty with Gore-Tex for voice restoration secondary to glottal incompetence: indications and observations. Ann Otol Rhinol Laryngol. 2003;112(2):180-4.
28. Hirano S, Bless DM, del Río AM, et al. Therapeutic potential of growth factors for aging voice. Laryngoscope. 2004;114(12):2161-7.
29. Ohno T, Yoo MJ, Swanson ER, et al. Regeneration of aged rat vocal folds using hepatocyte growth factor therapy. Laryngoscope. 2009;119(7):1424-30.
30. Gugatschka M, Ohno S, Saxena A, et al. Regenerative medicine of the larynx. Where are we today? A review. J Voice. 2012;26(5):670.e7-13.
31. Thibeault SL, Duflo S. Inflammatory cytokine responses to synthetic extracellular matrix injection to the vocal fold lamina propria. Ann Otol Rhinol Laryngol. 2008;117(3):221-6.

8

Voice Therapeutic Approaches

Usha Rani

INTRODUCTION

Voice therapy is an attempt to bring back the voice to a level and that will fulfil the occupational and social needs of the patient. Stemple[1] has classified voice therapy approaches as belonging to one of the four major categories—(1) hygienic, (2) symptomatic, (3) psychogenic, and (4) physiologic.[1] Voice therapy has been traditionally divided into two categories:

1. *Indirect voice therapy* involves vocal hygiene, voice rest, increasing awareness of potentially abusive vocal behaviors, respiratory retraining for breath support, and relaxation.
2. *Direct voice therapy* involves alteration of the patients speaking technique in an effort to improve voice. It constitutes of symptomatic and physiological voice therapy approaches.

SYMPTOMATIC VOICE THERAPY

It includes specific approaches to voice therapy where techniques are selected to target a set of signs or symptoms of a voice disorder. The focus of symptomatic voice therapy is to help the client optimally to use the systems of respiration, phonation, and resonance for easiest produced and best-sounding voice possible. Dr Daniel Boone[2] has systematically compiled the "facilitating approaches" to alter the method of voice production some of which were originally described in literature by Boone;[2] Aronson;[3] Coltan and Casper;[4] Stemple, Gerdeman, and Glaze.[5,6] They can be used with various voice disorders—organic, neurogenic or functional. These approaches are thus highly individualized and are trial- and error-based decisions. Boone[2] lists 25 classic facilitating techniques which include the following:

- *Auditory feedback*: Real-time amplification on instrument like facilitator, auditory metronome can be used in Parkinson patient and auditory modeling (loop playback) using recorders.
- *Change of loudness*: Decreasing the loudness in children by developing awareness of different voices, The Boone Voice Program for children,[2] or practice of quiet voice by using instruments that give feedback specific to intensity such as vocal loudness indicator and Visi-Pitch. For increasing loudness again Visi-Pitch or practice at pitch levels and respiration training with exercises that increase subglottal pressure can be used. Reading or speaking against increasing competing noise can also be done.
- *Chant talk*: It is characterized by increasing the pitch, prolonging the vowels, reducing syllable stress and softening of the glottal attacks during speech and used for hyperfunctional voice disorders.[7]
- *Chewing*: It is helpful for reducing unnecessary tension and hard glottal attacks. Initially awareness is developed of tension and an exaggerated chew is established with wide mouth opening. Later phonation is added to chewing and is continued and words, sentences and during conversational speech. Finally, the exaggerated chewing is eliminated with a normal jaw movement.
- *Digital manipulation*: The three digital manipulation procedures used in voice therapy are distinct from one another in procedural steps and also kind of voice problems for which they are used.
  - *Procedures:*
    1. *For lowering the pitch*: This is particularly effective for postadolescent males whose pitch levels remain at preadolescent levels. Light pressure anteriorly

on thyroid cartilage shortens the overall length of vocal folds and results in low Fo during vowel prolongation. The low pitch should be maintained and retained even after the fingers are removed.

2. *For monitoring vertical movements of larynx*: For most patients with excessive pitch variability and hyperfunctional voice disorders, the larynx is in elevated position with significantly decreased thyrohyoid space. Placing the fingers within thyrohyoid space, encircling the hyoid bone with middle finger and thumb. Begin gently with downward pressure and slight lateral movements to lower the larynx. With this, ask the patient to prolong the vowel and lower the pitch one note at a time to the lowest note in his or her pitch range. Then ask him to prolong one note up and should feel and monitor the lowering and rising of larynx at extremes of pitch range. Oral reading and speaking should be developed with little or no vertical movements.

3. *Unilateral digital pressure for unilateral vocal fold paralysis*: It is established that finger pressure on lateral thyroid lamina often produces better vocal fold approximation, resulting in stronger phonation. Begin by having the patient to posture the head straight forward (looking slightly down rather than upward), and phonating and extending a vowel. During phonation, the clinician exerts medium finger pressure on lateral thyroid wall on side of paralysis. If louder and firmer voice is produced with this various phonation tasks are continued. If louder voice is not achieved clinician exerts lateral pressure on the side opposite to vocal fold paralysis. If lateral pressure on either thyroid lamina has not produced an improvement in voice, lateral pressure is provided by head turned to one side (left head turn pressure on left thyroid lamina; if unsuccessful, left head turn pressure on right lamina). Similarly, if firm voice is not achieved then head turned to right side and each side pressed is tried to find better voice.

- *Eliminating vocal abuse*: Vocal abuse comprises of various behaviors and events that have some deleterious effect on the larynx and voice. Identification and reduction of vocal abuses and misuses are the primary goals of voice therapy. Initially, the identified abuses are discussed with patient and need to reduce their frequency is emphasized through awareness.

- *Establishing a new pitch*: A tape recording should be made of the patient producing various pitches by extending vowel /i/, including feedback of old pitch and target pitch. Instruments like PM 100 Pitch analyzer, phonatory function analyzer, Visi-Pitch and Bruel and Kjaer (B&K) real-time frequency analyzer can be used to display any deviation below or above the target Fo by providing immediate feedback. Establishing new pitch is facilitated by working on single words beginning with vowels in a pitch monotone (at target pitch). Later phrases and short sentences are introduced and when success is achieved a reading passage is assigned to read well in monotone.

- *Yawn-sigh approach*: The yawn-sigh is one of the most effective voice therapy techniques for minimizing the tension effects of vocal hyperfunction developed by Boone, 1971.[2] During yawn-sigh, the larynx drops to a low position, the tongue is more back, there is slight opening between the vocal folds, and the pharynx is usually dilated. It is frequently combined with other therapy approaches for problems as functional dysphonia, spasmodic dysphonia, thickening, nodules, and polyps.

  - *Procedure:* Explain the general physiology of yawn, i.e. a yawn represents a prolonged inspiration with maximum widening of the supraglottal airway, by demonstrating a yawn and how it feels like. Patient does the yawn and another yawn after that and breathes out with little voicing. After that patient says words with /h/ or vowels spoken with mouth open. The number of words is slowly increased. Next step yawning is stopped. Open mouth inhalation is done followed by long sigh with open mouth. Then next step is to say ha after the sigh.

- *Inhalation-phonation*: The high-pitched vocalization produced during inhalation is always produced by true vocal fold vibration. This technique is useful in patients who are aphonic or in ventricular dysphonia or functional aphonia.[2] Reverse phonation viewed by fiber-optic endoscopy shows vibrating vocal folds well.

  - *Procedure:* Demonstrate inhalation phonation by phonating high-pitched hum while elevating the shoulders. The elevation of shoulders shows the contrast between inhalation and exhalation. Inhale raising the shoulders and simultaneously humming in a high pitch, then dropping the shoulders on exhalation and producing the same voice. Repeat the inhalation-exhalation matched phonation several times. Ask the patient to make an inhalation-phonation and repeat it several times. After patient produced the matching hum, demonstrate the continuation of the high pitch, sweeping down from the falsetto to the regular chest register on one long continuous expiration. Repeat this several times. After some practice, use monosyllabic words for practice, and reduce the pronounced shoulder movements. Practice should be continued at single word practice until normal voicing is established.

- *Laryngeal adduction exercises*: These exercises can be used in patients with poor vocal fold adduction (hypoadduction) like laryngeal trauma (may result in recurrent laryngeal nerve paralysis), vocal fold bowing and vocal fold weakness or paralysis, neurological diseases [Parkinson's disease (PD), multiple sclerosis (MS), closed head injury, stroke, congenital conditions such as sulcus vocalis that is vocal fold furrow]. Pushing and pulling exercises should not be used with patients who have uncontrolled high blood pressure—Pushing or pulling, Holding breath, Glottal attack, Pseudo-supraglottic swallow.[8]

  - *Purpose:* To facilitate improved vocal fold closure by increasing the muscle activity in larynx during voice production, swallowing and to reduce breathiness, low intensity, hoarseness, swallow safety and airway protection or to improve overall vocal quality.[9] There are two sets of exercises. The series of exercises in each set should be completed in 5–7 sets about five times daily. The whole series of exercises should be repeated three times.[9]

    1. *Set 1*
       Exercise 1
       Instructions: Ask the patient to sit. He pushes down the chair while holding his breath (Fig. 1).
       Exercise 2
       In a sitting position and pushing the chair with one hand voicing is done (Fig. 2).
       Exercise 3
       "Ah" is repeated 5 times Ah... Ah...ah...ah...ah...
       Patients should practice this series every day for 1week. A follow-up swallow evaluation should be completed to assess improvements in airway protection from the larynx. If no improvements are noted, the exercises should be changed to those in set 2.[9]
    2. *Set 2*
       Exercise 1
       Ask the patient to try pull the chair while vocalizing with both hands while prolonging phonation (Fig. 3).
       Exercise 2
       Ah is vocalized with hard glottal attack and phonating.
       Exercise 3
       Pseudo-supraglottic swallow—Ask the patient to take a breath, hold it, and cough as strongly as possible.

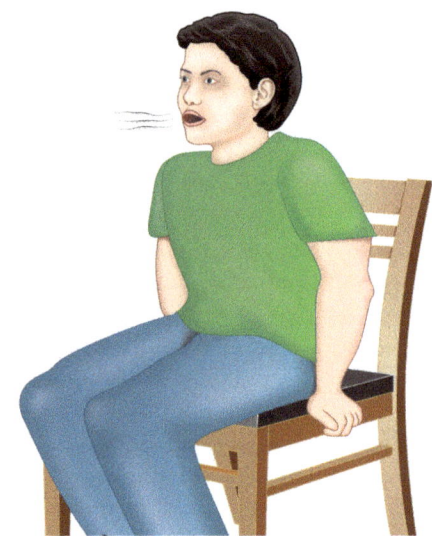

Fig. 2 Sitting position with one hand voicing

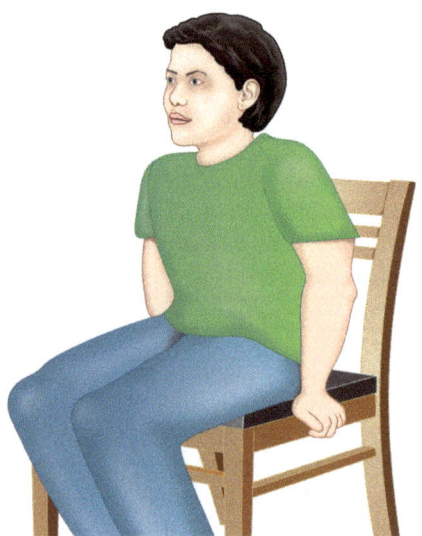

Fig. 1 Sitting position while holding breath

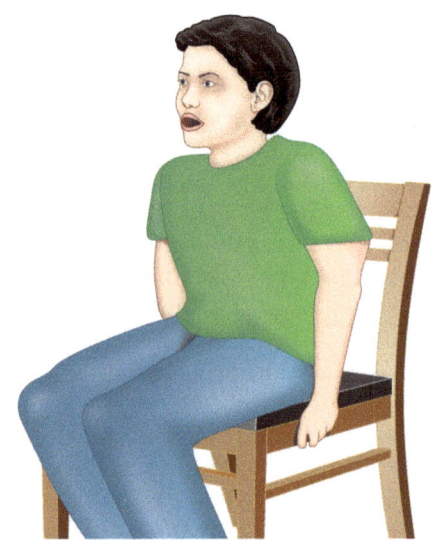

Fig. 3 Prolonging phonation

Improvement should be seen within 2 weeks. Occasionally, it will take 6–8 months with some patients to attain adequate airway protection or vocal quality for those who have had more serious conditions (i.e. extended supraglottic laryngectomy).[9] Results from these exercises depend on the gap between the vocal cords.

- *Efficacy:* There are extremely few efficacy studies concerning vocal fold adduction exercises, few speech language pathologists (SLPs) currently use the pushing and pulling type of exercises. Yamaguchi et al.[10] reported that three patients who had paralysis of the vocal folds improved following voice treatment with pushing exercises. Two improved 20 dB (statistically significant increase in intensity), and one improved 7 dB (clinically significant increase in intensity).

- *Half-swallow Boom method*: This technique is more useful in patients who have one-sided cord immobility, bowed vocal cords or falsetto. All of these patients have low loudness level and air wastage.
  - *Procedure:* Here we ask the patient not to swallow completely and say boom rather say boom during the swallow. We ask them to say a low-pitch boom. After 2–3 attempts, the boom is said in a louder and less breathy voice. Record this voice and show the dramatic improvement in voice. Usually, we do this with the head turned to one side and the other. Also we do this with the chin lowered and tucked in. Once the best boom is produced ask the patient to say boom one, etc. Gradually increase the length of the phrase after the boom and then phase out boom. Then phase out the swallow and then move the head back to the midline and raise the chin to the normal position. The swallow produces as much closure of the larynx as possible. The word "boom" is composed of voiced sounds that can all be produced as the air is produced from the constricted larynx. The head turning assist in mechanical sense.

- *Head positioning*: The production of normal voice is sometimes facilitated by changing the position of the head. Several distinct head positions can be tried to find the one that facilitates better voice.
  - Normal straight forward head
  - Neck extends forward with head tilted down, face looking up
  - Neck flexed downwards with head tilted downward, face looking down
  - Neck flexed unilaterally with head tilted to either the left or right, with tilted face looking forward
  - Head upright and rotated towards left or right, face looking in either direction.

Any one position may change the pharyngeal-oral resonating structures in such a way that a change in vocal quality may occur. These positioning can be used in combination with other facilitating techniques.

- *Procedure:* Introduce the approach by demonstrating various head positions. A simple explanation of the technique should accompany the demonstration. Prolongation of vowels like /I//o/u/ can be used as the best voicing task to search for the head position. Whenever a change is noted in a particular position of head, the head should be kept at that position and the activities have to carry out. Neurologically impaired patients may have some oropharyngeal asymmetry from their disease. A particular lateral movement of the head may make a sudden and noticeable improvement in the voice in such patients. Then ask the patient to practice voice material with the head in the lateral position. In case of vocal hyperfunction, the patients profit from the neck flexion with the chin tucked down toward the chest. This downward carriage seems to promote greater vocal tract relaxation.

- *Open mouth approach*: It reduces generalized vocal hyperfunction. This helps vocal folds to come together and correct problems of loudness, pitch, and quality.
  - *Procedure:* Patient sees himself in the mirror with open mouth and focus on areas of tension. Tutor him to have his mouth open and slight drop in the head whenever he is listening.

- *Redirected phonation*: Boone[2] described a method by which vegetative functions, such as throat clearing, cough, and laughing could be used to facilitate voicing at the level of true vocal folds. Boone used light coughs to elicit vocal fold contact and they were further modified and extended into sustained phonation. He added redirected phonation in facilitation approaches in 2005 which can be used for functional aphonia individuals in combination with inhalation and phonation.

- *Humming*: It was described by Colton and Casper,[3] and involves the use of hum to train easy, relaxed phonation. Humming gives increased proprioceptive feedback from oronasal resonances and decreased feedback from laryngeal resonances. This results to a more relaxed manner of production.

PHYSIOLOGICAL OR HOLISTIC VOICE THERAPY

Physiological or holistic voice therapy deals with voice condition in a holistic manner with the aim of altering the overall physiology of voice production and evidence suggests that physiological method received greater scientific support.

Physiologic voice therapy presumes that a measurable voice disturbance is present which can be directly modified and monitored through physical exercise of the laryngeal and respiratory system. Physiological voice therapy is used for functional voice disorders and the below six approaches fall under the physiologic umbrella.

Resonant Voice Therapy

It was developed by Dr Daniel Boone and Dr Morton Cooper.[11] It involves chant talk and Humming. A systematic approach to resonant voice therapy (RVT) was developed by Dr Katherine.[11] Verdolini[11] has developed a systematic, programmatic approach to RVT partly based on Dr Arthur Lessac's work in theater and Mark Madsen in singing. The Lessac-Madsen RVT (LMRVT) is well known.[11] This is an expansion of the moto-kinesthetic feedback offered by enhanced supraglottic vibrations on the lips, palate, nose, and face. The opposite of resonant voice is pharyngeal focus or throaty and patients with voice problems often develop it

because they are pushing to get the voice out. The use is in hyperfunctional voice disorders (Fig. 4).

Purpose

To achieve easy and clear voice with barely abducted or adducted vocal fold configuration with least vocal effort in order to avoid vocal fold injury. Dr Verdolini Abbott and Dr Titze[12] state that larynx has an equilibrium position where it functions more effectively and RVT trains this posture across speech production. Specific muscle tension in head, neck, throat, and larynx can be eliminated with RVT. The oral output can be increased by almost 6 dB without increasing subglottal pressure.

In the Lessac approach,[13] the consonant "y" and nasal consonants ("m," "n," and "ng") are used to facilitate training. Cooper's approach utilizes the utterance "m-hmmm" during conversation as a guidepost for resonant voice during ongoing speech. In Verdolini's approach, the Lessac work is used as a cue for a systematic, programmatic training. This resonant

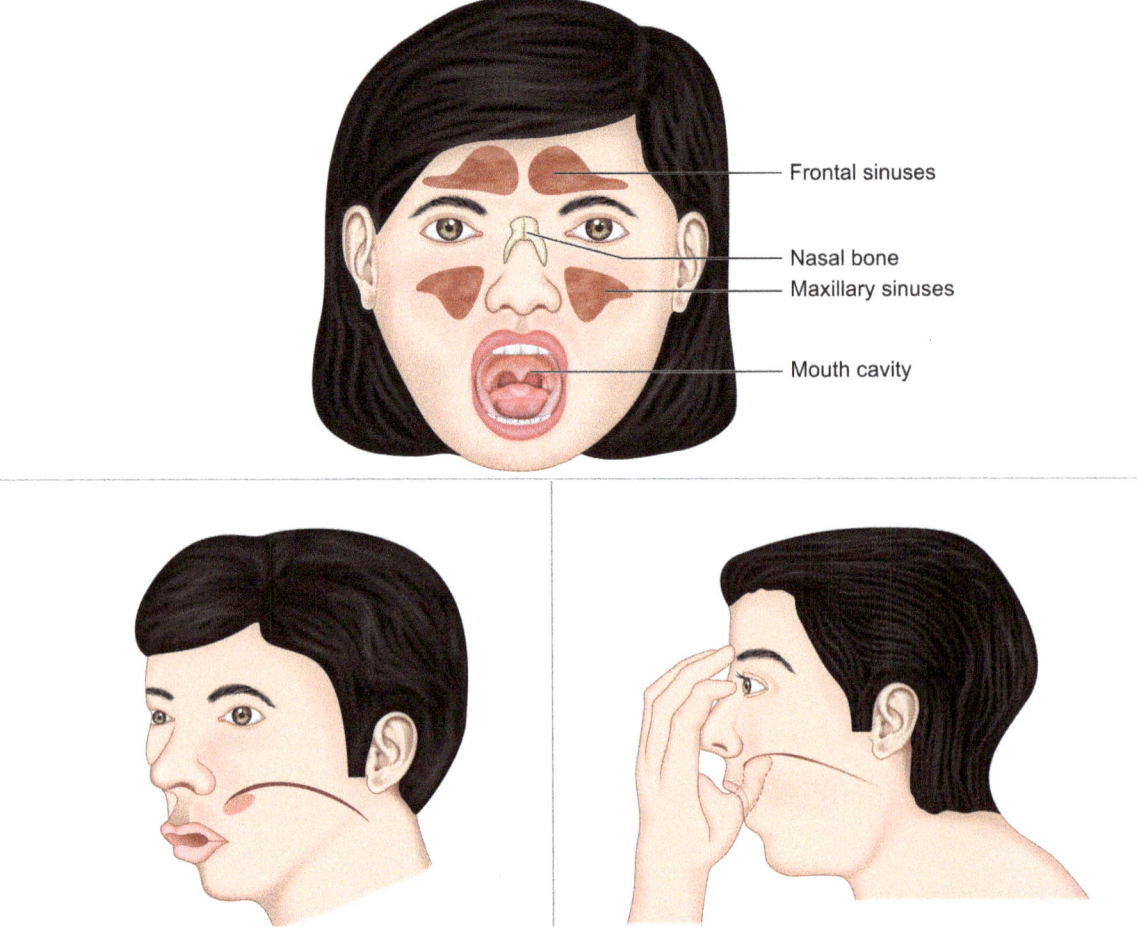

Fig. 4 Resonant voice therapy

"tone" is achieved, stabilized in sustained vowels, word, phrases, and connected speech through vocal tract widening and expansion of oral cavity postures.

Total duration is once in a week for 8 weeks. Each session involves stress on the "basic RVT gesture," a special type of humming, and application to functional phrases and finally speaking or singing.

1. Step number one is stretching massage. All the associated body parts are stretched.
   - *Shoulders*: Elbow is made to touch back and and arms are moved in front and stretched.
   - *Neck*: Head is dropped down slowly. Rotate head up until right on top and the neck muscles are felt.
   - *Jaws*: Masseter muscle is massaged and thumb is pulled into masseter muscle.
   - *Floor of the mouth*: Press thumb into floor of the mouth, first make no sound, and then produce a vowel with no tongue stiffness.
   - *Lips*: Movement of lips is made alternately with no voice or with voicing.
   - *Tongue*: Next tongue trill is done first with no voice and then with continuous voice.
   - *Pharynx*: Pharyngeal stretching is done by yawn and yawn-sigh with vocalizing.
   - *Breathing*: Say "f" and breathe out, when requirement for breathing comes just release the stomach. This can be done first without voicing and then with voicing.
2. Let patient say Hum-um-um-um. It should be done in a relaxed way.
3. Hummmmmmmmmmm is vocalized on a sustained comfort pitch and feels the vibration.
4. *Next voiced exercises are done on a comfortably pitch chant:* mi-mi-mi-mi-mi, ma-ma-ma-ma-ma, mo-mo-mo-mo-mo, mu-mu-mu-mu-mu.
5. Produce sentences with voice having more articulation and forward resonance at normal voicing levels.
6. *Voiced or voiceless:* Chant on a comfortable pitch—Go from slow or soft to louder or faster to slow or soft.
7. Then do sentences and paragraph reading.

Efficacy

Extensive research supports efficacy of RVT, Chen et al. 2007[14] reported that in voice disordered teachers the voice quality, vocal function and functional communication have improved following RVT.

Vocal Function Exercises

These exercises were developed by Dr Bertram Briess and Joseph Stemple, Glaze, and Gerdeman-Klaben,[15] adapted this therapy program into a series of vocal function exercises (VFEs). These exercises are a series of systematic vocal cord alterations manipulations similar in theory to physical therapy of vocal folds. These exercises can be used in vocal hyperfunctional or hyperfunctional voice disorder like benign laryngeal lesions, i.e. vocal nodules, polyps, cysts, singers, and aging voice.

Purpose

The laryngeal mechanism, like other muscle systems, may become imbalanced and/or strained. The VFEs improve glottal efficiency, i.e. the muscular and respiratory effort to maintain phonation.

There are a set of four exercises in the program. Each exercise should be practiced twice a day two times each.[16] They should be produced as softly as is possible with an easy start and forward placement of the tone.

1. *Exercise 1*
   Warm-up: Ask the patient to sustain the vowel /i/ for as long as possible. It may be modified based on patient's vocal range. Can use lip trill, tongue forward trill, hum, or forward vowel whichever works for the patient (easiest effort).
2. *Exercise 2*
   Stretching: Let the patient say the word "Knoll", or a tongue or lip trill, and change from lowest note to highest note in vocal range. Should complete it without voice breaks and the word "knoll", encourages a forward vocal focus and an open pharynx. Lips should be rounded and the patient should feel vibration on the lips. During this exercise, vocal folds are stretched and muscle control and flexibility is improved (Fig. 5).
3. *Exercise 3*
   Contraction: Let the patient say the word "Knoll" and glide from highest note to lowest note in vocal range. Patient should complete it without voice breaks and the word "knoll" encourages a forward vocal focus and an open pharynx complements the previous stretching exercise by contracting the laryngeal muscles (Fig. 6).

Fig. 5 Muscle stretching

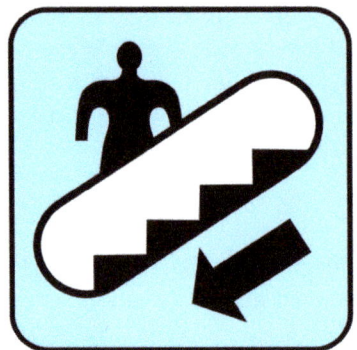

Fig. 6 Muscle contraction

4. *Exercise 4*
   Low impact adductor power exercise: Sustain voice on "Oll" ("knoll" without "kn") as long as possible on musical notes C, D, E, F, and G above middle C for women and children and below middle C for men, modify based on patient's vocal range.
   Improvement should be seen within 6–8 weeks.

Manual Circumlaryngeal Techniques

Dr Arnold Aronson and Dr Nelson Roy[17] developed, used, and described a specific technique called the "manual laryngeal muscle tension reduction procedure".[18] It is used for functional voice disorders, muscle tension dysphonia (MTD), and organic lesions. Dr Murray Morrison and Rammage elaborated it as circumlaryngeal massage also called as manual cirumlaryngeal therapy (MCT), laryngeal manual therapy (LMT), manual laryngeal tension reduction, and manual laryngeal reposturing maneuvers. This is done by placing thumb and forefinger over hyoid and applying pressure in a circular manner to the thyrohyoid space and thyroid cartilage posterior border and suprahyoid muscles (Fig. 7). It involves doing this to try pull down larynx. Areas of focal pain are identified and therapist moves from superficial to deep areas while patient phonates a vowel. Changes in vocal quality will be evident during sustained vowels, as tension is relieved.

Purpose

- To evaluate and assess the maladaptive compensatory habits of laryngeal musculoskeletal system
- For relaxation of the excessively stiff muscles of larynx and
- To lessen the excessive tension and pain and try to remove the vocal strain.

In focal palpation, moderate pressure is directed with hands over anterior border of sternocleidomastoid muscle, suprahyoid muscles, over hyoid, and superior border of thyroid cartilage to determine the tenderness, mobility [range of motion (ROM)], tonicity, extent of laryngeal elevation and

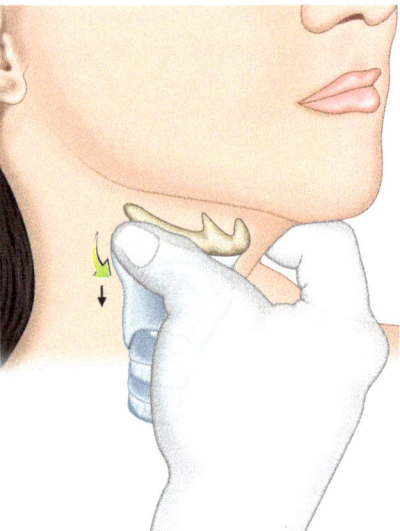

Fig. 7 Circumlaryngeal massage

lateralization, size of thyrohyoid space, resting position and the presence of taut muscle bands, knots.

Laryngeal Reposturing Maneuvers

They are direct hands-on strategy in which the voice box is repositioned during phonation while observing the changes in voice quality.

- *Pushback maneuver*: Digital compression in posterior direction within hyoid bone varying the height and pressure.
- *Pull down maneuver*: Impede the laryngeal elevation by applying downward pressure over the superior border of thyroid cartilage.
- *Medial compression and downward traction*: Pressure directed over the posterior aspect of thyroid cartilage and within the thyrohyoid space. It is often helpful for nonadducted hyperfunctional disorders.

The most completely described type of massage, developed by Aronson,[17] is called the "manual laryngeal muscle tension reduction procedure".[18] In this procedure, the clinician massages the laryngeal area, starting with the hyoid bone at the angle of the chin, and moving to the thyroid cartilage. The larynx is moved from side to side as well as downward, and various types of rotary and other movements are used. Protocol of laryngeal massage includes masseters muscle, the tongue base muscles (genio, mylo, and stylohyoid muscles), suprahyoid, perihyoid, thyrohyoid, cricothyroid stretch, strap muscles, and lateral larynx.

Efficacy

It is effective in patients with elevated laryngeal position, increased laryngeal muscle tension, and MTD as significant difference between the objective overall voice quality before and after MCT was reported by Van Lierde et al. In patients with laryngeal cancer following radiation treatment often exhibit stiffness that can become fibrotic if not treated and they benefit from laryngeal massage treatment evidenced by reduced muscular tension. Evidence also shows laryngeal massage is effective as a supplement to traditional treatment methods for disorders such as paradoxical vocal fold movement (PVFM), hyperphonic voice disorders secondary to neurologic disease, and chronic cough.

Confidential Voice Therapy

Dr Janina Casper[19] developed and first used "confidential voice" which refers to an easy, quiet, and breathy voice. It is useful for recent vocal fold injury or after surgery on the vocal cords, benign lesions, MTD, and voice fatigue. It is usually used in therapy for only a few weeks following an acute injury. During confidential voice therapy (CVT), the vocal folds have small amplitudes of vibration and they do not strike each other very forcefully when they vibrate. This helps in protecting the vocal cords in the period of healing.

Purpose

To reduce the vocal cords rubbing against each other and reducing laryngeal hyperfunction during voicing. Studies have shown that RVT and CVT produce almost equal benefits.[20]

Accent Method

Accent method is a holistic approach to voice therapy that utilizes a series of rhythmic beats in coordination with respiratory, phonatory, and articulatory "pulses" in increasing tempo and complexity. It was developed by Dr Svend Smith, Dr Kirsten Thyme-Frokjaer (1978), Dr Borge Frokjaer-Jensen, and Dr M N Kotby.[21] It can be used for organic and nonorganic voice disorders, disorders of speech (stuttering and dysarthria). Even singers and actors can utilize accent method to achieve strong and flexible voice.

Purpose

To develop good and effective breathing pattern. To develop and strengthen the normal functions of the voice by giving a secure foundation for voice use.

It consists of: Teaching patients to vocalize using easy abdominal breathing and relaxed neck. There is stress on steady, stable, and rhythmic movements of the body. Later speech is introduced till speaking level and as therapy goes on rhythmic movements are reduced.

Accent method relies on three principles:
1. *Breathing exercises*: The abdominal-diaphragmatic oro/nasal breathing patterns are established with quick and deep inspirations and controlled and phasic expirations.
2. *Phonatory exercises (vowel play) at accentuated rhythms*:
   - Preparatory phase where patient will be made to phonate vowels and voiced fricatives /z/ and /v/ replacing the unvoiced fricatives /f/, /s/, /h/ /i/
   - Phonatory phase: The exercises proceed in a hierarchy of accented beats (largo, andante, and allegro) with vowel play to create a dynamic balance between voice production subsystems—breath, phonation, and articulation
   - Stabilization of the newly acquired vocal behavior by interplay of different rhythms with variations in loudness and pitch
   - Transfer from vowel play into connected speech gradually by repetition of utterances, reading, monologue, and dialogue.
3. *Movement exercises*: Body and arm movements.

Efficacy

Vocal cord position trained in accent method is similar to that in RVT. Vocal cords in close position should maximize output while preventing injury. (Berry et al., in revision; Verdolini and Titze, 1995). Kotby and colleagues[21] reported improved voice quality and Smith and Thyme report harmonics increase in voice with accent method.

Lee Silverman Voice Treatment

The credit for developing Lee Silverman voice treatment (LSVT) goes to Dr Lorraine Ramig and her colleagues.[22] They also developed techniques for voice and speech problems with Parkinson's disease, which shared some similarities with LSVT. LSVT was developed to address hypokinetic voice issues associated with Parkinson's disease. It consists of increasing loudness for 4 consecutive weeks at 4 sessions a week.

Aim is to increase overall loudness with little ignoring other associated speech issues commonly associated with Parkinsonism (e.g. dysarthria). Patients are trained to "recalibrate their habitual speaking volume to the one level louder than what they are used to speak". Loud speaking leads to better closure of the vocal cords and speech improves.

Voice therapist must also focus on:
- Respiration any abnormality
- Pitch changes
- Tension in oral and neck muscles
- Problems with initiating voice
- Stress must be on correct abdominal breathing.

Pitch Limiting voice treatment is another modification of LSVT.

Efficacy

A study[23] investigated the effect of two forms of intensive speech treatment, respiration and voice and respiration (LSVT), on the speech and voice deficits associated with idiopathic Parkinson's disease. Ramig et al.[23] reported that patients who received LSVT had more improvement in voice and speech than who had respiratory training. This study concluded that intensive voice and respiration (LSVT) treatment, focusing on increased vocal fold adduction and respiration, is more effective than respiration treatment alone for improving vocal intensity and decreasing the impact of Parkinson's disease on communication.

REFERENCES

1. Stemple JC, Hapner ER. Voice therapy: Clinical case studies, 4th edition. Canada: Singular publishing; 2006. pp. 41-6.
2. Boone DR, McFarlane SC. The voice and voice therapy, 6th edition. Boston: Allyn & Bacon; 2000.
3. Aronson AE. Clinical voice disorders: An interdisciplinary approach, 3rd edition. New York, NY: Thieme Publishers; 1990.
4. Colton RH, Casper JK, Leonard R. Understanding voice problems: A physiological perspective for diagnosis and treatment. Philadelphia: Williams & Wilkins; 2006.
5. The national center for voice and speech. 2009. Vocal function exercises [online]. Available from *www.ncvs.org/freebooks/ vocologyguide.pdf [Accessed January 2017]*.
6. Stemple JC, Glaze LE, Gerdeman BK. Clinical voice pathology: Theory and management, 3rd edition. Canada: Singular Publishing; 2000.
7. Van Lierde KM, Claeys S, De Bodt M, et al. Long-term outcome of hyper functional voice disorders based on a multiparameter approach. J Voice. 2007;21(2):179-88.
8. Ramig LO, Verdolini K. Treatment efficacy: Voice disorders. J Speech Lang Hear Res. 1998;41:101-16.
9. Management of the patient with oropharyngeal swallowing disorders. In: Logemann JA (Ed). Evaluation and treatment of swallowing disorders. Austin, TX: Pro-Ed; 1998.
10. Yamaguchi H, Watanabe Y, Hajime H, et al. Pushing exercise program to correct glottal incompetence. Ann Bull Res Ins Logoped. 1990;24:223-34.
11. Yiu EM, Lo MC, Barrett EA. A systematic review of resonant voice therapy. Int J Speech Lang Pathol; 2016. pp. 1-13.
12. Titze IR, Abbott KV. Vocology: The science and practice of voice habilitation. Salt Lake City, UT: The National Center for Voice and Speech; 2012.
13. Arthur L. The use and training of the human voice, 3rd edition. New York: Mc Graw Hill; 1997. pp. 140, 159, 264.
14. Chen SH, Ssiao TY, Hsiao LC, et al. Outcome of resonant voice therapy for female teachers with voice disorders. J Voice. 2007;21(4):415-25.
15. Stemple JC. Voice therapy: Clinical studies. Canada: Delmar; 2000.
16. Andrews ML. Manual of voice treatment: Pediatrics through geriatrics. Canada: Thomson; 2006.
17. Aronson AE. Clinical voice disorders, 3rd edition. New York: Thieme Stratton; 1990.
18. Roy N, Leeper HA. Effects of the manual laryngeal musculoskeletal tension reduction technique as a treatment for functional voice disorders: Perceptual and acoustic measures. J Voice. 1993;7:242-9.
19. Casper JK. From the urine of sacred cows to the laying on of hands and beyond-G. Paul Moore lecture. J Voice. 2007;21(1):2-11.
20. Verdolini KM, Burke MK, Lessac A, et al. Preliminary study of two methods of treatment for laryngeal nodules. J Voice. 1995;9(1):74-85.
21. Kotby MN, Shiromoto O, Hirano M. The accent method of voice therapy: effect of accentuations on F0, SPL, and airflow. J Voice. 1993;7(4):319-25.
22. Ramig LO, Fox C, Sapir S. Parkinson's disease: speech and voice disorders and their treatment with the Lee Silverman voice treatment. Semin Speech Lang. 2004;25(2):169-80.
23. Ramig LO, Countryman S, Thompson LL, et al. Comparison of two forms of intensive speech treatment for Parkinson disease. J Speech Hear Res. 1995;38(6):1232-51.

Voice and Medicines

KK Handa

INTRODUCTION

There is a very close relationship between use of medicines and voice. Medicines may be used to restore and improve voice. However, some drugs being used for systemic conditions may have deleterious effects on the voice. A good knowledge of the medicines in question, in both the situations, is required.

STEROIDS IN ACUTE LARYNGEAL CONDITIONS

Corticosteroids are quite often used for acute laryngeal conditions, e.g. acute laryngitis. This is quite common situation, especially for professional voice users who are in urgent need for a good voice for their next performance. The author prefers to use tablet prednisolone in a dose of 1 mg/kg body weight tapering over 7 days. Methylprednisolone has also been used with good results.[1] Short use of steroids usually does not have significant side effects. Rarely patients may have change in mood, acidity and reflux, dryness of mouth and vocal tract, and occasionally changes in vision.

Long-term use of corticosteroids can cause muscle wasting and weakness. It can also cause Cushing's syndrome and later Addisonian-like crisis.

SEX HORMONES

There are significant androgen and estrogen receptors in the larynx.[2] Hormones can affect the fluid content or the structure of the vocal folds.

Androgen-containing drugs can affect the fundamental frequency of voice and cause permanent lowering. These drugs are commonly used for number of gynecological conditions, including cancer and endometriosis.[3]

Hormonal replacement therapy given very commonly had come under scrutiny after the million women study[4] stated that there is an increased risk of developing breast cancer. It is often given for aging voice and has been found to be beneficial in delaying age-related voice changes.[5] However, the side effects have to be kept in mind and monitored.

Oral contraceptives contain estrogen and can cause fluid retention.

Thyroid

Both hypothyroidism and hyperthyroidism can affect voice. Hypothyroidism causes mucopolysaccharide depositions in the body, and also causes the vocal folds to thicken. Voice can get muffled. It is correctable by correct thyroxine replacement. Similarly hyperthyroidism can also affect voice.

Beta Blockers

These are used in certain situations to allay anxiety, especially before performances. They lower the heart rate and blood pressure and are a variety of antihypertensives. They can increase salivation and also induce asthma. If taken in high doses to cause a calming effect, they can affect the performance negatively.[6]

DRUGS USED FOR GASTROESOPHAGEAL AND LARYNGOPHARYNGEAL REFLUX

Both conditions have a very strong association with voice. However, this is not properly understood and appreciated by many laryngologists and otorhinolaryngologists. Half of the study population by Kaufmann et al., were found to have objective evidence of laryngopharyngeal reflux (LPR) and only one-third of these LPR present patients had heartburn.[7]

The four types of drugs used are:
1. *Antacids*: They cause drying of the vocal tract and occasionally cause diarrhea or constipation.
2. *Histamine (H$_2$) receptor antagonists*: They include drugs like ranitidine, cimetidine, etc. They block H$_2$-mediated release of gastric acid. They also cause dryness of vocal tract apart from gastrointestinal (GI) disturbances, confusion and hypersensitivity reaction.
3. *Proton pump inhibitors*: They are today the standard of care and most commonly used drugs for treating gastroesophageal reflux and LPR. They include drugs like rabeprazole, omeprazole and pantoprazole. They are more effective in older groups and with possibly lesser side effects.
4. *Prokinetic agents*: These are supportive drugs used to modify gastroesophageal sphincter function and to increase the stomach emptying time. They increase contractions of lower esophageal sphincter.

The two common drugs in this category are metoclopramide and cisapride; however recently has been found to cause cardiac arrhythmias.

DRUGS USED FOR COUGH AND THICK MUCUS

Probably the simplest way to treat cough and thick mucus is steam inhalation. It causes humidification and reduces the laryngeal irritation. Compounds with aromatic properties are often added but it is not clear as to how useful they are.

Cough Suppressants

Cough suppressants are used in case the cough is very aggressive and coughing may damage the vocal cords.

Opiate-based suppressants, e.g. codeine act on the higher centers while antihistaminic suppressants act due to their antihistaminic and anticholinergic actions. Opiate-based suppressants are more effective; however, both group of cough suppressants cause sleepiness and dryness of vocal tracts. There are combinations which contain pseudoephedrine which further causes dryness of vocal tract and raised pulse rate and cardiac effects. Dextromethorphan is often recommended in professional voice users.

Saline sprays are very useful for reversing the dried upper respiratory airway. However, the saline sprays should not contain propellants which irritate the upper airway.

Some expectorants in low doses can also increase mucus production.

There are some other drugs like carbocisteine and acetylcysteine which are mucolytic and modify the thick mucus to a thinner form.[8] Steam is again a very good mucolytic.

Angiotensin-converting Enzyme Inhibitors

Angiotensin-converting enzyme (ACE) inhibitors may induce a cough or excessive throat clearing in as many as 5–35% of patients.[9] ACE inhibitors, such as captopril, ramipril, enalapril, and benazepril, are recommended for people with heart failure and are the drugs of choice for treating high blood pressure in people with diabetes. In some studies, the drugs also are associated with a lower risk for heart attack or stroke. Coughing or excessive throat clearing can contribute to vocal cord lesions.

DRUGS USED IN ALLERGIC RHINITIS

Antihistaminics

These are very commonly prescribed medicines, especially for allergic rhinitis and cold. These drugs can cause dryness of the vocal tract by increasing the viscosity of mucosal blanket. They also cause sedation[10] and can affect the performance. They can have more side effects in association with sympathomimetic agents. The older generation ones like chlorpheniramine have more side effects than the newer generation ones like cetirizine, loratadine, and fexofenadine.

These are very effective and essential drugs for allergic rhinitis. However, they should not be added to all prescriptions with upper respiratory tract infection and nonspecific conditions.

Topical Steroid Sprays

These are used commonly for number of nose and upper airway conditions. These are one of the most effective drugs for allergic rhinitis.

In some of the older ones like betamethasone, systemic absorption does occur and hence they should be used with caution in children.[11] They can also cause oral thrush (candidiasis).

Some newer ones like mometasone have less side effects because of less bioavailability.[12]

Proper techniques should be followed while inhaling the sprays including use of spacers, holding of breath after inhalation, and rinsing and swallowing after inhalation.[13]

Vasoconstrictors

Topical vasoconstrictors, e.g. oxymetazoline, are used commonly to open the nasal passages during an acute episode.

However, their use should not be prolonged and can lead to raised blood pressure and also a condition called rhinitis medicamentosa where because of prolonged addictive use of these drugs, the nose becomes paradoxically blocked.

Commonly used medicines for asthma administered by spray can also cause hoarseness by getting deposited on the vocal cords and causing hoarseness.

Anti-inflammatory/Analgesics

Aspirin can cause platelet dysfunction and submucosal vocal cord hemorrhage. One should be careful in patients on long-term low-dose aspirin and also over-the-counter aspirin containing prescriptions.

DRUGS ACTING ON AUTONOMIC NERVOUS SYSTEM

The common ones being used are pseudoephedrine and phenylephrine.[14] They can cause dryness of vocal tract and hazy vision.

Pseudoephedrine

Pseudoephedrine is indicated for the treatment of—nasal congestion, sinus congestion, Eustachian tube congestion, vasomotor rhinitis, and as an adjunct to other agents in the optimum treatment of allergic rhinitis, croup, sinusitis, otitis media, and tracheobronchitis.

Pseudoephedrine is a sympathomimetic amine. Its principal mechanism of action relies on its direct action on the adrenergic receptor system. The vasoconstriction that pseudoephedrine produces is believed to be principally an α-adrenergic receptor response.

Phenylephrine

Phenylephrine is used as an alternative for pseudoephedrine in decongestant medicines due to pseudoephedrine's use in the illicit manufacture of methamphetamine. Its efficacy as an oral decongestant has been questioned with multiple studies not being able to come to an agreement.[15] Its main side effect is hypertension.

PSYCHOTROPIC AGENTS

Monoamine oxidase inhibitors can cause sedation, insomnia sedation, and dry mouth. Tricyclic antidepressants can cause dry vocal tract, reflux, dry mouth, and constipation. Serotonin-reuptake inhibitors can cause dry mouth, blurred vision, and sedation.

Anticoagulants and Blood Thinners

They are very commonly used in cardiac patients often in the post-heart surgery or after stent insertions. The common ones are aspirin (often low dose) and clopidogrel. They can cause vocal cord hemorrhage and voice change. The incidence of hemorrhage after clopidogrel is increased if coadministered with aspirin.[15]

Clopidogrel

Clopidogrel (INN) is an oral, thienopyridine-class antiplatelet agent used to inhibit blood clots in coronary artery disease (CAD), peripheral vascular disease (PVD), cerebrovascular disease (CVD), and to prevent myocardial infarction (heart attack) and stroke.

Clopidogrel is used to prevent heart attack and stroke in people who are at high risk of these events, including those with a history of myocardial infarction and other forms of acute coronary syndrome, stroke, and those with peripheral artery disease.

It is also used, along with acetylsalicylic acid (ASA, aspirin), for the prevention of thrombosis after placement of a coronary stent or as an alternative antiplatelet drug for people intolerant to aspirin.

The Food and Drug Administration (FDA) announced in November 2009 that clopidogrel should be used with caution in patients using the proton pump inhibitors omeprazole or esomeprazole, but pantoprazole appears to be safe.[16] The newer antiplatelet agent prasugrel has minimal interaction with omeprazole, hence might be a better antiplatelet agent (if no other contraindications are present) in patients who are on these proton pump inhibitors.

Herbal Medicines

Herbal medicines and over-the-counter drugs should be taken with caution as they can also affect the voice. Some of the common herbal medicines, which are known to affect voice, are given below:

Yellow Jasmine
Scientific name: Gelsemium sempervirens

Use: It is used to prevent stage fright that can affect voice due to strong effect on muscles.

Nettle

Scientific name: Urtica dioica

Uses: It has a diuretic action. It is used for allergies.

Dry mouth: It can cause dry mouth resulting in hoarseness, sore throat and voice changes. Dry vocal folds may be more prone to injuries such as nodules.

Jimson weed
Scientific name: Datura stramonium

Use: Asthma.

Effect(s) on voice: It could affect the voice due to strong effects on muscles.

Dry mouth: Dry mucous membranes can result in hoarseness, sore throat and voice changes. Dry vocal folds may be more prone to injuries such as nodules.

Burdock
Scientific name: Arctium lappa or *A. minus*

Use: Antibacterial.

Drug group: It has antibacterial effect on voice.

Dry mouth: Dry mucous membranes can result in hoarseness, sore throat and voice changes. Dry vocal folds may be more prone to injuries such as nodules.

Elderberry
Scientific name: Sambucus canadensis

Uses: Coughs appetite suppressant, diuretic effects on voice.

Dry mouth: Dry mucous membranes can result in hoarseness, sore throat and voice changes. Dry vocal folds may be more prone to injuries such as nodules.

Diuretics

Diuretics are commonly used to treat high blood pressure (hypertension) or increase excretion of excess fluid retention in body tissues by increasing urine output. They can also dry out the mucous membranes that line the throat and vocal cords.

REFERENCES

1. Harris TS, Kariyawasan HH, Rubin JS. The voice and medications. In: Rubin JS, Sataloff RT, Korovin GS (Eds). Diagnosis and Treatment of Voice Disorders, 4th edition. California, CA, USA: Plural Publishing; 2014. pp. 617-30.
2. Newman SR, Butler J, Hammond EH, et al. Preliminary report on hormone receptors in the human vocal fold. J Voice. 2000;14(1):72-81.
3. Pattie MA, Murdoch BE, Theodoros D, et al. Voice changes in women treated for endometriosis and related conditions: the need for comprehensive vocal assessment. J Voice. 1998;12(3):366-71.
4. Beral V. Million Women Study Collaborators. Breast cancer and hormone-replacement therapy in the million women study. Lancet. 2003;362(9382):419-27.
5. Lindholm P, Vilkman E, Raudaskoski T, et al. The effect of postmenopause and postmenopausal HRT on measured voice values and vocal symptoms. Maturitas. 1997;28(1):47-53.
6. Gates GA, Saegert J, Wilson N, et al. Effect of beta blockade on singing performance. Ann Otol Rhinol Laryngol. 1985;94(6 Pt 1):570-4.
7. Kaufmann JA, Cummins M. (2002). The prevalence and spectrum of reflux in laryngology: a prospective study of 132 consecutive patients with laryngeal and voice disorders. [online] Available from: *wfubmc.edu/voice/reflux_prev_study. html.* [Accessed November, 2016].
8. Sataloff RT, Hawkshaw M, Rosen DC. Medications: Effects and side effects in professional voice users. In: Sataloff RT (Ed). Professional Voice: Science and Art of Voice Care, 2nd edition. San Diego, CA, USA: Singular Publishing Group; 1997. pp. 457-69.
9. Dicpinigaitis PV. Angiotensin-converting enzyme inhibitor-induced cough: ACCP evidence-based clinical practice guidelines. Chest. 2006;129(1 Suppl):169S-73S.
10. Goodman AG, Rall TW, Nies AS, Tayor P (Eds). Goodman and Gilman's The Pharmacological Basis of Therapeutics, 8th edition. New York, NY, USA: Pergamon Press; 1990. p. 658.
11. Homer JJ, Gazis TG. Cushing's syndrome induced by betamethasone nose drops. BMJ. 1999;318(7194):1355-6.
12. Schenkel EJ, Skoner DP, Bronsky EA, et al. Absence of growth retardation in children with perennial allergic rhinitis after one year of treatment with mometasone furoate aqueous nasal spray. Pediatrics. 2000;105(2):E22.
13. Dolovich M, Ruffin R, Corr D, et al. Clinical evaluation of a simple demand inhalation MDI aerosol delivery device. Chest. 1983;84(1):36-41.
14. Horak F, Zieglmayer P, Zieglmayer R, et al. A placebo-controlled study of the nasal decongestant effect of phenylephrine and pseudoephedrine in the Vienna Challenge Chamber. Ann Allergy Asthma Immunol. 2009;102(2):116-20.
15. Diener HC, Bogousslavsky J, Brass LM, et al. Aspirin and clopidogrel compared with clopidogrel alone after recent ischaemic stroke or transient ischaemic attack in high-risk patients (MATCH): randomised, double-blind, placebo-controlled trial. Lancet. 2004;364(9431):331-7.
16. Food and Drug Administration (FDA). (2009). Public Health Advisory: Updated Safety Information about a drug interaction between Clopidogrel Bisulfate (marketed as Plavix) and Omeprazole (marketed as Prilosec and Prilosec OTC). [online] Available from: *www.fda.gov/Drugs/DrugSafety/ PostmarketDrugSafetyInformationforPatientsandProviders/ ucm190825.htm.* [Accessed November, 2016].

10

Vocal Fold Immobility

Mausumi N Syamal, Michael S Benninger

INTRODUCTION

Vocal fold immobility is a broad term used to describe vocal folds that are restricted in motion either due to mechanical fixation or neurologic insult. Mechanical fixation may result from dislocation or fixation of the arytenoid, edema, or inflammation of the glottis, or neoplastic invasion on the vocal folds themselves or surrounding structures.[1] Such a fixation can also develop from scar band or web formation either congenitally or from trauma and instrumentation. Neuropathic immobility may occur with lesions in the motor cortex or compromise of the recurrent laryngeal nerve at any point along its course from the jugular foramen to the carotid sheath, mediastinum, and either around the subclavian artery on the right or the aortic arch on the left, to the tracheoesophageal groove.

Vocal fold movement may be partially limited or a paretic. For the otolaryngologist, the term "vocal fold paresis" represents a spectrum of motion impairment that can range from being nearly imperceptible to complete and obvious paralysis. However, the term "paresis", denotes the preservation of some degree of mobility, thereby making it a discrete clinical entity from paralysis.[2,3] Vocal motion impairment may also be unilateral or bilateral. The distinction between hypomobile or immobile and unilateral or bilateral is important in workup and management because of the implications that these factors have on the potential etiology and prognosis. This chapter reviews the varying etiology of vocal fold immobility, its clinical presentation including evaluation and diagnostic tools, and management encompassing recent operative trends.

ETIOLOGY

The etiology vocal fold paralysis (VFP) or immobility is vast spanning a myriad of conditions and diseases. Congenital causes of VFP include hydrocephalus, Arnold-Chiari malformation, tracheoesophageal fistula, vascular ring, other vascular anomalies, dysmorphic syndromes (Mobius, Goldenhar), syndromes involving brainstem dysfunction, and neuromuscular disorders such as Charcot-Marie-Tooth.[4-6] While it is likely that the presence of a full paralysis will be diagnosed early due to respiratory distress, the presence of congenital syndromes or anomalies vary in severity and course and should be considered.

Infectious causes have largely been attributed to post-viral neuropathy. While "post-viral" and "idiopathic" VFP are often lumped together, it is important to discern in the history and physical exam if current or active viral infection is present as treatment of the underlying virus may result in improvement or prevention of progression. Vocal fold palsies have been associated with herpes simplex virus, Epstein-Barr virus, varicella-zoster, cytomegalovirus, human immune deficiency virus (HIV) and even West Nile virus.[7-12] While not well-documented in the literature, but seen more commonly in a clinical setting, is the onset of a paresis or a paralysis following an upper respiratory infection (URI).[13] Of particular note, bacterial infections such as syphilis and Lyme disease have also been identified as causes.[14,15]

The most common causes of immobility include malignancies, tumors, and traumatic causes frequently following intubation, surgery (thyroidectomy, spine surgery, or carotid endarterectomy) or neck trauma (Fig. 1). In a

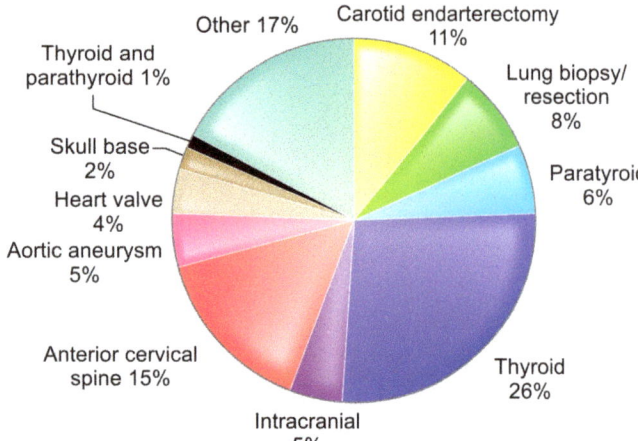

Fig. 1 Surgical causes of unilateral vocal fold immobility, 1996–2005[1]

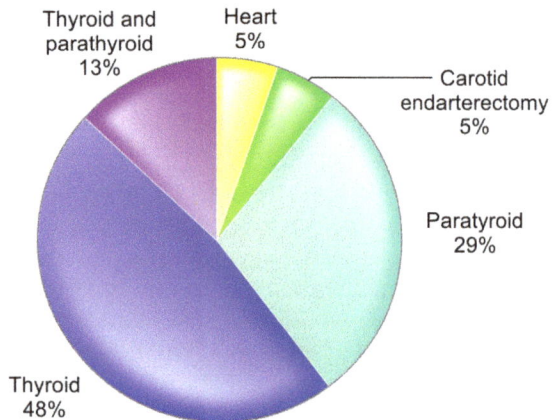

Fig. 2 Surgical causes of bilateral vocal fold immobility, 1996–2005

longitudinal study of 827 patients spanning 20 years, vocal fold immobility was most commonly associated with a surgical procedure (46%).[16] This study examined the etiologies of vocal fold immobility and noted that they are "changing, with extralaryngeal malignancies and nonthyroidectomy surgical trauma having become more common causes". Thyroid surgeries, including thyroidectomy and parathyroidectomy, accounted for the majority (33%) of all surgical causes of immobility. The surgical procedures most likely to cause unilateral vocal fold immobility are shown in Figure 2. The most common nonthyroid surgery to cause vocal fold immobility was anterior cervical spine corpectomy and fusion (15%). The next most common surgical cause of unilateral vocal fold immobility was carotid endarterectomy (11%). Newer surgical procedures such as traumatic paresis following recent vagal nerve stimulator implantation have been noted as well.[17] The presence of endocrinologic diseases such as hypothyroidism, goiter, thyroiditis should also be a part of the working differential. In a series of 308 patients, 146 (47.4%) patients with vocal fold paresis were diagnosed with concurrent thyroid disease.[18]

Systemic neurologic diseases such as myasthenia gravis, Charcot-Marie-Tooth, multiple sclerosis, spinocerebellar atrophy should be investigated in addition to systemic rheumatological diseases such as sarcoidosis, rheumatoid and scleroderma as a paresis may be an initial presenting sign for all these disorders.[6,19-26] Additionally, the possibility of a paresis or immobility due to botulinum neurotoxin injection whether intentional or due to diffusion of injection into the strap musculature or cricopharyngus should also be considered in the initial assessment.[27,28]

When the causes for bilateral vocal cord immobility are compared with those of unilateral vocal fold immobility, there are not significant differences. The two exceptions are: (1) idiopathic immobility, which is more common for unilateral (23%) than for bilateral (12%), and (2) intubation trauma, which counted for only 3% of cases of unilateral vocal fold immobility but 12% of cases of bilateral vocal fold immobility.[29] Patients with a number of psychogenic disorders will also appear to have stridor and bilateral vocal cord paralysis. These include malingerers, patients with true conversion disorders with paradoxical vocal fold motion and closure, and patients with neurologic disease exacerbated by psychogenic factors. The conversion disorders are more common in young female patients.[30,31]

Another entity, termed spasmophilia or pseudotetany, may cause stridor and produce a picture simulating bilateral weakness or paralysis. This usually has a psychogenic origin in which patients hyperventilate and become alkalotic. This causes a flux of Ca^{++} ions, causing hyperreactivity and pseudotetany.[32] It should be noted that true bilateral immobility rarely occurs in the absence of a clear cause and given the high percentage of vocal fold paralyses that are caused by chest or mediastinal neoplasms, further investigation is often needed.[30]

CLINICAL PRESENTATION

Recurrent Laryngeal Nerve versus Superior Laryngeal Nerve

For the purpose of this chapter, our discussion will mainly be limited to vocal fold immobility or motion abnormalities due to neurologic insult to the recurrent laryngeal nerve. While the superior laryngeal nerve provides both motor innervation (cricothyroid muscle) and sensory innervation to the larynx, injury to this nerve alone has not been shown to result in gross vocal fold immobility. A superior laryngeal nerve paralysis is primarily thought to affect ability to produce higher vocal registers, thereby decreasing pitch and vocal projection.[33-35]

For a patient presenting with such complaints, it is important to consider that while a gross motion abnormality or immobility may not be present on exam, a superior laryngeal nerve paralysis may still be present.

Unilateral Vocal Fold Paralysis

Unilateral vocal fold paralysis (UVFP) inhibits adequate closure of the vocal folds, causing breathy dysphonia frequently accompanied by symptoms of aspiration.[29,36] In some cases, the underlying glottal insufficiency results in more subtle complaints such as vocal fatigue due to hyperfunction as a compensatory measure. Compensatory measures are described as abnormal or compensatory muscle tension patterns (MTPs) that have developed as a result of an organic voice disorder.[37,38] The sheer effort of MTPs can often account for a loss in vocal stamina. Patients may state that they feel that baseline speech or singing is simply more effortful despite achieving what appear to be adequate tone, pitch, and timbre. Difficulty vocalizing over distances or outdoors, fading over prolonged use, or even difficulty in rapidly changing pitch may all serve as clues of underlying vocal fold immobility.[2] However, if compensation or position of the immobile vocal fold is favorable, some patients may even have a near-normal or normal voice.

Vocal Fold Paresis

In patients with some preservation of vocal fold motion, the clinical presentation can be even more subtle as their compensatory measures may truly mask their motion deficits. The concept that a "hypokinetic" disorder may present with "hyperkinetic" facets is one that is critical to understanding and recognizing vocal fold paresis.[37] A patient who sounds "hyperfunctional" may be overlooked for a potential paresis.[39,40] These patients may present after failing what appears to be a compliant course of voice therapy as they may have been initially diagnosed with a functional dysphonia. Similarly, the seemingly dismissive complaint of diplophonia outside of prepubescent or adolescence (puberphonia) warrants closer investigation. Koufman and colleagues make particular mention of the presence of diplophonia as a "red flag" for vocal fold paresis as "diplophonia implies differential tension or mass between the two vocal folds" stating that "diplophonia implies paresis unless proved otherwise".[37]

It is also important to keep in mind that the symptoms of paresis are often "common" and nonspecific. Not surprisingly so, hoarseness is the most common chief complaint in vocal fold paresis.[37,38] Additionally, a paresis may involve sensory deficits (suggesting superior laryngeal nerve pathology) alone or in addition to motor deficits. Thus, odynophonia, globus sensation, dysphagia, chronic cough and laryngospasm have all been identified as symptoms present in laryngeal neuropathies.[38,41]

Bilateral Vocal Fold Paralysis

In contrast to the dysphonic clinical presentation of a UVFP or paresis, bilateral VFP usually presents in the setting of dyspnea or airway obstruction. It can be life-threatening for some while others, who have an open glottic chink, may have a breathy dysphonia, intermittent dyspnea, and stridor.[30] In a review of patient's with bilateral VFP presenting to a tertiary-care clinic, the most common presentation was dyspnea and airway obstruction (75%), followed by dysphonia (13%) and aspiration (4%).[42] It is an important discern however, the difference between a patient presenting with signs of bilateral vocal fold immobility versus laryngospasm, which is intermittent but may be confused with bilateral paralysis because of the presentation of stridor.[30]

EVALUATION OR WORKUP

Laryngoscopy or Videostroboscopy

Laryngoscopy and stroboscopy are powerful and essential adjuncts to evaluate any patient presenting with vocal or laryngeal complaints. While transoral rigid stroboscopy in experienced hands may be comparable in view, some feel that transoral examination may alter the laryngeal biomechanics thereby obscuring subtle motion abnormalities.[38] Rigid endoscopy also inhibits rapid and repetitive vocalizations and various pitches and vowel sounds. An assessment cannot be made in running speech or while singing. All of these limit the ability to assess the impact of significant vocal fold asymmetrical movements or identification of subtle movement impairments. An obvious paralysis can be readily identified as gross vocal fold immobility.

Identifying a paresis is often more involved. Most of the authors identify vocal fold paresis in the literature utilizing visual clues such as vocal fold bowing (especially in a patient <50-year-old), decreased abduction or adduction, axial tilt of the larynx, vertical height mismatch, phase lag, and asymmetric mucosal wave amplitudes and frequencies.[2,3,14,37,43] Another finding that can suggest paresis is anterior positioning of the paretic arytenoid anterior to the nonparetic in recurrent laryngeal injury or a tilt of the posterior larynx to the side of the paresis in superior laryngeal nerve paresis.

The presence of overt lesions such as granulomas, contact ulcers, localized or unilateral Reinke's edema called "podules", vocal nodules or even free-edge leukoplakia (due to shear-force trauma) may be signs of a paresis.[44-46] Yet, it is when the findings are more subtle or masked, that identifying a paresis becomes more challenging. Recalling the presentation of hypokinesis as a hyperkinetic disorder, the presence of supraglottic compression anteroposterior vocal fold shortening and side-to-side false vocal fold compression (plica ventricularis) are often more clinically apparent and can mask an underlying paresis.[47] These signs may be present without obvious visual and motion asymmetries or even in situations where there may be bilateral paresis.

To aid in recognition, some authors have developed techniques to be used during videolaryngostroboscopy. Rubin and colleagues outlined three specific repetitive phonatory tasks (RPTs): (1) "alternating a sniff with the /i/ vowel repeatedly", (2) /i/-/hi/-/i/-/hi/-/i/-/hi/, and (3) /pɑ/-/tɑ/-/kɑ/-/pɑ/-/tɑ/kɑ/-/pɑ/tɑ/kɑ/" that were used to assess 96 patients with suspected laryngeal movement abnormalities.[48] Even in the presence of an obvious immobility, these tasks are helpful for training the eye to readily identify motion asymmetries.

Laryngeal Electromyography

With the advent of laryngeal electromyography (LEMG) in 1944, LEMG has become an increasingly useful tool in the assessment of patients with suspected neurological injury. While EMG is often stated as the "gold standard" for diagnosis of paresis and is touted as the only method to determine if a subtle vocal fold motion asymmetry is due to a neurologic insult, recent retrospective reviews reveal that most otolaryngologists use LEMG as a confirmatory diagnostic test.[49,50] Such an observation is not surprising, since symptomatology is often what prompts endoscopy or stroboscopy to be performed first with scope findings, in turn, prompting further studies. Yet arguably, the subtleties of stroboscopic findings are subject to interpretation just as the subtleties of electromyographic findings, thereby making neither modality a clear "gold standard".

Laryngeal EMG is usually performed by a neurologist certified in electrodiagnostic testing who performs and then interprets the signs. In many practices, the needle is introduced by a laryngologist who is more familiar with the anatomy and then interpreted by the neurologist. The electromyography should examine the thyroarytenoid (TA) and both posterior cricoarytenoid (PCA) muscles. The presence of fibrillation potentials, positive sharp waves, polyphasic motor action potentials, and a neuropathic interference pattern are pathognomonic for neurological injury and clearly point to a diagnosis of paralysis".[36,49,50] Moreover, LEMG can be very useful in discerning between actual neurologic trauma and arytenoid dislocation or cricoarytenoid joint fixation.[51]

However in paresis, the LEMG signs may not always be clear cut. This can be due to an inherently mild neurologic pathology or due to normally functioning muscles that may compensate for the relative weakness of the paretic nerves.

Of the many LEMG features, it appears a decreased recruitment pattern is present most reliably in paresis.[14] The degree of recruitment is subjective and having an experienced laryngeal electromyographical team who has performed many procedures will help to optimize the interpretation. It should be noted that most studies evaluating LEMG for diagnosis of VFP to date are unblinded and/or retrospective with a level IV category of evidence.[49] Thus, while the information obtained from an LEMG can be helpful, it is rarely, in a clinical setting, used as a stand-alone tool for diagnosis.

Imaging

The use of adjunct imaging in the initial evaluation of vocal fold immobility is often motivated by a search for the underlying cause. Ultrasound, chest radiograph [chest X–ray (CXR)], computed tomography (CT), magnetic resonance imaging (MRI), and esophagram have all been recommended in varying studies.[52] Yet the cost of these studies can quickly become staggering. In a 2013 study of patients with idiopathic UVFP, CT scanning had an initial 1.7% yield, suggesting that "chest and neck CT may not be clinically beneficial provided the patient has good otolaryngologic and medical follow-up".[53] Yet in another 2013 study of patients with idiopathic UVFP, CT revealed the case in 23.5% of patients.

While the utility of CT is debatable, often starting with a routine CXR may help direct the judicious use of further imaging. In fact, many patients may already have a recent routine chest radiograph at the time of assessment. A positive CXR can lead to expedient and directed pulmonary, thoracic, or vascular evaluation. A negative CXR, can then be followed with a CT scan of the neck from the skull base to the thoracic inlet [for right-sided unilateral vocal fold immobility (R-UVFI)] or to the aortic triangle (for left-sided UVFI) can then solidify the diagnosis.[53] Other diagnostic studies such as a swallow study or esophagram are directed by signs and symptoms (i.e. aspiration signs). It is noteworthy to mention that often a CT scan should be ordered to aid in surgical planning which will be discussed further in the chapter.[54]

UNILATERAL VOCAL FOLD IMMOBILITY MANAGEMENT

The primary goal of treatment for unilateral vocal fold immobility (UVFI) is to medialize the affected vocal fold, allowing better approximation to the opposite vocal fold. This can be achieved by four main strategies: (1) reinnervation of the vocal fold, (2) injection of connective tissue or biomaterial lateral to the affected vocal fold (injection laryngoplasty), (3) rotation or repositioning of the arytenoid, or (4) placement of a prosthetic implant via a surgical window in the thyroid cartilage [medialization laryngoplasty (ML)].[55-57]

Voice Therapy

Voice therapy by speech-language pathologists (SLPs) specializing in voice is often the first step in managing a patient with vocal fold immobility. Heuer and colleagues studied 19 female patients and 22 male patients with unilateral recurrent nerve paralysis and found that 68% of the female patients and 64% of the male patients considered their voices satisfactory and elected not to undergo surgery.[58]

Even in patients with gross glottal incompetence, voice therapy can often address the undesirable compensatory hyperfunctional behaviors and can train and prepare patients for optimal postoperative phonation.[59] A recent longitudinal study found that voice therapy for UVFP not only effective but its benefits are sustained.[60] Moreover, while early referral for voice therapy seems to be associated with greater benefit, the quality of life still improves for patients with delayed treatment.[60]

Injection Medialization

Injection laryngoplasty has been used to medialize vocal folds for almost 100 years. First described in 1919, by Bruennings using paraffin, injection laryngoplasty (IL) with temporary injectable materials is a well-established technique for managing glottial insufficiency from laryngeal pathology including vocal fold immobility, UVFP or paresis.[61-64] Temporary laryngoplasty is particularly beneficial in the setting of idiopathic vocal fold immobility or iatrogenic recurrent laryngeal nerve trauma when spontaneous recovery of the injured nerve may occur. Early injection has been shown to potentially reduce the need for surgery should the nerve not recover, and therefore, many are advocating for early injection in patients with VFP, whether or not there is likelihood of recovery.[65,66]

There is general agreement that the ideal material for injection should be biocompatible, easy to inject with minimal preparation, and possess a residence time that offers the patient a reasonable period of benefit before reabsorption.[61,64] Previously, Teflon was the most widely used injectable material; however, a well-established side effect of reactive granuloma formation has decreased its popularity.[67] Other materials currently in use for IL include calcium hydroxylapatite (Radiesse Voice), hyaluronic acid (HA) gels (Restylane), human- and bovine-based collagen products (Cymetra/Zyplast, respectively), bovine gelatin (Gelfoam), particulate silicone, and autologous adipose.[62] Of the materials available for injection, except for fat, HA gels most closely match the viscoelastic properties of the true vocal folds.[68-70] In the largest series to date, no hypersensitivity or granulomatous reactions were observed thus making it a safe and effective temporary material for office-based injection medialization with an average length of benefit of 12.2 weeks.[71]

In 1990, Mikaelian et al. described the use of autologous fat for vocal fold augmentation to treat UVFP and praised the "soft bulkiness" fat imparted to the treated fold.[72] Autologous adipose injection (AAI) utilizes abdominal adipose harvested during the same operation as the laryngoscopic injection as the injected substance to add bulk to the vocal fold(s) and afford some potential for permanent fat retention and long-term effect. While results can be variable as fat is thought of as "semipermanent" material due to some degree of resorption, our experience suggests benefit for AAI injections. Since there is at least some potential for long-term retention and clinical benefit and the procedure is relatively easy with low morbidity and complications.

Autologous adipose injection is a reasonable option for certain cases: patients who have had prior medialization laryngoplasty, VFP patients where motion recovery cannot as yet be determined, or those who do not want to have an open neck procedure but would like the potential of permanency. Adipose injections do not interfere with the pliability of the vocal folds in the event that a medialization is required. It is a useful option as an adjunct to other laryngeal procedures such as laryngeal reinnervation or procedures for scars and sulci. AAI successfully augments vocal folds in short-term outcomes with some gradual decrease in effectiveness. While limited, a retrospective review of 43 patients demonstrated objective long-term benefit may occur in more than 50% of patients.[73] Figures 3 and 4 show vocal folds before and after AAI.

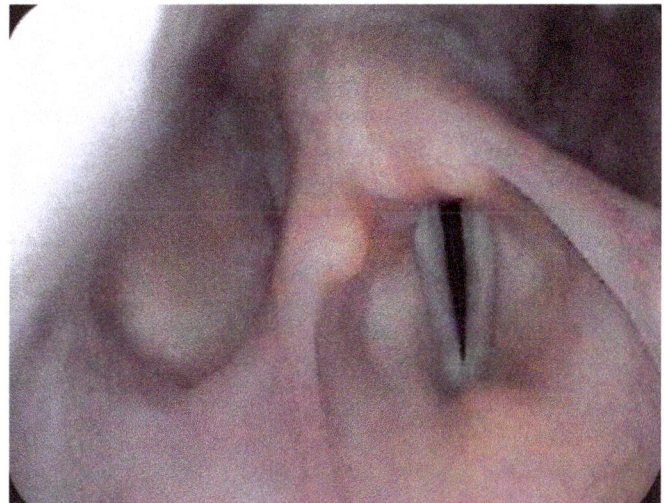

Fig. 3 Vocal folds on phonation in a patient with left vocal fold immobility

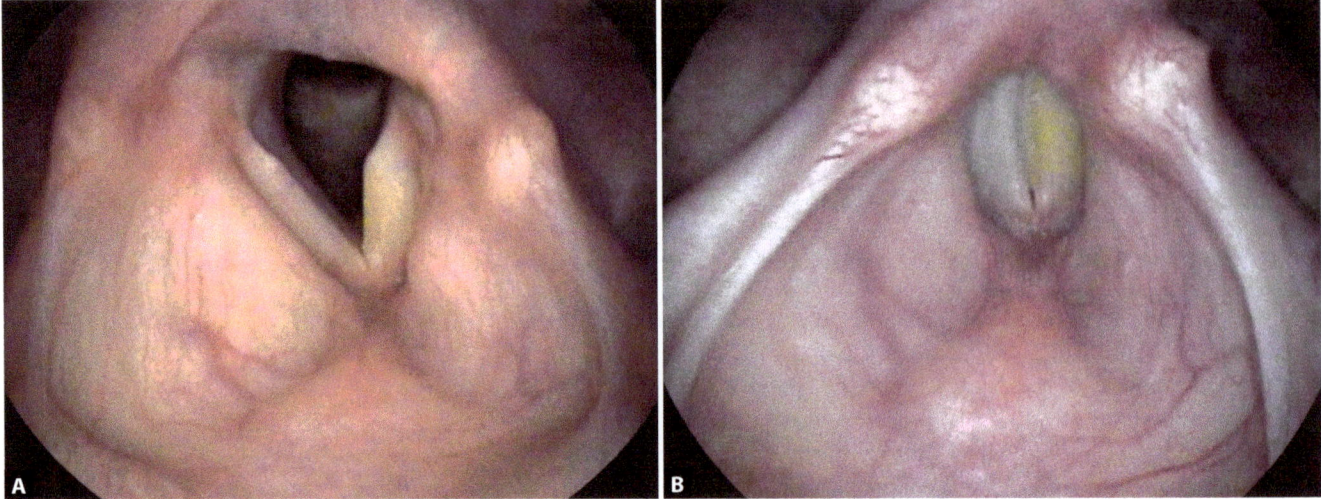

Figs 4A and B Vocal folds on phonation in a patient with left vocal fold immobility after autologous adipose injection. (A) Close-up after left vocal fold AAI (fat injection); (B) on phonation

Implant Medialization

Another more permanent medicalization procedure is the placement of an implant which was first described by Isikii in 1974.[56] Implants are typically created at the time of surgery from silastic or Gore-Tex (WL Gore and Associates, Incorporation, Flagstaff, AZ) or prefabricated implants. There are different advantages and disadvantages in using these different approaches.[57] Prefabricated prostheses, such as the Montgomery implant (Montgomery Implant System; Boston Medical Products, Boston, MA), come in a variety of sizes and are meant to fit most patients.[74] Montgomery implants demonstrate good outcomes; however, in one study, the authors noted that individual variation in thyroid cartilage anatomy led to difficulty in placing the implant in some patients.[75,76]

Carved prostheses made from silicone products have demonstrated successful outcomes.[77,78] They also offer a solution to many of the problems with prefabricated implants, although they are not without their own drawbacks. Proponents argue that they may be designed so that the laryngoplasty window is small, allowing for potential adjustment, and that the wedge of the implant may extend posteriorly for additional medialization. Unlike prefabricated prostheses, they can be modified intraoperatively to best optimize a patient's voice. The low cost of the carvable silicone and the ability to make real-time adjustments and customization to patient anatomy are significant benefits. The disadvantages of this method include the time it takes to carve the implant, which may increase the length of surgery, although with experienced surgeons this time is minimal. Carving implants may, however, prove difficult for surgeons unfamiliar or less nuanced with the technique.

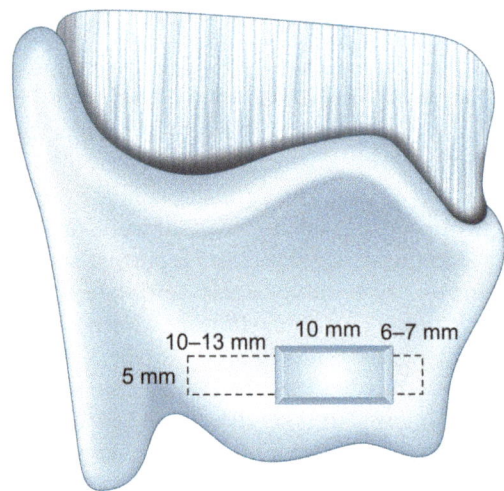

Fig. 5 Typical template for window for silastic medialization implant

Figures 5 and 6 illustrate a typical template for window for silastic medialization implant with a common design for the implant. Recent advent of an implant prediction model can often serve as a "starting point" for implant carving, utilizing a preoperative CT scan of the patient's larynx. Using triangulation and a linear regression model for tissue compression, it is possible to estimate and even prefabricate a customized implant thereby reducing intraoperative time (Figs 7A and B).[54]

Arytenoid Procedures

Arytenoid procedures are often used to address both unilateral and bilateral VFP. The concept behind to address the arytenoid complex lies in the belief that a longstanding paralysis can often cause ankylosis of the joint or scarring thereby fixing it in an unfavorable position. If the paralysis is unilateral, arytenoid adduction (AA) procedures can be done to medialize the complex and arguably improve the results of an implant medialization.[79] An AA arytenopexy can reconfigure the ipsilateral arytenoid for improved glottic closure, if needed.[1,80] For most patients with glottal insufficiency, implant medialization alone without an arytenoid rotation is sufficient. However, there are circumstances where addressing the arytenoid is beneficial.[81] For example, a large vertical plane mismatch would be difficult to manage with an implant alone and an arytenoid procedure may be necessary. In addition, fixed vocal folds with a significant glottal gap would require implant medialization, and an arytenoid procedure with disruption and resetting the joint, such as a posterior-lateral approach to an AA or an arytenoidopexy.[81]

BILATERAL VOCAL FOLD IMMOBILITY MANAGEMENT

In contrast to UVFI or paralysis, bilateral vocal fold immobility management is geared towards improving the airway as many of these patients have good voice quality. Bilateral vocal cord paralysis can be treated with three general classifications of procedures: (1) reinnervation, (2) electrical pacing, and (3) static procedures.

Laryngeal Reinnervation

Laryngeal reinnervation is aimed at providing some degree of neuronal input to the laryngeal musculature so as to prevent denervation atrophy or muscle wasting.[59] Numerous variations of the procedure have been noted using various grafts including the ansa cervicalis, phrenic nerve, and hypoglossal nerve.[82-84] Reinnervation of the TA muscle aims to restore tension to the vocal fold resulting while reinnervation of the PCA aims to prevent further prevents inferior displacement of the vocal process.[59] Animal studies have been done with varying degrees of success with some studies showing that reinnervation additionally improves synkinesis (aberrant reinnervation) after injury.[85] There have

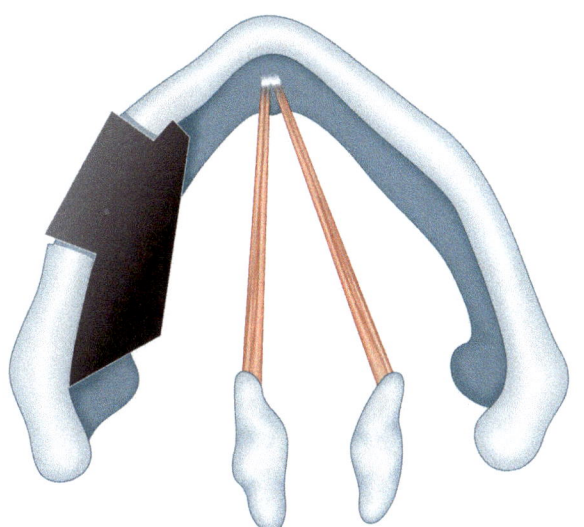

Fig. 6 Common design for medialization silastic prosthesis. Note large posterior segment of implant abutting against the vocal process of the arytenoid

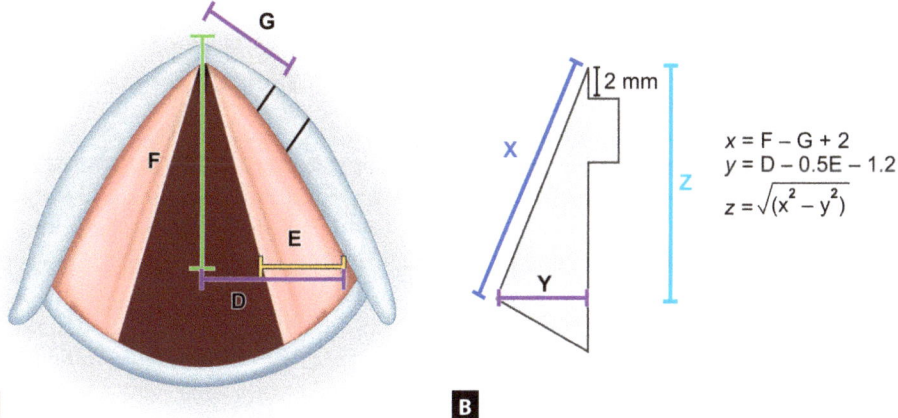

$$x = F - G + 2$$
$$y = D - 0.5E - 1.2$$
$$z = \sqrt{(x^2 - y^2)}$$

Figs 7A and B Schematic of axial computed tomography of larynx and silastic implant showing metrics required for prediction of implant dimensions. G is the distance from the anterior commissure to the anterior edge of the thyroplasty window. F is the distance from the anterior aspect of the thyroid cartilage to the point of planned medialization. E is the width of vocal fold at the point of planned medialization, and D is half the width of the thyroid cartilage at the point of the desired maximal medialization. These points can be used to determine x and y using the formula. All measurements are in millimeters[54]

also been isolated studies showing return of physiologic motion although no human studies exist to date.[86-88]

Electrical Pacing

Electrical pacing is a new and innovative approach to the problem of bilateral VFP. The concept behind laryngeal pacing is that electrical stimulation can be applied to the paralyzed PCA muscle and causes it to contract and open the airway. For a laryngeal pacer to stimulate denervated muscle, the technical requirements are more stringent than compared to other excitable tissue.[89] Particularly, denervated muscle requires high current pulses delivered throughout its volume to cause a full contraction which is feasible only when the electrode is near or in the muscle, but configured so that it will not injure the muscle.[30] In the largest recent human study, Zealear and colleagues implanted 6 patients with an Itrel II stimulator (Medtronic, Incorporation). In the study, PCA stimulation produced a large dynamic abduction (3.5–7 mm) in three patients and moderate abduction (3 mm) in one. Another patient showed a large but delayed response of 4 mm to stimulation with some lateralization of the vocal fold.[90] While larger human trials are yet to be reported, these findings are promising.

Static Procedures

Static procedures are designed to enlarge the airway permanently. These procedures attempt to create a stable airway at mild activity and in the event of vocal fold edema that can occur with upper respiratory infections. By the nature of their static design, these procedures necessitate an inverse balance between the airway and the voice. To date, all static procedures have been destructive of normal laryngeal tissue. One static procedure, arytenoidectomy has been a standard of care for many years. The surgical approach can be external, by laryngofissure, or endoscopic using laser or controlled ablation (coblation).[91,92] Often arytenoidectomy is accompanied by a lateralization suture to aid in the opening of the airway during the postoperative period.[30] Arytenoidectomy has the disadvantage of a large, permanent posterior gap with a relatively more breathy voice than more conservative alternatives. It is therefore rarely needed at this time.

Transverse cordotomy (Fig. 8) has also been used as an effective procedure to improve the airway.[93,94] This procedure has traditionally been done endoscopically and often with a CO_2 laser. However, the senior author has performed a large series of cordotomies under coblation (Figs 9 and 10). In this method, some patients can avoid intubation by simply having the procedure performed quickly with jet ventilation. In an animal study on canine vocal folds, coblation injury demonstrated complete epithelialization by postoperative

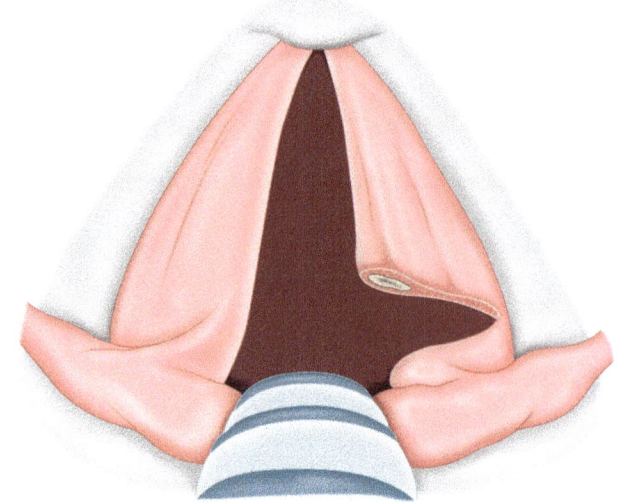

Fig. 8 Transverse cordotomy

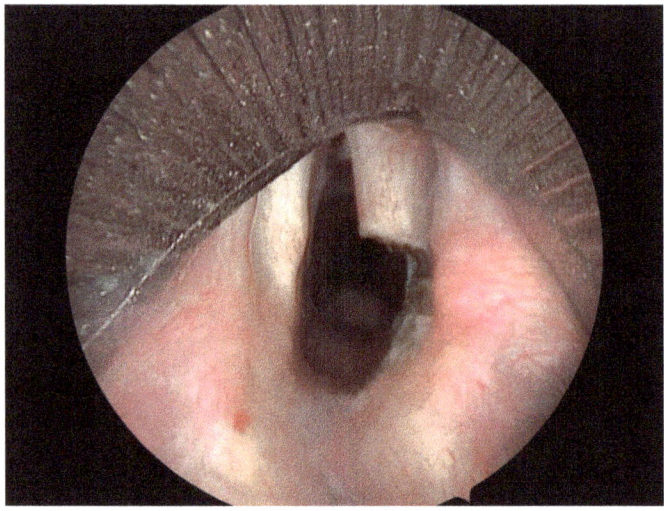

Fig. 9 Coblator cordotomy intraoperative

day 7 with no injury to the underlying vocalis muscle noted.[95] The study also noted that the inflammatory response demonstrates less inflammation than reported with CO_2 laser injury. Thus, coblation is a viable method for removal of tissue from the vocal fold resulting in minimal scar formation and a controlled depth of injury making this method to be not only expedient but immensely helpful at preserving voice quality while widening the airway.

One consideration in the surgical treatment of bilateral vocal fold immobility is whether or not the vocal folds are paralyzed or fixed. With a bilateral VFP, a unilateral posterior cordotomy (often with resection of the vocal process of the arytenoid) is adequate. The scar formation and contraction in the area of the surgical defect will help to slightly lateralize

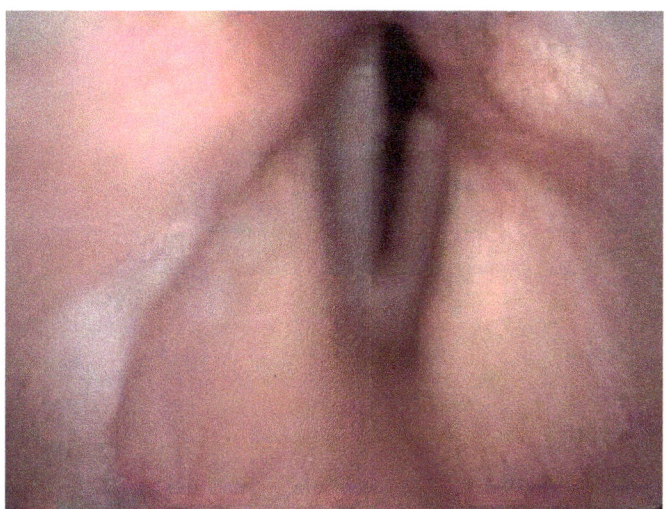

Fig. 10 Coblator cordotomy 2 weeks postoperative

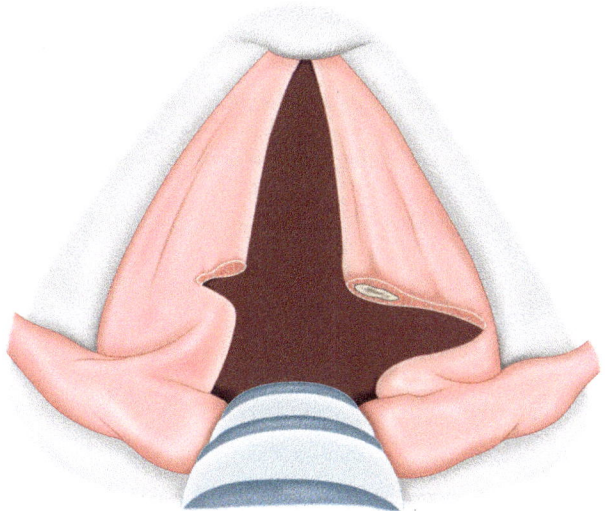

Fig. 11 Bilateral vocal fold fixation requiring a transverse cordotomy with a small cordotomy on the other side

the vocal fold, increasing the posterior glottis aperture. With bilateral vocal fold fixation, no movement can occur, so that the adequate initial opening may fill in and reduce over time. A small cordotomy on the other side is usually necessary (Fig. 11).

Tracheostomy

A final management option, which is often overlooked, is a simple permanent tracheotomy. It is rare that a tracheotomy is necessary for bilateral vocal fold immobility in the setting of a trained laryngologist since other options are available.

However, a tracheostomy offers the best and safest airway without sacrificing the voice. The main barriers are patient ability to provide routine diligent tracheostomy care, the limitations near water, and the social aspects. However, a permanent tracheotomy can be a very manageable condition for motivated patients.

REFERENCES

1. Rosenthal-Swibel L, Benninger MS, Deeb RH. Vocal fold immobility: a longitudinal analysis of etiology over 30 years. Laryngoscope. 2007;117:1864-70.
2. Sulica L. Vocal Fold Paresis: An evolving clinical concept. Curr Otorhinolaryngol Rep. 2013;1:158-62.
3. Wu AP, Sulica L. Diagnosis of vocal fold paresis: current opinion and practice. Laryngoscope. 2015;125:904-8.
4. Grundfast KM, Harley E. Vocal cord paralysis. Otolaryngol Clin North Am. 1989;22(3):569-97.
5. Miyamoto RC, Parikh SR, Gellad W, et al. Bilateral congenital vocal cord paralysis: a 16-year institutional review. Otolaryngol Head Neck Surg. 2005;133:241-5.
6. Lewis AF, Carron JD, Vedanarayanan V. Congenital bilateral vocal fold paralysis and Charcot-Marie-Tooth disease. Ann Otol Rhinol Laryngol. 2010;119(1):47-9.
7. Parano E, Pavone L, Musumeci S, et al. Acute palsy of the recurrent laryngeal nerve complicating Epstein-Barr virus infection. Neuropediatrics. 1996;27(3):164-6.
8. Randel RC, Kearns DB, Nespeca MP, et al. Vocal cord paralysis as a presentation of intrauterine infection with varicella-zoster virus. Pediatrics. 1996;97(1):127-8.
9. Small PM, McPhaul LW, Sooy CD, et al. Cytomegalovirus infection of the laryngeal nerve presenting as hoarseness in patients with acquired immunodeficiency syndrome. Am J Med. 1989;86:108-10
10. Bachor E, Bonkowsky V, Hacki T. Herpes simplex virus type 1 reactivation as a cause of a unilateral temporary paralysis of the vagus nerve. Eur Arch Otorhinolaryngol. 1996;253: 297-300.
11. Marie JP, Keghian J, Mendel I, et al. Post-intubation vocal cord paralysis: the viral hypothesis. A case report. Eur Arch Otorhinolaryngol. 2001;258(6):285-6.
12. Steele NP, Myssiorek D. West Nile virus induced vocal fold paralysis. Laryngoscope. 2006;116(3):494-6.
13. Rees CJ, Henderson AH, Belafsky PC. Postviral vagal neuropathy. Ann Otol Rhinol Laryngol. 2009;118(4):247-52.
14. Heman-Ackah YD, Barr A. Mild vocal fold paresis: understanding clinical presentation and electromyographic findings. J Voice. 2006;20:269-81.
15. Klein TA, Ridley MB. An old flame reignites: vagal neuropathy secondary to neurosyphilis. J Voice. 2014;28(2):255-7.
16. Benninger MS, Gillen JB, Altman JS. Changing etiology of vocal fold immobility. Laryngoscope. 1998;108(9):1346-50.
17. Zalvan C, Sulica L, Wolf S, et al. Laryngopharyngeal dysfunction from the implantable vagal nerve stimulator. Laryngoscope. 2003;113:221-5.
18. Heman-Ackah YD, Joglekar SS, Caroline M, et al. The prevalence of undiagnosed thyroid disease in patients with symptomatic vocal fold paresis. J Voice. 2011;25(4):496-500.

19. Teramoto K, Kuwabara M, Matsubara Y. Respiratory failure due to vocal cord paresis in myasthenia gravis. Respiration. 2002;69:280-2.

20. Mao VH, Abaza M, Spiegel JR, et al. Laryngeal myasthenia gravis: report of 40 cases. J Voice. 2001;15:122-30.

21. Sulica L, Blitzer A, Lovelace RE, et al. Vocal fold paresis of Charcot–Marie–Tooth disease. Ann Otol Rhinol Laryngol. 2001;110:1072-6.

22. Isozaki E, Naito R, Kanda T, et al. Different mechanism of vocal cord paralysis between spinocerebellar atrophy and multiple system atrophy. J Neurol Sci. 2002;197:37-43.

23. Rontal E, Rontal M, Wald J, et al. Botulinum toxin injection in the treatment of vocal fold paralysis associated with multiple sclerosis: a case report. J Voice. 1999;13(2):274-9.

24. Jaffe R, Bogomolski-Yahalom V, Kramer MR. Vocal cord paralysis as the presenting symptom of sarcoidosis. Respir Med. 1994;88(8):633-6.

25. Lally EV, Jimenez SA. Vocal cord palsy in systemic sclerosis. J Rheumatol. 1988;15(12):1876-7.

26. Merati AL, Halum SL, Smith TL. Diagnostic testing for vocal fold paralysis: survey of practice and evidence-based medicine review. Laryngoscope. 2006;116(9):1539-52.

27. Venkatesan NN, Johns MM, Hapner ER, et al. Abductor paralysis after botox injection for adductor spasmodic dysphonia. Laryngoscope. 2010;120(6):1177-80.

28. Benninger MS, Hanick A, Hicks DM. Cricothyroid Muscle Botulinum Toxin Injection to Improve Airway for Bilateral Recurrent Laryngeal Nerve Paralysis, A Case Series. J Voice. 2016;30(1):96-9.

29. Benninger MS, Crumley RL, Ford CN, et al. Evaluation and treatment of the unilateral paralyzed vocal fold. Otolaryngol Head Neck Surg. 1994;111(4):497-508.

30. Hillel AD, Benninger M, Blitzer A, et al. Evaluation and management of bilateral vocal cord immobility. Otolaryngol Head Neck Surg. 1999;121(6):760-5.

31. Patterson R, Schatz M, Horton M. Munchausen's stridor: nonorganic laryngeal obstruction. Clin Allergy. 1974;4:307-10.

32. Younger D. Neuromuscular diseases. In: Blitzer A, Brin M, Sasaki C (Eds). Neurological disorders of the larynx. New York: Thieme; 1992. pp. 240-7.

33. Orestes MI, Chhetri DK. Superior laryngeal nerve injury: effects, clinical findings, prognosis, and management options. Curr Opin Otolaryngol Head Neck Surg. 2014;22(6):439-43.

34. Barczynski M, Bellantone R, Brauckhoff M, et al. External branch of the superior laryngeal nerve monitoring during thyroid and parathyroid surgery: International Neural Monitoring Study Group standards guideline statement: IONM During Thyroid Surgery. Laryngoscope. 2013;123:S1-14.

35. Sulica L. The superior laryngeal nerve:function and dysfunction. Otolaryngol Clin North Am. 2004;37:183-201.

36. Sataloff RT, Praneetvatakul P, Heuer RJ, et al. Laryngeal electromyography: clinical application. J Voice. 2010;24: 228-34.

37. Koufman JA, Postma GN, Cummins MM, et al. Vocal fold paresis. Otolaryngol Head Neck Surg. 2000;122:537-41.

38. Koufman JA. Evaluation of laryngeal biomechanics by fiberoptic laryngoscopy. In: Rubin JS, Sataloff RT, Korovin GS (Eds). Diagnosis and treatment of voice disorders. New York: Igaku-Shoin; 1995. pp. 122-34.

39. Morrison MD, Nichol H, Rammage LA. Diagnostic criteria in functional dysphonia. Laryngoscope. 1986;96:1-8.

40. Koufman JA, Blalock PD. Functional voice disorders. Otolaryngol Clin North Am. 1991;24:1059-73.

41. Amin MR, Koufman JA. Vagal neuropathy after upper respiratory infection: a viral etiology? Am J Otolaryngol. 2001; 22(4):251-6.

42. Brake MJ, Anderson J. Bilateral vocal fold immobility: a 13 year review of etiologies, management and the utility of the empey index. J Otolaryngol Head Neck Surg. 2015;44(1):27.

43. Woo P, Parasher AK, Isseroff T, et al. Analysis of laryngoscopic features in patients with unilateral vocal fold paresis. Laryngoscope. 2016;126(8):1831-6.

44. Koufman JA, Belafsky PC. Unilateral or localized Reinke's edema (pseudocyst) as a manifestation of vocal fold paresis: the paresis podule. Laryngoscope. 2001;111:576-80.

45. Carroll TL, Gartner-Schmidt J, Statham MM, et al. Vocal process granuloma and glottal insufficiency: an overlooked etiology? Laryngoscope. 2010;120(1):114-20.

46. Halum SL, Miller P, Early K. Laryngeal granulomas associated with superior laryngeal nerve paresis. J Voice. 2010;24(4):490-3.

47. Belafsky PC, Postma GN, Reulbach TR, et al. Muscle tension dysphonia as a sign of underlying glottal insufficiency. Otolaryngol Head Neck Surg. 2002;127:448-51.

48. Rubin AD, Praneetvatakul V, Heman-Ackah Y, et al. Repetitive phonatory tasks for identifying vocal fold paresis. J Voice. 2005;19(4):679-86.

49. Meyer TK, Hillel AD. Is laryngeal electromyography useful in the diagnosis and management of vocal fold paresis/paralysis? Laryngoscope. 2011;121(2):234-5.

50. Simpson CB, Cheung EJ, Jackson CJ. Vocal fold paresis: clinical and electrophysiologic features in a tertiary laryngology practice. J Voice. 2009;23(3):396-8.

51. Rontal E, Rontal M, Silverman B, et al. The clinical differentiation between vocal cord paralysis and vocal cord fixation using electromyography. Laryngoscope. 1993;103:133-7.

52. Altman JS, Benninger MS. The evaluation of unilateral vocal fold immobility: is chest X-ray enough? J Voice. 1997;11(3):364-7.

53. Badia PI, Hillel AT, Shah MD, et al. Computed tomography has low yield in the evaluation of idiopathic unilateral true vocal fold paresis. Laryngoscope. 2013;123(1):204-7.

54. Benninger MS, Chota RL, Bryson PC, et al. Custom implants for medialization laryngoplasty: a model that considers tissue compression. J Voice. 2015;29(3):363-9.

55. Dursun G, Boynukalin S, Ozgursoy OB, et al. Long-term results of different treatment modalities for glottic insufficiency. Am J Otolaryngol. 2008;29:7-12.

56. Isshiki N, Morita H, Okamura H, et al. Thyroplasty as a new phonosurgical technique. Acta Otolaryngol. 1974;78:451-7.

57. Damrose EJ, Berke GS. Advances in the management of glottic insufficiency. Curr Opin Otolaryngol Head Neck Surg. 2003;11:480-4.

58. Heuer R, Sataloff RT, Rulnick R, et al. Unilateral recurrent laryngeal nerve paralysis: the importance of "preoperative" voice therapy. J Voice. 1998;11(1):88-94.

59. Rubin AD, Sataloff RT. Vocal fold paresis and paralysis. Otolaryngol Clin North Am. 2007;40(5):1109-31, viii-ix.

60. Busto-Crespo O, Uzcanga-Lacabe M, Abad-Marco A, et al. Longitudinal voice outcomes after voice therapy in unilateral vocal fold paralysis. J Voice. 2016;30(6):767.e9-e15.

61. Bruennings W. Uber eine neue behandlungsmethode der rekurrensslahmung. Ver Deutsch Laryng. 1911;18:93-151.

62. Mallur PS, Rosen CA. Vocal fold injection: review of indications, techniques, and materials for augmentation. Clin Exp Otorhinolaryngol. 2010;3(4):177-82.

63. Kwon TK, Buckmire R. Injection laryngoplasty for management of unilateral vocal fold paralysis. Curr Opin Otolaryngol Head Neck Surg. 2004;12:538-42.

64. King JM, Simpson CB. Modern injection augmentation for glottic insufficiency. Curr Opin Otolaryngol Head Neck Surg. 2007;15:153-8.

65. Friedmann AD, Burns JA, Heaton JT, et al. Early versus late injection medialization for unilateral vocal cord paralysis. Laryngoscope. 2010;120:2042-6.

66. Prendes BL, Yung KC, Likhterov I, et al. Long-term effects of injection laryngoplasty with a temporary agent on voice quality and vocal fold position. Laryngoscope. 2012;122:2227-33.

67. Sataloff RT. Teflon granuloma—complications of surgical procedure to correct vocal disorder—Brief Article. Ear Nose Throat J. 2000.

68. Borzacchiello A, Mayol L, Garskog O, et al. Evaluation of injection augmentation treatment of hyaluronic acid based materials on rabbit vocal folds viscoelasticity. J Mater Sci Mater Med. 2005;16: 553-7.

69. Hertegard S, Dahlqvist A, Goodyer E. Viscoelastic measurements after vocal fold scarring in rabbits-short-term results after hyaluronan injection. Acta Otolaryngol. 2006;126:758-63.

70. Choi JS, Kim NK, Klemuk S, et al. Preservation of viscoelastic properties of rabbit vocal folds after implantation of hyaluronic acid-based biomaterials. Otolaryngol Head Neck Surg. 2012;147:515-21.

71. Halderman AA, Bryson PC, Benninger MS, et al. Safety and length of benefit of restylane for office-based injection medialization—a retrospective review of one institution's experience. J Voice. 2014;28(5):631-5.

72. Mikaelian DO, Lowry LD, Sataloff RT. Lipoinjection for unilateral vocal cord paralysis. Laryngoscope. 1991;101(5):465-8.

73. Benninger MS, Hanick AL, Nowacki AS. Augmentation Autologous Adipose Injections in the Larynx. Ann Otol Rhinol Laryngol. 2016;125(1):25-30.

74. Montgomery WW, Montgomery SK. Montgomery thyroplasty implant system. Ann Otol Rhinol Laryngol Suppl. 1997;170:1-16.

75. McLean-Muse A, Montgomery WW, Hillman RE, et al. Montgomery thyroplasty implant for vocal fold immobility: phonatory outcomes. Ann Otol Rhinol Laryngol. 2000;109:393-400.

76. Laccourreye O, Benkhatar H, Menard M. Lack of adverse events after medialization laryngoplasty with the montgomery thyroplasty implant in patients with unilateral laryngeal nerve paralysis. Ann Otol Rhinol Laryngol. 2012;121:701-7.

77. Lundy DS, Casiano RR, Xue JW, et al. Thyroplasty type I: short- vs long-term results. Head Neck Surg. 2000;122:533-6.

78. Netterville JL, Stone RE, Luken ES, et al. Silastic medicalization and arytenoid adduction: the Vanderbilt experience. A review of 116 phonosurgical procedures. Ann Otol Rhinol Laryngol. 1993;102:413-24.

79. Isshiki N, Tanabe M, Sawada M. Arytenoid adduction for unilateral vocal cord paralysis. Arch Otolaryngol. 1978;104:555-8.

80. Spector BC, Netterville JL, Billante C, et al. Quality-of-life assessment in patients with unilateral vocal cord paralysis. Otolaryngol Head Neck Surg. 2001;125:176-82.

81. Benninger MS, Manzoor N, Ruda JM. Short- and long-term outcomes after silastic medicalization laryngoplasty: are arytenoid procedures needed? J Voice. 2015;29(2):236-40.

82. Crumley R. Update: ansa cervicalis to recurrent laryngeal nerve anastomosis for unilateral laryngeal paralysis. Laryngoscope. 1991;101:384-8.

83. Baldissera F, Cantarella G, Marini G, et al. Recovery of inspiratory abduction of the paralyzed vocal cords after bilateral reinnervation of the cricoarytenoid muscles by one single branch of the phrenic nerve. Laryngoscope. 1989;99:1286-92.

84. Paniello R, Lee P, Dahm D. Hyposglossal nerve transfer for laryngeal reinnervation: a preliminary study. Ann Otol Rhinol Laryngol. 1999;108:239-44.

85. Crumley RL. Laryngeal synkinesis revisited. Ann Otol Rhinol Laryngol. 2000;109:365-71.

86. Secarz J, Nguyen L, Nasri S, et al. Physiologic motion after laryngeal nerve reinnervation: a new method. Otolaryngol Head Neck Surg. 1997;116(4):466-74.

87. Van Lith-Bijl J, Stolk R, Tonnaer J, et al. Selective laryngeal reinnervation with separate phrenic and ansa cervicalis nerve transfers. Arch Otolaryngol Head Neck Surg. 1997;123:406-11.

88. Hogikyan N, Johns M, Kileny P, et al. Motion specific laryngeal reinnervation using muscle-nerve-muscle neurotization. Ann Otol Rhinol Laryngol. 2001;110(9):801-20.

89. Sanders I. Electrical stimulation of laryngeal muscle. Otolaryngol Clin North Am. 1991;24:1253-74.

90. Zealear DL, Billante CR, Courey MS, et al. Reanimation of the paralyzed human larynx with an implantable electrical stimulation device. Laryngoscope. 2003;113(7):1149-56.

91. Ossoff RH, Sisson GA, Duncavage JA, et al. Endoscopic laser arytenoidectomy for the treatment of bilateral vocal cord paralysis. Laryngoscope. 1984;94(10):1293-7.

92. Googe B, Nida A, Schweinfurth J. Coblator arytenoidectomy in the treatment of bilateral vocal cord paralysis. Case Rep Otolaryngol. 2015;2015:487280.

93. Dennis D, Kashima H. Carbon dioxide laser posterior cordectomy for treatment of bilateral vocal cord paralysis. Ann Otol Rhinol Laryngol. 1989;98:930-4.

94. Kashima H. Bilateral vocal fold motion impairment: pathophysiology and management by transverse cordotomy. Ann Otol Rhinol Laryngol. 1991;100:717-21.

95. Divi V, Benninger M, Kiupel M, et al. Coblation of the canine vocal fold: a histologic study. J Voice. 2012;26(6):811.e9-13.

Laryngeal Framework Surgery

KK Handa

INTRODUCTION

It was the pioneering work of Professor Isshiki[1] from Japan which revitalized the concept of laryngeal framework surgery. He did a set of experiments on dogs and devised a set of procedures called "laryngeal framework surgery". The procedures had been described before Payr,[2] a German surgeon, gave the first description of laryngoplasty as early as 1915. Isshiki's work was followed by Koufmann who also published case series[3] and by other workers.[4]

The principle of external laryngeal framework surgery lies in trying to alter the voice working through the skeleton of the larynx rather on the vocal cords directly. There were four procedures described:

1. Type 1 thyroplasty (medialization).
2. Type 2 thyroplasty (lateralization).
3. Type 3 thyroplasty.
4. Type 4 thyroplasty.

   Subsequently there have been some modifications in the procedures, e.g. European Laryngological Society nomenclature.

It is preferable to perform most of the procedures under local anesthesia so that the voice can be monitored on the table. Patient is kept under sedation.

ADVANTAGES OF THE LARYNGEAL FRAMEWORK SURGERY

Some of the advantages of the laryngeal framework surgery are:

- The medial vibrating edge is not manipulated at all

- There is direct control on improvement in voice and the amount of medialization
- If required, the procedure can be reversed
- It is mostly possible to do the procedure under local anesthesia so as to monitor the voice
- The procedures are generally very safe without any significant complications.

PROCEDURES UNDER LOCAL ANESTHESIA

Type 1 Thyroplasty

Today type 1 thyroplasty is the international standard for management of unilateral vocal fold paralysis. The aim is to medialize the vocal fold so that glottis closure is achieved. A patient with unilateral vocal fold paralysis is first assessed to ascertain a cause of the cord paralysis. Now-a-days a contrast-enhanced computed tomography (CT) scan of the neck and chest is done instead of the classical panendoscopy done previously. In case no cause is found we wait for 4–6 months before doing thyroplasty. Apart from unilateral immobile cord, type 1 thyroplasty can also be done for atrophic cord, severe sulcus, aspiration, and scarred cord.

Surgical Procedure

Mostly local anesthesia is preferred so that intraoperatively voice can be monitored and modulated during surgery. However, in case of noncompliant patients general anesthesia can be given. The neck is positioned in neutral position without undue flexion or extension so that natural voice is maintained (Fig. 1). Subplatysmal flaps are elevated.

Strap muscles are split to expose the thyroid cartilage. The most important step of the surgery is making the window at the correct place.[5]

Few tips for making the window are:

- The superior border of the window and the placed implant has to be at the level of true cord
- The lower border should be 2–3 mm from the lower border of the thyroid cartilage
- The superomedial angle of the window should be 5 mm from the midpoint between superior and inferior thyroid notch
- At times cartilage is ossified then drill can be used.

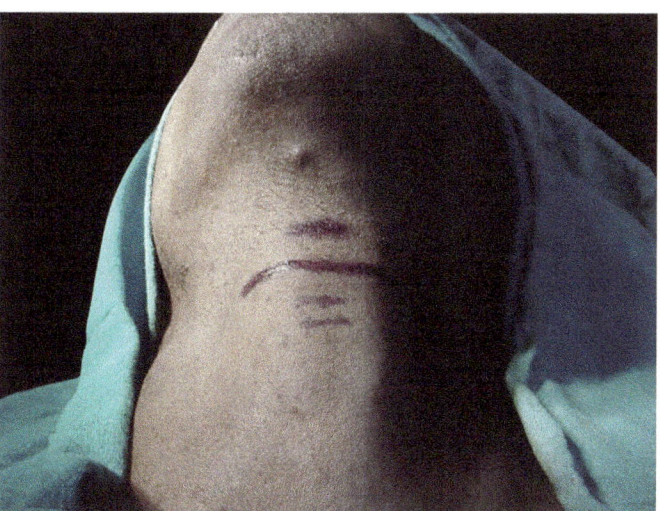

Fig. 1 Incision marked showing different landmarks. Neck is in neutral position

Inner perichondrium should not be traumatized as this will lead to hematoma forming in the thyroarytenoid muscle. However, author makes a linear cut in the inner perichondrium along the borders of the window. This helps in implant appropriately medializing the vocal cord.

Implant

The author's first choice is TVFMI [titanium vocal fold medializing implant (Friedrich design; company Kurtz)]. This prosthesis is made of titanium (Figs 2A and B).

It is easy to insert, biocompatible and secure prosthesis. It is inserted and the optimum position at which the patient has best voice improvement is marked on the posterior flange. The posterior flange is bending with the plier at the marking and the implant is reinserted.

Alternatively, a prosthesis can be carved out from silicon block[6] or a preformed prosthesis, e.g. Netterville prosthesis can be used (Fig. 3). Gore-Tex is another material which can be used. The other materials being used are hydroxyapatite and autologous cartilage. Gore-Tex strip is easy to insert but being in a strip form can change shape (Fig. 4).

Intraoperatively the appropriate medialization can be monitored either by the voice of the patient or by doing a flexible endoscopy.

Arytenoid Adduction

In selected cases, the procedure of arytenoid adduction is combined with type 1 thyroplasty (Figs 5 and 6). Isshiki described this for cases where there is a big posterior glottic defect.[7] The procedure consists of identifying muscular process of arytenoid and passing a Figure of 8 suture through it and anchoring to the thyroid cartilage anteriorly.

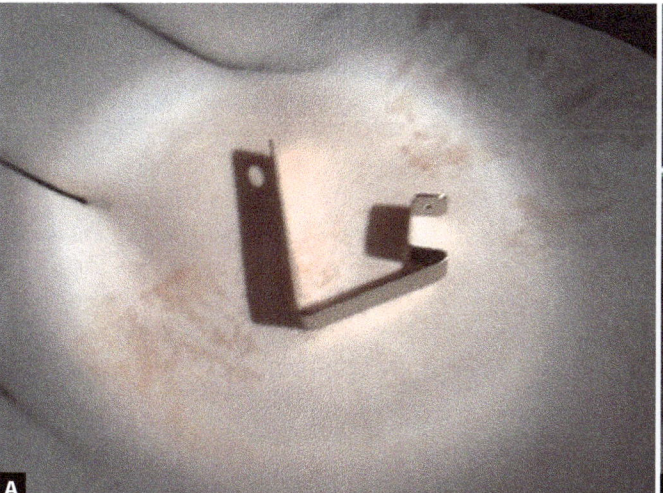
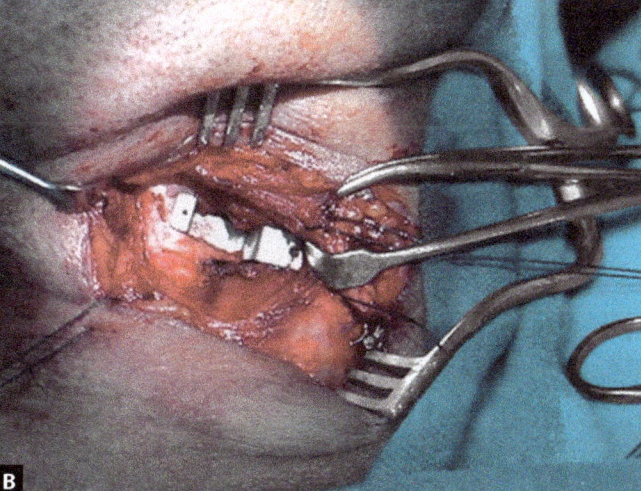

Figs 2A and B TVFMI [titanium vocal fold medializing implant (Friedrich design)]

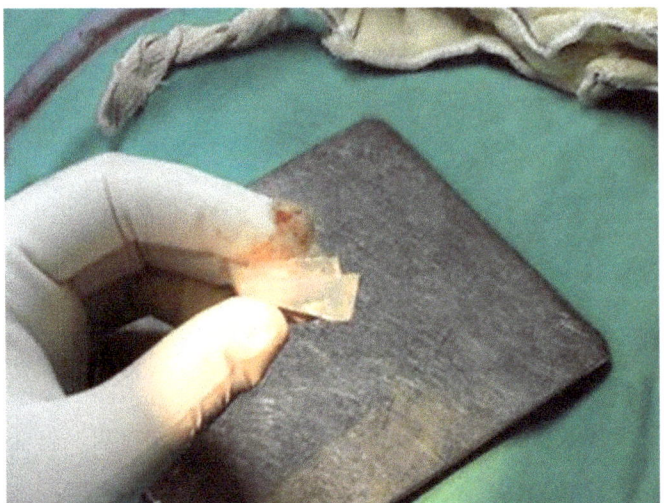

Fig. 3 Netterville's silastic preformed implant

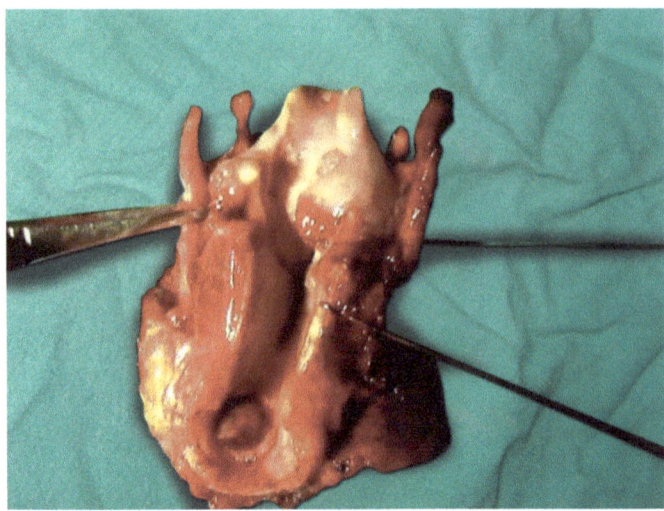

Fig. 5 A postlaryngectomy specimen is very good to practise arytenoid adduction

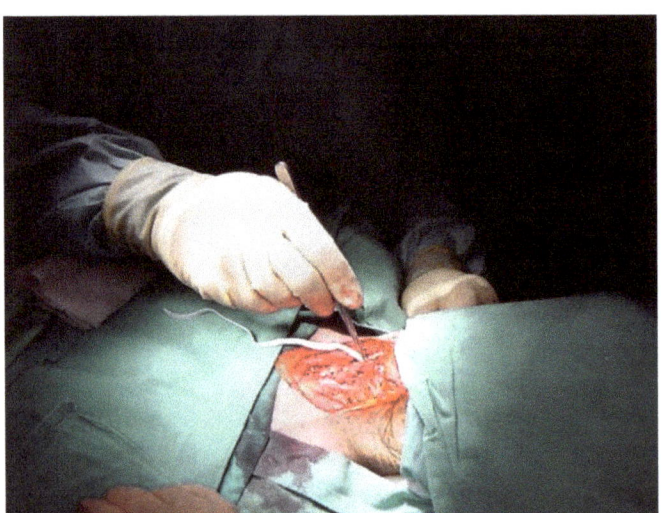

Fig. 4 Gore-Tex strip as medialization prosthesis

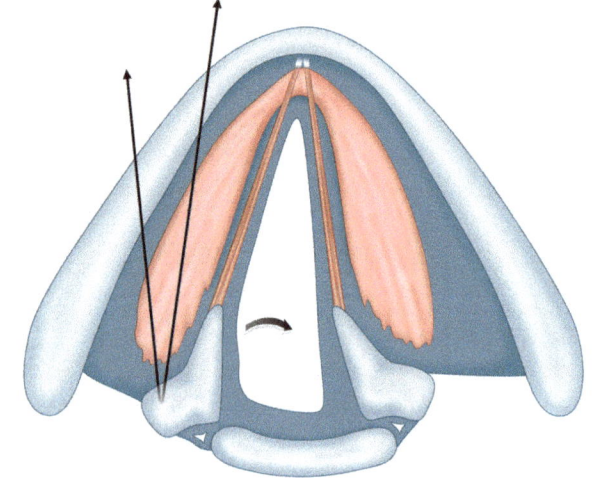

Fig. 6 Concept of arytenoid adduction. A suture passed through muscular process of arytenoid cartilage

This pulls the muscular process laterally, in turn, turning the vocal process medially and closing the posterior gap. Now it is believed that arytenoid adduction does more than just closing the posterior gap. It increases the tension in the vocal cord also. In certain cases where the vertical level of the two cords is different arytenoid adduction is also helpful.

A modification of arytenoid adduction has been described by Zeitels. This consists of arytenoid adduction and cricothyroid subluxation.[8] Here full arytenoid cartilage is exposed through an extended incision. The muscle attachments of the arytenoid are divided and it is fixed in the midline. A suture is further passed between the inferior horn of the thyroid cartilage and cricoid cartilage.

Thyroplasty can be combined with type 4 thyroplasty.

Patient may be told that voice will only stabilize after 1 week because of postoperative edema. Patient may need postoperative voice therapy.

Type 1 thyroplasty is a fairly safe procedure and the incidence of extrusion or displacement of the implant into the laryngeal lumen is rare. Postoperative bleeding and infection are very rare.

Patients who have atrophic or scarred cords may get/give very good results, especially after postlaser resection. A local muscle flap may be used to create space between medial scar and the cartilage so as to enable implant insertion and reduce chances of extrusion of the implant.

Type 1 thyroplasty gives fairly consistent results provided the patient selection is correct.[9]

Type 2 Thyroplasty

This was originally described for bilateral abductor cord paralysis; however, with time better procedures have evolved for that indication. Now it is used as surgery for adductor spasmodic dysphonia. Botox is the treatment of choice for adductor spasmodic dysphonia; however, the duration of action is limited to about 4–6 months. It is offered to patients if they do not want to repeat botox injections. In this procedure, the thyroid ala is vertically split in the midline. Caution is to be exercised so as not to open in the laryngeal lumen as anteriorly there is no muscle and only Broyles' ligament. Two to three silastic shims about 2 mm × 3 mm are inserted to get both the thyroid ala apart (Fig. 7). In place of silastic shims, 4 mm titanium plates can be used. The operation has the effect of keeping both thyroid ala apart and reducing the hyperadduction and choking in the voice.

Type 3 Thyroplasty

This surgery is used to lower the pitch. It was originally based on the concept that a change in the anteroposterior diameter of the thyroid ala will result in a change in the vocal cord tension. Later modifications were made. Most common indication is puberphonia. Puberphonia in majority of cases is correctable by voice therapy. It is only in about 10% cases

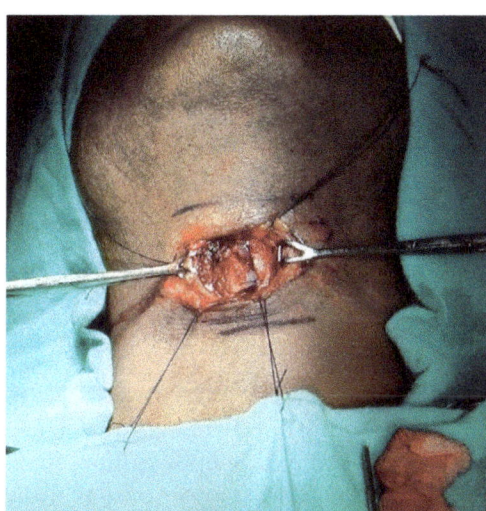

Fig. 7 Type 2 thyroplasty; 3 mm × 2 mm silastic shims used to separate thyroid ala divided in the midline

that surgery is required. In this procedure, again vertical cuts are given in the thyroid ala about 5 mm from the midline and this medial segment of thyroid cartilage is mobilized on both sides to make it free. Some surgeons put a retrusion sutures, however in our experience, just making the medial segment free is enough to change the pitch from high pitch to low pitch.

Type 4 Thyroplasty

This procedure is done to increase the pitch from low pitch to high pitch. The request to do so usually comes in sex change operations from male to female. This procedure is also useful for superior laryngeal paralysis. Here cricothyroid approximation is done by passing few 2-0 Prolene sutures over silastic shims or titanium miniplates. The results are more unpredictable as compared to type 3 thyroplasty. The operation also results in a prominent Adam's apple and some patients require achondroplasty for the same.

REFERENCES

1. Isshiki N, Okamura H, Ishikawa T. Thyroplasty type 1 (lateral compression) for dysphonia due to vocal cord paralysis or atrophy. Acta Otolaryngol. 1975;80(5-6):465-73.
2. Payr E. Plastik am Schildknorpelzur Behebungder Folgeneinsteiger Stimmbandlahmung. Dtsch Med Wochenschr. 1915;41:1264-70.
3. Koufman JA. Laryngoplasty for vocal cord medialization: an alternative to Teflon. Laryngoscope. 1986;96(7):726-31.
4. McCulloch TM, Hoffman HT. Medialization laryngoplasty with expanded polytetrafluoroethylene. Surgical technique and preliminary results. Ann Otol Rhinol Laryngol. 1998;107(5 Pt 1):427-32.
5. Harries M, Morrison M. Phonosurgery and microlaryngeal surgery. In: Bleach N, Milford C, Van Hasselt A (Eds). Operative Otorhinolaryngology. Oxford, UK: Blackwell Science; 1997. pp. 315-25.
6. Mahieu HF. Correction of dysphonia using laryngeal framework surgical techniques. Indian J Otorhinolaryngol Head Neck Surg. 1997;49(3):247-57.
7. Isshiki N, Taira T, Tanabe M. Surgical correction of the vocal pitch. J Otolaryngol. 1983;12(5):335-40.
8. Zeitels SM, Hochman I, Hillman RE. Adduction arytenopexy: a new procedure for paralytic dysphonia with implications for implant medialization. Ann Otol Rhinol Laryngol Suppl. 1998;173:2-24.
9. Dursun G, Boynukalin S, Ozgursoy OB, et al. Long-term results of different treatment modalities for glottic insufficiency. Am J Otolaryngol. 2008;29(1):7-12.

Pediatric Voice Disorders

KK Handa, M Haq

INTRODUCTION

Voice disorders in children are common although overlooked at times. A normal child's voice should be pleasing in quality and have an appropriate balance of oral and nasal resonance, intensity and fundamental frequency level. Disorder of voice must be distinguished from disorder of speech, articulation, and language, in which usually laryngeal function is normal. Voice disorder may be due to organic abnormality or may be functional disorder. However, even when voice disorder is due to primarily from organic reason, there is often a psychological overlay.[1]

Childhood hoarseness is not an uncommon entity. Although, it is an underdiagnosed entity, its prevalence may be as high as 23.4% in school going children with boys affected more than girls.[2] The causes may be benign vocal cord lesions, infections, inflammations, congenital, neurological, or traumatic. Voice problems in children may impair quality-of-life. Children with vocal nodules, vocal fold paralysis and paradoxical vocal cord movements had a statistically significant pediatric voice-related quality-of-life impairment as compared to their age-matched normal counterparts as per study conducted in 2008 by Merati et al.[3]

PEDIATRIC LARYNX

Pediatric larynx is different from adult larynx. To effectively manage childhood disorders, it is important to consider the difference between the two and transition from pediatric to adult larynx during adolescence.[4]

In pediatric age group:
- Larynx is relatively smaller

- Higher up in position cricoid at level of fourth cervical vertebra as compared with sixth cervical vertebra in an adult
- Epiglottis is more tightly curled shape. Mucosa of the subglottis is more reactive and prone to edema.

Epidemiology

Prevalence of voice disorder in child is 6–9% and mostly reported in 5–18-year-old children.[3] The range of voice problems varies from those child performers with normal conversational voice but concern about loss in upper range of their singing voice to those with severe laryngeal pathology and no voice at all.

There are enough literature that shows impact of voice disorder in children both in terms of child's perception of themselves and how they are perceived by others.[4]

Development of Larynx

It is important to understand changes that take place in the human larynx during development to understand the disease and start correct management. Some disorder may be congenital and related to embryological development of larynx, e.g. glottic web resulting from incomplete recanalization of embryonic larynx at approximately 10 week of gestation.[5]

Length of Vocal Cord

According to Hirano, up to 10 years of age length of vocal fold is about 6–8 mm in both gender but at puberty, marked growth occur in vocal fold length in both gender but more marked in male as compared to female. Membranous fold increases up to 15–18 mm in male which is more than double increment and in female increase up to 8.5–9 mm an increasing in length of third. Cartilaginous portion also grows but less as compared to membranous fold so ratio between membranous to cartilaginous fold which is 1.5:1 in new born became 5.5:1 in adult male, and 4:1 in adult female.

Hirano also gave the concept of anterior glottis as phonatory glottis and wider posterior portion as respiratory glottis. This concept can be useful in planning phonosurgery like arytenoidectomy to increase airway passage with minimal impact on the voice outcome.[6]

Change in Vocal Fold Laminar Structure

The knowledge of the layered structure of vocal cord is important to understand disease and phonosurgery. Adult vocal fold has five layers which are not differentiated at birth but rather to start during first few months of life and continued throughout childhood and adult form attained at puberty.[7] This is the reason why phonosurgery is more challenging in younger children.

Change in Pitch

Pitch is an important feature in pediatric voice which drops throughout infancy and childhood in both male and female with mark change occur at puberty particularly in males. The change in pitch occurs due to anterior growth of thyroid cartilage in response to testosterone. The drop in pitch is approximately proportional to the growth of membranous vocal fold.

Assessment

A systematic approach is required to evaluate the child with voice disorder. Child may need to be evaluated by specialist from other specialties including pediatrician, pulmonologist, psychologist apart from laryngologist, and voice therapist.

Vocal abuse plays a major role causing hoarseness in pediatric age group. It is more commonly observed in boys, in view of more aggressive nature as compared to girls.

The various causes of hoarseness in children are:
- Benign vocal cord lesions like vocal nodule, polyp
- Vocal cord cysts, sulcus vocalis
- Juvenile laryngeal papillomatosis
- Vocal fold paresis
- Laryngopharyngeal reflux
- Acute or chronic laryngitis
- Foreign body inhalation
- Malignant lesions of larynx

- Systemic illness like hypothyroidism
- Postsurgery (Iatrogenic).

History

History including birth history, growth and development, medical, speech and language history should be taken followed by detailed voice history to distinguish whether child has voice disorder rather than problem with speech, articulation or language; where possible information should be taken from both child and parents. History of endotracheal intubation may suggest laryngeal stenosis, cricoarytenoid joint dislocation, fibrosis, intubation granuloma or vocal cord cyst formation.

An intermittent dysphonia is less likely due to discrete vocal cord lesion. It is common that later onset intermittent symptoms may be due to an upper respiratory tract infection with associated laryngitis with persistence of symptoms exacerbated by voice misuse.

Stridor and reduced exercise intolerance suggest an obstructive pathology such as laryngeal stenosis or papillomas.

In case of vocal fold paralysis, there may be history of swallowing problem, persistent cough, corticosteroid inhaler used to treat asthma or throat clearing habit may be the reason for vocal fold trauma and voice disorder.[8] Some disease like hearing problem indirectly can affect voice indirectly. It may encourage child to shout leading to voice misuse-related symptoms.

Examination

Basic ear, nose, and throat (ENT) examination should be performed. Voice should be assessed thoroughly. Combination of subjective and objective voice analysis measure can be used to assess voice (For detailed description kindly refer to Chapter 2, Voice Evaluation). Videostroboscopy is an established method of assessing the fine vibratory-edge of the vocal cords (Fig. 1).

SPECIFIC DISORDERS

Vocal Nodules

Vocal nodule is the most common cause of dysphonia in children and it is regarded as organic manifestation of laryngeal hyperfunction.[9] Other conditions that can lead to predisposition to vocal nodules include gastroesophageal reflux and velopharyngeal insufficiency.[10] Nodules are more common in boys and most often seen when a child enters group activity. On stroboscopic examination, there is

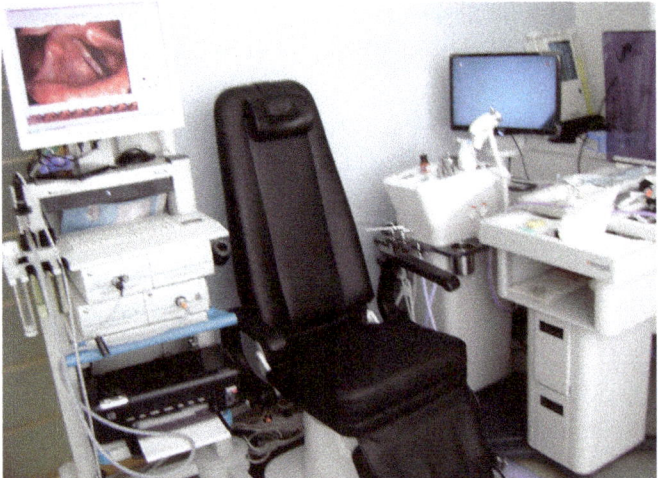

Fig. 1 Videostroboscopic unit for examination of the vocal cords. Even in children whenever possible an attempt should be made to examine the vocal folds

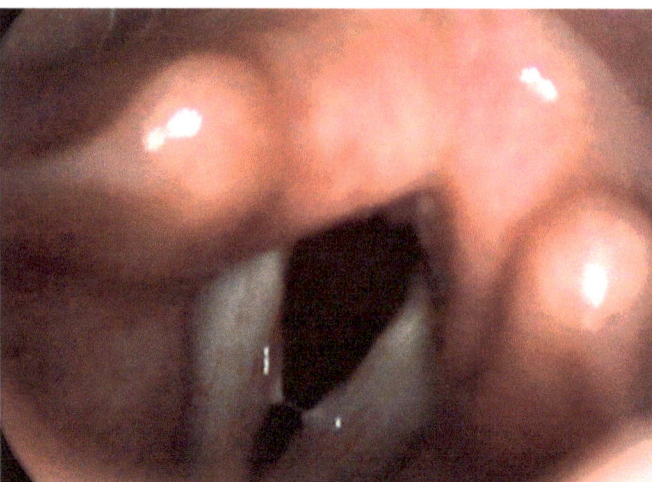

Fig. 2 Bilateral vocal cord nodules

decreased mucosal wave and incomplete approximation of the free edges of vocal cord.[11]

Mostly vocal nodules are usually bilateral (Fig. 2), but unilateral nodule can occur. Vocal nodule arises due to the mechanical trauma, injury and with secondary hyalinization at the free edge of vocal cords.

There are three stages of development of vocal nodules.[12]

1. First stage is an inflammatory phase with increase vascularity and protein accumulation.
2. In the second stage, there is localized swelling on the edge of vocal fold that appear as grayish translucent thickening. Vocal nodules are reversible within 24–48 hours if underlying trauma is eliminated.
3. In the last stage, there is replacement of thickening by fibrotic tissue that appears gray or white.

Voice therapy is the mainstay of treatment. Here main emphasis is on the reduction of vocal strain. Various techniques can be employed to reduce shouting, coughing, and throat clearing.

The fact based on clinical experience that vocal nodules in children often resolve spontaneously by puberty can also influence management.[1]

According to Von-Laden, most nodules resolve or show significant improvement within 3–6 months of initiation of voice therapy.[11] Surgery is rarely recommended in those children who fail to show improvement with voice therapy and severe hoarseness interferes with the daily activity.

Bouchayer and Cornut found cyst, sulci, and polyps at microlaryngoscopy in children with prior diagnosed vocal nodule and not responding to voice therapy.[13]

Surgery is only reserved for a small number of cases who do not respond to speech therapy and have fibrotic

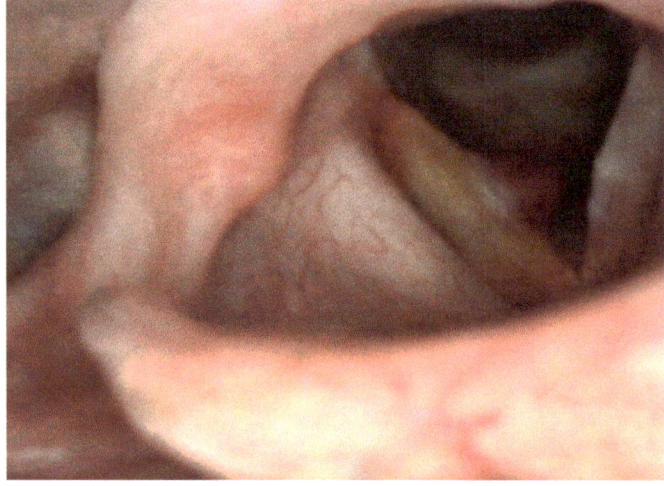

Fig. 3 Telangiectasia polyp right vocal cord

nodules. Bilateral nodules can be removed in same sitting; however, some surgeons prefer to remove bilateral nodules in two sittings that are at least 4 weeks apart.[14] Voice rest is recommended for 7–10 days. Recurrence is frequent without voice therapy and vocal hygiene. The patient must be counseled to alter his vocal behavior.

Vocal Polyp

Mostly vocal polyps developed after chronic abuse of larynx but can often develop after single episode of trauma (Fig. 3).

Polyps may be pedunculated, fusiform, or generalized.[15]

Surgical removal is the mainstay of treatment. Pedunculated polyps are removed from the base using CO_2

laser or cold instrumentation,[16] e.g. laryngeal microscissors. In case of large polyp with wide base fibrous exudates are suctioned out or vaporized after giving incision over superior surface of vocal fold.[15] Postoperative voice quality depends upon the degree of irreversible damage to superficial layer of lamina propria. Voice therapy is advised before and after surgery to prevent recurrence.[17]

Functional Dysphonia

When no anatomical or organic cause is found, dysphonia can be labeled as functional voice disorder. Child may have dysphonia or even aphonia secondary to psychological factors. The underlying psychological problems may be related to or part of tension symptoms, adjustment, anxiety, problems at school or with siblings or personality disorder.[18] In these children, voice therapy may be helpful in combination with psychological assessment.

Puberphonia

This is the condition when prepubertal voice presents in adolescence or adulthood. High pitch, hoarseness, and voice breaks are the characteristics symptoms. This can be associated with psychological disturbance or endocrinopathy.[5] Voice therapy along with counseling by the psychologist is the mainstay of management. Majority of the cases respond very well to voice therapy. Type 3 thyroplasty is an option in a small percentage of cases who do not respond to voice therapy. Here a vertical incision is given on the thyroid ala 5 mm from midline on each side and this segment is mobilized. This has the effect of reducing the pitch. This surgery has dramatic results and change in voice can be demonstrated on the table.

Laryngeal Papillomatosis

Laryngeal papillomatosis (recurrent respiratory papillomatosis) patient can present either with hoarseness or airway obstruction which can be fatal, so diagnosis should be as early as possible. Tracheostomy is needed in about 14–21% of cases of recurrent respiratory papillomatosis.[19] However, any attempt should be made to avoid tracheostomy to avoid stromal recurrence which happens because of loss of protective mucosal blanket (Fig. 4).

Commonly affected site in larynx are midzone of laryngeal surface of epiglottis, upper and lower margin of ventricles, and under surface of vocal fold.[20] Recurrent respiratory papillomatosis is caused by human papillomavirus (HPV) 6 and 11.[21] Transmission is maternofetal and thought to be related to passage through the birth canal but cases have been found in child born by cesarean section suggesting a more complex route of transmission *in utero* (Fig. 5).[22]

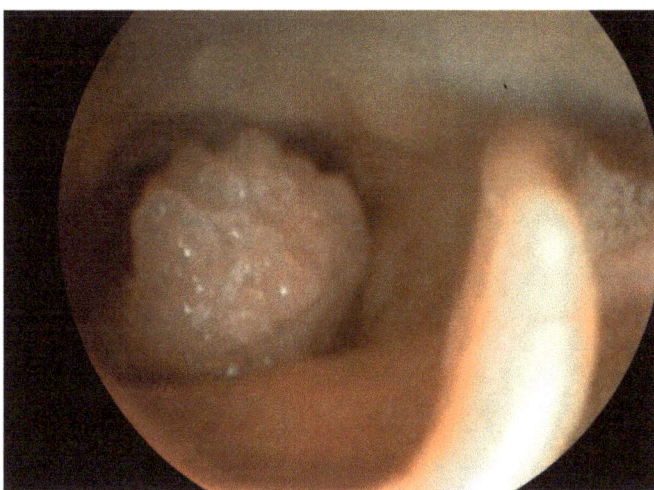

Fig. 4 Endoscopic view of recurrent respiratory papillomas arising from supraglottis

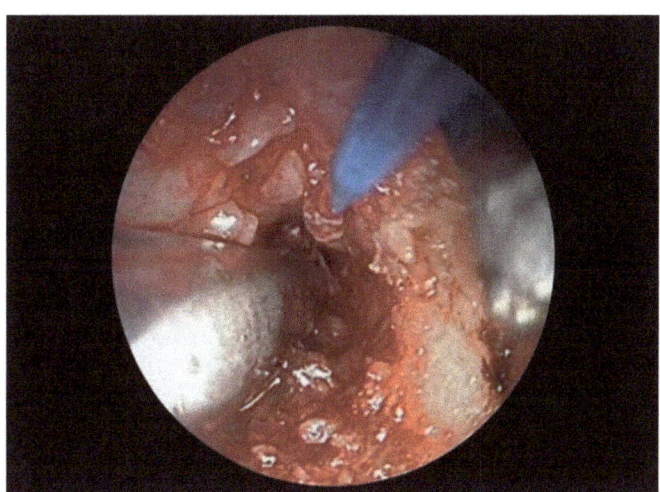

Fig. 5 Case of extensive recurrent respiratory papillomatosis. Fiber laser being used for tracheal papillomas

Surgery is the treatment of choice. Surgery may be needed multiple times because recurrence is the natural history of recurrent respiratory papillomatosis. Aim of surgery is to establish stable airway and serviceable voice. Surgery can be done either by CO_2 laser, microlaryngoscopy with forceps removal or by microdebrider technique. Microdebrider can be used for debulking while laser is used for removing lesions in close proximity to vocal folds.[23] During surgery, attention should be given not to damage deeper muscle and ligament. More precaution should be taken in removing papilloma from anterior and posterior commissure area because irreversible scaring can occur.

Adjuvant medical treatment has been tried with some success.

Leventhal and other recommended the use of interferon in any patient requiring surgery every 2–3 month.[24] Therapy should be given for 6 months. There is high chance of rebound effect and papilloma recurrence at an increased rate on cessation of therapy.[25]

There are several study showing good response with intralesional cidofovir injection but there has been recent concern raised regarding possible carcinogenic effect observed *in vitro* studies.[26] Other therapies including acyclovir, ribavirin, isotretinoin, indole-3-carbnol, and photodynamic are infrequently used.

Laryngeal Web

Actual incidence of laryngeal web is debatable. According to Smith and Caitlyn, glottic web and atresia account for 5% of congenital anomalies.[27]

On the basis of severity, it can be classified as:[28]

- *Type I*: Anterior web involving 35% or less of the glottis with little or no subglottic extension. Voice dysfunction without airway obstruction may be the only complaint.
- *Type II*: Anterior web involving up to 50% of glottis, true vocal cord visible within web, subglottic involvement is minimal. Voice disorder is common presenting symptom but at the time of upper respiratory tract infection patient can complaint of respiratory difficulty.
- *Type III*: Glottic web involves up to 75% of glottis. Anterior portion of web is thick and extend into subglottic. Patient present with symptom of both dysphonia and airway obstruction which may be moderate to severe in nature.
- *Type IV*: Involve up to 90% of glottis and web is uniformly thickened and extends into subglottic area. Infant may have dysphonia and severe airway compromise.

Management depends upon thickness of web. In case of thin web, web can be divided endoscopically either with a knife or CO_2 laser with temporary placement of keel to prevent adhesions. Open approach is better if web is thick. Web is reached through midline thyrotomy and excess tissues are removed with placement of mucosal graft which is fixed with fibrin glue and stenting[29] may also be done.

Vocal Cord Granuloma

Vocal fold granulomas commonly affect voice. Most of the time granuloma occurs after intubation trauma. Other causes may be habit of throat clearing, excessive glottal attack and reflux esophagitis.[30] Laryngopharyngeal reflux is a common cause of granuloma. Child should be evaluated for laryngopharyngeal reflux and gastroesophageal reflux disease.

Management of underlying laryngopharyngeal reflux is the primary management of vocal fold granuloma. Most granulomas resolve with medical management and lifestyle modifications. Granuloma causing airway obstruction may need surgical removal. Recurrence is frequent regardless of surgical technique.

Posterior Glottic Stenosis and Cricoarytenoid Joint Fixation

Most common cause of posterior glottic stenosis is airway trauma from intubation, but can be congenital also. Posterior glottic stenosis in pediatric population is classified into four types by Irring and associate.[31]

1. *Type I*: Vocal process adhesion.
2. *Type II*: Posterior commissure or interarytenoid scar.
3. *Type III*: Congenital or acquired unilateral cricoarytenoid fixation with or without interarytenoid scar.
4. *Type IV*: Congenital or acquired bilateral cricoarytenoid fixation with or without interarytenoid scar.

Both abduction and adduction are affected in case of cricoarytenoid joint fixation while in case of interarytenoid scar mainly abduction is affected that is why in case of interarytenoid scaring child may have normal voice, but in case of cricoarytenoid joint fixation patient have dysphonia.[32]

Palpation of cricoarytenoid joint at rigid endoscopy is necessary to distinguish from vocal fold paralysis. In case of doubt, a laryngeal electromyography (EMG) may differentiate vocal cord paralysis from cricoarytenoid fixation.

Benjamin and Mair[32] recommended that wait and watch policy for interarytenoid web unless any obstructive symptoms exits in which case tracheotomy may be needed. Arytenoidectomy should be avoided to prevent aspiration and voice deterioration. If necessary, anterior and posterior cricoidotomy with posterior graft is considered the procedure of choice.[33]

Vocal Fold Paralysis

Vocal fold paralysis represents 10% of all congenital anomalies of larynx.[34] Birth trauma or congenital anomalies of central nervous system, heart, and great vessels can cause vocal fold paralysis. Acquired right side and unilateral paralysis has better prognosis for spontaneous recovery.[35,36] In more than 50% children paralysis is bilateral.[37,38] Electromyography of larynx is most sensitive and specific test to diagnosed vocal fold paralysis and also differentiate it from cricoarytenoid joint fixation.

In unilateral paralysis voice is hoarse, weak, and breathy, and rarely required airway intervention. Surgical intervention should be considered after 10–12 months, if spontaneous recovery not occurs.

Unilateral vocal fold paralysis, usually improves over 6–12 months by contralateral vocal fold compensation.

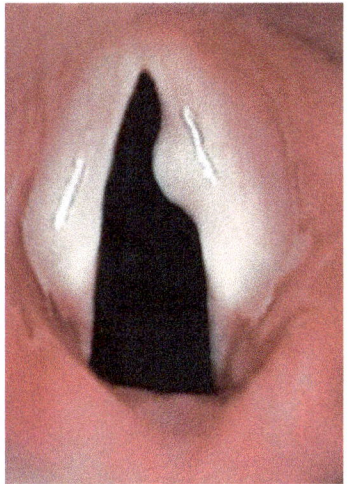

Fig. 6 Vocal cord cyst

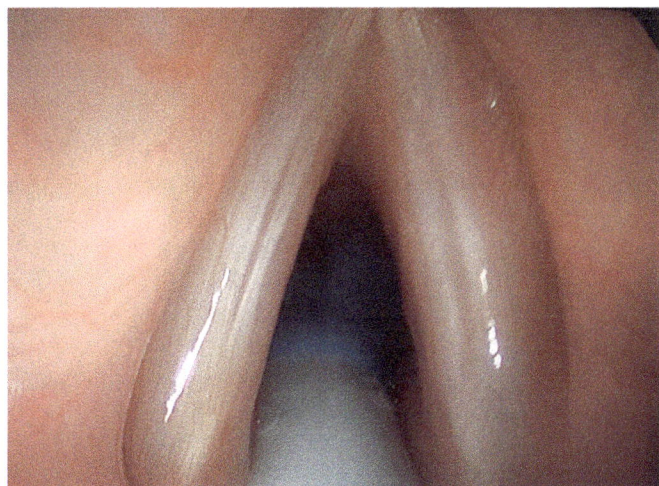

Fig. 7 Bilateral sulcus vocalis

Voice therapy helps in early recovery. Surgical intervention required in few patients where dysphonia or aspiration persists. Surgical option includes vocal fold injection, surgical medialization or reinnervation. Voice therapy is must in both preoperative and postoperative period in case surgery is done.

In bilateral paralysis, voice is usually not affected significantly. It is the airway that causes symptoms, and requires treatment. Approximately 50% of the children required tracheostomy.

Surgical principle in case of bilateral vocal fold paralysis is to increase space in the posterior glottis to improve the airway while preserving anterior glottic closure to maintain voice.

Surgical options include:
- Cordotomy
- Lateralization procedure
- Arytenoidectomy (through posterolateral external approach)
- Endoscopic arytenoidectomy
- Reinnervation of posterior cricoarytenoid muscle with nerve muscle flap can also be done but is not universally successful.

Vocal Fold Cyst

They are either mucosal retention cysts or epidermoid cysts. It is still not clear if vocal fold cysts are congenital or acquired.[39,40] Epidermoid cysts are lined with stratified keratinized squamous epithelium and contain keratin debris. Hoarseness, voice break, and vocal fatigue are symptoms of vocal fold cyst (Fig. 6).

Surgical intervention is the primary management of vocal fold cyst. In cyst management mucosal incision is given parallel to free-edge on superior surface of vocal fold and cyst is dissected. Woo and colleagues[41] reported improved result using 6–0 chromic ENDOKNOT® suture to close microflaps of the vocal fold. Postoperative voice therapy is important and recommended for at least 3–6 months.

Sulcus Vocalis

The word sulcus means a furrow or cleft. In sulcus vocalis, surface epithelium invaginates into Reinke's space and adheres to vocal ligament resulting in longitudinal furrow parallel to the edge of vocal fold and glottic chink. Some authors consider sulcus vocalis as acquired disorder and others as congenital.[39] Sulcus vocalis is often missed or underdiagnosed (Fig. 7).

Sulcus vocalis causes hoarseness of voice on effortful talking.

Treatment option included surgery and speech therapy. Results of surgery are not dramatic. The surgical technique consists of giving mucosal incision on the superior edge of the sulcus, and the sulcus is dissected from vocal ligament. Then autologous fat harvested from the outer abdominal wall is either implanted or injected in the cord. This is an attempt to separate the epithelium and the vocal ligament and obliterate the sulcus.

REFERENCES

1. Toohill RJ. The psychosomatic aspects of children with vocal nodules. Arch Otolaryngol Head Neck Surg. 1975;101:591-5.
2. Silverman EM. Incidence of chronic hoarseness among school-age children. J Speech Hear Disord. 1975;40(2):211-5.
3. Merati AL, Keppel K, Braun NM, et al. Pediatric voice related quality of life: findings in healthy children and in common laryngeal disorders. Ann Otol Rhinol Laryngol. 2008;117(4):259-62.

4. Dalal PG, Marray D, Messner AH, et al. Pediatric laryngeal dimensions: an age based analysis. Anesth Analg. 2009;108: 1475-9.

5. Wilson DK. Management of voice disorders in children and adolescents. Semin Speech Lang. 1983;4:245.

6. Hirano M, Kurita S, Nakashima T. Growth, development and aging of the human vocal folds. In: Bless DM, Abbs JH (Eds). Vocal fold physiology: contemporary research and clinical issues. San Diego (CA): College Hill Press; 1983. pp. 22-43.

7. Hirano M, Kurita S, Kiyokawa K. Posterior glottis. Morphological study in excised human larynges. Ann Otol Rhinol Laryngol. 1986;95:576-81.

8. Roland NJ, Bhalla RK, Earis J. The local side effects of corticosteroids. Chest. 2004;126(1):213-9.

9. Koufman JA, Blalock PD. Functional voice disorders. Otolaryngol Clin North Am. 1991;24:1059-73.

10. Gray SD, Smith ME, Schneider H. Voice disorders in children. Pediatr Clin North Am. 1996;43:1357.

11. Von Leden HV. Vocal nodules in children. Ear Nose Throat J. 1985;64:473.

12. Vaughan CW. Current concepts in otolaryngology: diagnosis and treatment of organic voice disorders. N Engl J Med. 1982;307:863.

13. Campisi P, Tewfik TL, Manoukian JJ, et al. Computer-assisted voice analysis: establishing a pediatric database. Arch Otolaryngol Head Neck Surg. 2002;128:156-60.

14. Benjamin B, Croxson G. Vocal nodules in children. Ann Otol Rhinol Laryngol. 1987;96:530.

15. Kleinsasser O. Pathogenesis of vocal cord polyps. Ann Otol Rhinol Laryngol. 1982;91:378.

16. Bouchayer M, Cornut G. Microsurgical treatment of benign vocal fold lesions: indications, technique, results. Folia Phoniatr (Basel). 1992;44:155.

17. Wilson DK. Voice problems of children, 3rd edition. Baltimore: Williams & Wilkins; 1987.

18. Morrison MD, Nichol H, Rammage LA. Diagnostic criteria in functional dysphonia. Laryngoscope. 1986;94:1-8.

19. Cole RR, Myer CM, Cotton RT. Tracheotomy in children with recurrent respiratory papillomatosis. Head Neck. 1989;11:226.

20. Kashima HK, Mounts P, Leventhal B, et al. Sites of predilection in recurrent respiratory papillomatosis. Ann Otol Rhinol Laryngol. 1993;102:580-3.

21. Abramson AL, Steinbert BM, Winkler B. Laryngeal papillomatosis: clinical, histopathologic and molecular studies. Laryngoscope. 1987;97:678.

22. Kosko JR, Derkay CS. Role of cesarean section in prevention of recurrent respiratory papillomatosis—is there one? Int J Pediatr Otorhinolaryngol. 1996;35(1):31-8.

23. El-Bitar MA, Zalzal GH. Powered instrumentation in the treatment of recurrent respiratory papillomatosis: an alternative to the carbon dioxide laser. Arch Otolaryngol Head Neck Surg. 2002;128:425-8.

24. Leventhal B, Kashima HK, Mounts P. Long-term response of recurrent respiratory papillomatosis to treatment of lymphoblastoid interferon alpha-N1. N Engl J Med. 1991;325:613.

25. Healy GB, Gelber RD, Trowbridge AL, et al. Treatment of recurrent respiratory papillomatosis with human leukocyte interferon: results of a multicenter randomized clinical trial. N Engl J Med. 1988;319:401.

26. Donne AJ, Hampson L, He XT, et al. Potential risk factors associated with the use of cidofovir to treat benign human papillomavirus-related disease. Antivir Ther. 2009;14(7):939-52.

27. Smith RJ, Caitlin FI. Congenital anomalies of the larynx. Am J Dis Child. 1984;138:35.

28. Cohen SR. Congenital glottic webs in children: a retrospective review of 51 patients. Ann Otol Rhinol Laryngol. 1985;14:2-16.

29. Isshiki N, Taira T, Nose K, et al. Surgical treatment of laryngeal web with mucosa graft. Ann Otol Rhinol Laryngol. 1991;100:95.

30. Ward PH, Zwitman D, Hanson D, et al. Contact ulcers and granulomas of the larynx: new insights into their etiology as a basis for more rational treatment. Otolaryngol Head Neck Surg. 1980;88:262.

31. Irving RM, Bailey CM, Evans JN. Posterior glottic stenosis in children. Int J Pediatr Otorhinolaryngol. 1993;28:11.

32. Benjamin B, Mair EA. Congenital interarytenoid web. Arch Otolaryngol Head Neck Surg. 1991;117:1118-22.

33. Zalzal GH. Posterior glottic fixation in children. Ann Otol Rhinol Laryngol. 1993;102:680.

34. Holinger PH, Brown WT. Congenital webs, cysts, laryngoceles and other anomalies of the larynx. Ann Otol Rhinol Laryngol. 1967;76:744.

35. Dedo DD. Pediatric vocal cord paralysis. Laryngoscope. 1979;89:1378.

36. Dedo DD, Dedo HH. Neurogenic diseases of the larynx. In: Bluestone CD, Stool SE, Scheetz MD (Eds). Pediatric Otolaryngology, 2nd edition. Philadelphia: WB Saunders; 1990.

37. Holinger LD, Holinger PC, Holinger PH. Etiology of bilateral abductor vocal cord paralysis: a review of 389 cases. Ann Otol Rhinol Laryngol. 1976;85:428.

38. Cohen SR, Geller KA, Birns JW, et al. Laryngeal paralysis in children: a long-term retrospective study. Ann Otol Rhinol Laryngol. 1982;91:417.

39. Ishii H, Baba T, Kawabata J. Clinical observations on the sulcus vocalis. J Otolaryngol (Japan). 1967;70:911.

40. Itoh T, Kawasaki H, Morikawa I, et al. Vocal fold furrows: a 10 year review of 240 patients. Auris Nasus Larynx. 1983;10:S17.

41. Woo P, Casper J, Griffin B, et al. Endoscopic microsuture repair of vocal fold defects. J Voice. 1995;9:332.

13

Office-based Laryngeal Procedures

KK Handa

INTRODUCTION

Office-based laryngeal procedures mean doing laryngeal procedures under local anesthesia in the outpatient setting and mostly in an upright position. The switchover from the secure operative room settings to the outpatient settings have been propelled by improved technology in the form of distal chip fiberoptic endoscopic cameras and the fiber lasers. The concept of office-based procedures is not new and even in 19th century such procedures were performed in the surgeon's office or outpatient suite under local anesthesia. However, with advent of general anesthesia, microscope, endotracheal intubation, jet ventilation, and lasers the focus shifted to doing these procedures under general anesthesia. However, in recent times with improvement in technology and development of chip tip endoscopes, high-speed imaging, transnasal esophagoscopy (TNE) with thin caliber esophagoscopes, fiber lasers, and more and better injection materials the focus has again shifted to the office. These procedures have the advantage of not only cutting down the cost but also avoiding general anesthesia and hospital stay. These procedures are very useful in patients who are not fit for general anesthesia for various reasons. Most important in laryngology, the patient can phonate during the procedure and his voice can be tested and monitored during surgery. Many laryngologists have revived the old tradition of doing these interventions in office. However, for lesions like polyps, nodules, varices cysts, etc. where precise removal is required still removal under general anesthesia is preferred and the advantage of microscopic magnification, operating in a still field and ability to use both hands can never be replaced.

ANESTHESIA AND PATIENT SELECTION FOR OFFICE PROCEDURES

Correct patient selection and appropriate anesthesia is very important for success of these office-based procedures.[1] Patient needs to be informed about the procedure and also involved during the procedure including monitor visualization. In fact, for more specialized procedures including injections, laser initially ideal patients who are not apprehensive, have no gag, have good pain tolerance, and are able to stay quiet should be taken. As the clinicians learning curve gets better than more complex patients can be taken.

Some criteria helpful in patient selection are:

- Roomy nasal cavity with patent airway is desirable. Slight more space is required for transnasal esophagoscope
- Excessive gag should not be there on routine flexible laryngoscopy
- A very fidgety patient who continuously moves, has posture problems or has excessive tremor is a very difficult candidate for office-based procedures
- Care needs to be exercised in patients who are on anticoagulants or blood thinners
- Nervous patients with anxiety disorders are better avoided. However, during the procedure intravenous (IV) alprazolam is helpful in some patients.

Most of the procedures are adequately managed with topical anesthesia. In some patients, superior laryngeal block is given by blocking the superior laryngeal nerve where it enters the thyrohyoid membrane. External landmark is about 1 cm below and medial to greater horn of hyoid bone. About 3 mL of 2% Xylocaine is injected. A pop is felt as the thyrohyoid membrane is breeched. Bilateral superior laryngeal block can be given (Figs 1 and 2).

Topical anesthesia for larynx and trachea may involve:

- Xylocaine 10% spray to nose and oral cavity along with decongestion of the nose with oxymetazoline
- Xylocaine 4% drip on tongue base and larynx either through Abraham cannula or through the side channel of the fiberoptic laryngoscope. For this, patient should be in a sniffing position to maximize laryngeal exposure. 2–4 cc of the solution is sprayed onto the vocal folds producing the laryngeal gargle.[2] If there is no laryngeal gargle it means that patient has swallowed the anesthetic and more dose is required.[1]
- For transtracheal anesthesia about 2 cc of 2% Xylocaine solution is injected through the cricothyroid membrane. The 4% Xylocaine can also be given via a nebulizer or a

special catheter placed through the working channel of the laryngoscope. This allows anesthetic to be given in a more controlled manner. The anesthesia achieved allows 20–25-minute procedure comfortably. If procedures are longer then anesthesia may have to be repeated.

- For transnasal esophagoscopy only topical nasal anesthesia along with spraying of oropharynx is required.
- Normally doing office-based procedures under local anesthesia is safe and drug reactions are rare. The 4% Xylocaine can be given to a maximum dose of 7–8 cc, i.e. 300 mg in 70 kg patient. Allergic reactions consisting of rash and urticaria often occur. Very rarely methemoglobinemia can occur. Excessive dose can cause cardiac and neurological side effects. Sometimes a vasovagal syncope occurs which is normally self-limiting and management consists of putting the patient in a reclining position and monitoring vitals. Post office-based procedures patient is instructed not to eat anything for 1 hour to reduce chances of aspiration.

AIRWAY EVALUATION

Flexible awake endoscopy of laryngotracheal tree has many advantages over rigid assessment.[3] It allows dynamic and static obstruction to be assessed. Carretta et al.[4] found the difference between clinical and operative endoscopy. Computed tomography (CT) scan was not useful in assessing the length of stenosis, however, it was useful in assessing stenosis distal to a tight stenosis.[4]

Office-based fiberoptic endoscopy is useful in studying the whole airway till the carina including the vocal cord movements which cannot be assessed in an anesthetized patient. It is also helpful in assessing bilateral cord mobility including posterior glottis stenosis. The 4% Xylocaine is instilled through the tracheostomy tube and patient is asked to cough so that the anesthetic is spread. Then the tracheostomy tube is removed and the scope is passed assessing the glottis, subglottis, and trachea and past the stoma. Retrograde scopy is done through the stoma to visualize the subglottis, posterior commissure, and inferior aspect of the vocal cords. It is important to diagnose and differentiate the type of posterior glottis stenosis.[5]

Cricoarytenoid Fixation

Distinguishing cricoarytenoid fixity from neurological impairment is always a challenge. "Jostle sign" where mobile but neurologically denervated arytenoid will move on adduction from the other side while in case of cricoarytenoid fixation there will not be any movement.[6] The common causes of cricoarytenoid fixation are during intubation or due to prolonged intubation and rheumatoid arthritis. Cricoarytenoid fixation can also be assessed during awake

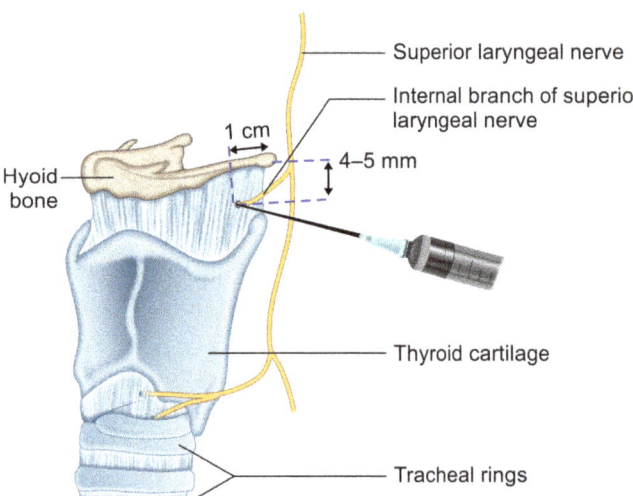

Fig. 1 Superior laryngeal nerve block lateral view

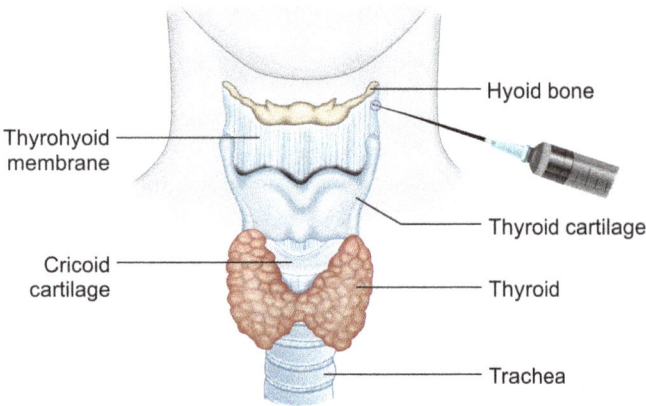

Fig. 2 Superior laryngeal block anterior view

fiberoptic laryngoscopy by visualizing the larynx with 90° telescopy and trying to test mobility of the cricoarytenoid joint with a curved forceps.

Paradoxical Vocal Cord Movement Disorder
This is a challenging condition faced by laryngologist and voice therapist. The synonym is vocal cord dysfunction. In this condition, there is untimely and excessive adduction of vocal cords during inspiration and expiration leading to breathlessness. The cause is still not known. Flexible laryngoscopy is the initial way to assess these disorders. One way to diagnose is to let the patient climb up and go down stairs till he is short of breath. Then a laryngoscopy is performed and cord movement during inspiration is assessed. An alternative is to make the patient count in one breath without stopping till patient experiences some breathlessness and then assessment is done. Exercise laryngoscopy can be performed in athletes who are being assessed for this disorder. Vocal cord dysfunction is best managed by voice therapist who is experienced in this area.[7,8] Correct diagnosis of this disorder apart from management helps in reassuring the patient and family about the nature of the disorder.

Laryngotracheal Stenosis

Diagnosis

Laryngotracheal stenosis after prolonged intubation and tracheostomy accounts for a large number of patients. The incidence ranges from 0.9% to 8.3%.[9,10] Narrowing of airway may remain asymptomatic for some time. It is only when 30% of lumen is involved that the patient becomes symptomatic.[11]

Endoscopic assessment is very important for these patients for assessment of the site, length, and type of obstruction. The main indication of office-based surgery in case of airway is stenosis treatment. The most common cause of stenosis is idiopathic subglottic stenosis, followed by acquired airway stenosis, glottic webs, and supraglottis stenosis.

Preoperative Counseling

This procedure should be avoided in anxious patients where general anesthesia or IV sedation should be preferred. Patient should be explained all the steps before the procedure and even during the procedure communication should be maintained. There should be monitoring during the procedure. These procedures can induce hemodynamic changes and also exacerbate airway diseases like asthma. Care must be taken while doing these procedures in patients with cardiopulmonary disease and risks weighed against risks of IV sedation or general anesthesia (Fig. 3).

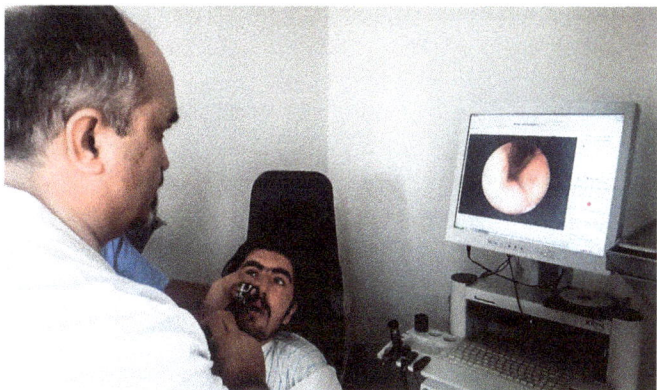

Fig. 3 Diagnostic office-based procedure with visualization on the monitor

Procedure

The requirements for the procedure are adequate anesthesia, correct and good quality endoscopes, and assistant to help during the procedure. Preferred scopes are ultrathin distal chip scopes with chip-tip camera. The anesthesia with 4% Xylocaine can be given with a nebulizer and then 10% Xylocaine local spray is also done. The tip of the scope is lubricated with Xylocaine viscous. An extra 2 mL of 2% Xylocaine is given by the working channel of the scope into trachea and another 1 mL is sprayed onto the vocal folds as the patient performs the laryngeal gargle by saying a prolonged vowel during administration of an anesthetic. If longer duration anesthesia is required, then bilateral superior laryngeal nerve block can also be given. The total amount of Xylocaine cannot exceed more than 5 mg/kg.

Diagnostic procedure: The most common procedure is diagnostic evaluation of the airway beyond the vocal cords.[12] Here additional anesthesia delivered by techniques as described above is given if longer procedure is required. If only a short visualization is required, then the scope is passed beyond the cords when cords are abducted without any extra anesthesia.

Balloon Tracheoplasty

This procedure is commonly done for dilatation of the grade 1 or grade 2 tracheal stenosis and is showing a lot of promise.[13]

The laryngoscope is passed through the larynx into trachea. The stenosis is assessed and a guidewire is passed through the working channel of the scope and past the stenosis. The endoscope is removed while the guidewire is kept distal to the stenosis. The endoscope is again placed side-by-side to the guidewire. Once tip of guidewire is visualized balloon is passed over the guidewire. The guidewire is withdrawn as the balloon is advanced. The center of the balloon is placed at the midpoint of the stenosis. Patient is now explained that procedure is going to take place. He is asked to take a deep breath, exhale, and then hold his breath. The balloon is now inflated with saline or air to correct pressure and kept inflated for 30 seconds. It is deflated and advanced distally so that the patient can breathe. Procedure can be repeated if required. Continuous communication with the patient is very essential for a successful procedure. Postdilatation steroids can also be injected.

Balloon selected should have a diameter about 5 mm greater than the stenosis. A multidiameter hydrostatic radial expansion balloon is used for dilatation.[14] The length used is either 3 mm or 5 mm and required pressure ranges from 3 atm to 8 atm depending on the balloon size.

Office-based Laser Procedures for Airway

Fiber laser can be put through the channel of the fiberoptic laryngoscope and used for treatment of number of conditions like laryngeal webs, papilloma's, or early stenosis. Lasers which can be used are potassium titanyl phosphate (KTP), CO_2 fiber, neodymium-doped yttrium aluminium garnet (Nd:YAG), and pulse dye laser.

It is useful in early subglottic or tracheal stenosis and can be used along with balloon tracheoplasty. Laser fiber is used to make 4 quadrant radial incisions and then balloon dilatation is done.

These are safe procedures and it is only rarely that superficial tears, vaso vagal reaction and bronchospasm can occur.[12] Episodes of bronchospasms occur in less than 1% procedures.[13] Bronchospasm can be prevented by adequate anesthesia and if it occurs, oxygen and nebulization are of help. Airway rupture is a very rare but serious complication.[15]

Postoperative monitoring is required for about 4 hours. Patient is advised nil orally after the procedure for about 5 hours and is observed for tachycardia, cough, breathing problem, bleeding, and pain.

Surprisingly the patient tolerance of these airway office-based procedures is high.[2,16] These procedures give good results,[1] but have little complications. Two series[17,18] establish the utility of office laser (Nd:YAG) to treat laryngotracheal stenosis in spontaneously breathing patients. One of the reasons for the popularity of these procedures is cost saving.[19]

VOCAL CORD INJECTIONS

One of the best and most commonly performed indications for office-based procedures is vocal cord injection in cases of unilateral vocal cord paralysis. These patients have breathiness of voice, weak cough, and aspiration. Similar injections can be done in patients with phonatory gap, presbylaryngis, vocal cord atrophy, sulcus vocalis, and

laryngeal scar. The office-based injection laryngoplasty is very convenient, appealing to the patient, and cheap.

Majority of these procedures are performed for vocal fold augmentation but it can also be used for injecting materials like steroids and acyclovir which is done into superficial layers. The success of the procedure depends on a compliant patient who knows about what is being done and who can phonate, cough and swallow during the procedure. Anxious patients with an excessive gag may not be good candidates. Most of the available materials can be injected by this technique except autologous fat. However, care needs to be exercised in injecting permanent materials as wrong placement of materials into subepithelial layers can increase hoarseness instead of improving voice.[20]

These office-based injections are particularly useful for prompt temporary relief especially after major surgery including esophagectomy, skull base surgery like glomus jugulare resection, carotid endarterectomy and also in patients with end-stage malignancy. At times when the surgeon is not sure about the results a temporary injection can be done to see the likely result.[21] In vocal cord atrophy injections are bilateral. However, scar management is more difficult. Here apart from glottis insufficiency mucosal stiffness is also an issue. In fact, in certain vocal scar cases hoarseness may be made worst by injection. Here trial injection is of immense help.[21] In certain cases, where gap is focal, it may be handled better by direct laryngoscopy.[22]

These injections can be given by either:
- Side channel of fiberoptic scope
- Transoral route
- External approach which is either trans-cricothyroid, trans-thyroid, or trans-thyrohyoid membrane approach.

Visualization has improved with scopes with better optics including distal chip tip technology. Help may also be taken from the patient who can hold his own tongue forward especially for transoral injections.

Anesthesia is the key to a successful injection. Initially, nasal decongestion is done with pledgets of Xylocaine and oxymetazoline. For percutaneous approaches, the overlying skin also needs to be anesthetized. Topical 4% Xylocaine anesthesia is given either by nebulization or spray. Sometimes bilateral superior laryngeal blocks may be required.

Materials commonly used are Restylane (hyaluronic acid), hydroxyapatite, and collagen. However, till today there is no perfect injection material. Second issue is some expertise is required so as not to inject long-lasting injectable materials into subepithelial space. This can increase hoarseness. As a rule, in all office-based procedures injection should be in the muscle lateral to vocal ligament. More lateral injection causes no harm but voice improvement may not be optimum. In case of large posterior gap, the injection should be lateral to the vocal process of the arytenoid. In case of patients with paresis or atrophy, the injection should be mid-membranous. Too much anterior injection should be avoided.

The amount injected varies from patient-to-patient and depends on amount of gap, breathiness, appearance of the vocal fold, and physical traits of the patient. Most materials require some over correction. At an average 0.5 mL of the injection suffices in a normal adult male. The biggest advantage of office-based injection laryngoplasty is that voice quality and the vocal cord gap can be monitored during the procedure.

Transoral Approach

It is technically demanding as the needle has to travel a long distance to reach the larynx through a number of structures. The anesthesia has to be really good. But the effort is worth as the precision is more as the visualization of needle is there along the entire tract to the larynx. The best position is sniffing position which means patient leans in front with chin thrust forward. The first step in learning this technique is by delivering local anesthetic through Abraham Cannula.

One way is to let the patient holds his tongue, while the clinician holds Hopkins scope in one hand and does the injection through the other hand or an assistant can put the flexible scope while the main clinician holds the tongue and does the injection seeing on the monitor. The injection substance should be preloaded into the needle from the syringe before injection so as to avoid air entering and causing a swelling in the vocal cord.

Transcricothyroid Approach

This approach is very familiar to those doing botulinum injections. A 25-gauge needle bend at 45° about 1 cm from the tip is inserted about 3 mm from the midline. The needle trajectory is toward 1 o'clock on the patient's left side and 11 o'clock on the patient's right side. The entire path of needle is submucosal. Assistant does a flexible laryngoscopy and visualizes the glottis on the monitor. The position of the needle in the cord is checked by moving the needle and visualizing the needle motion. Then the injection is done.

In case the needle is not visualized, it is inserted in the midline and then redirected into the vocal cord after visualizing on the monitor.

Transthyroid Cartilage Approach

Skin over the site needs to be anesthetized. A 23-gauze needle is inserted parallel to the thyroid cartilage at the midpoint of the thyroid ala at the perceived vertical level of the membranous vocal cord. A good cue is to enter about 5 mm above the inferior border. Transmitted movement of the needle should be visible on the monitor. A cartilage plug may obstruct the needle but can be cleared with gentle pressure on the plunger. Casiano needle made by Meditronics is able to overcome the plugging problem.[23]

Transthyrohyoid Approach

Here good mucosal anesthesia is required. Again a 23-gauze needle is used and made to enter through the thyrohyoid membrane near the thyroid notch. It should be guided sharply downwards. The assistant is helping with a fiberoptic laryngoscope and visualization on the monitor. The advantage of this technique is good visualization of the needle.

Postoperatively, the patients are kept under observation for 1 hour and observed for any breathing problem or bleeding. They may not eat anything for 2–3 hours if topical anesthesia has been given to prevent aspiration. Immediate postoperative period the voice may not be good and it may take 2 weeks for the voice to stabilize. Patients on blood thinners are better avoided.

LARYNGEAL BIOPSY

This is again one of the most commonly performed and useful application of office-based procedures. One way which was being done previously is per oral while visualizing with a rigid telescope or a fiberoptic laryngoscope. Nowadays a better method has been developed which consists of inserting a biopsy force through the working channel of fiberoptic laryngoscope. A 2 mm flexible cup forceps is used. First the lesion is visualized with the fiberoptic laryngoscope and the forceps inserted and opened some distance away from the lesion. Then both the endoscope and force in the channel are advanced and biopsy taken. Channel can be removed and put back again if more tissue is required. It can be combined with TNE and bronchoscopy and substitute the conventional panendoscopy which used to be done under general anesthesia. The literature supports that awake laryngeal biopsy is as effective as biopsy under general anesthesia.[24,25]

SECONDARY TRACHEOESOPHAGEAL PUNCTURE

Transnasal esophagoscope or flexible fiberoptic laryngoscope can be used to aid in making a tracheoesophageal puncture (TEP) in a staged setting or where TEP needs to be changed. Transnasal esophagoscope is passed through nose and its illumination is used to visualize the puncture site in the tracheostoma. Local anesthesia is given. Incision is made with a 15 number blade and a 14 number Ryle's tube is put through the stoma. This avoids a general anesthesia (Figs 4A to C).

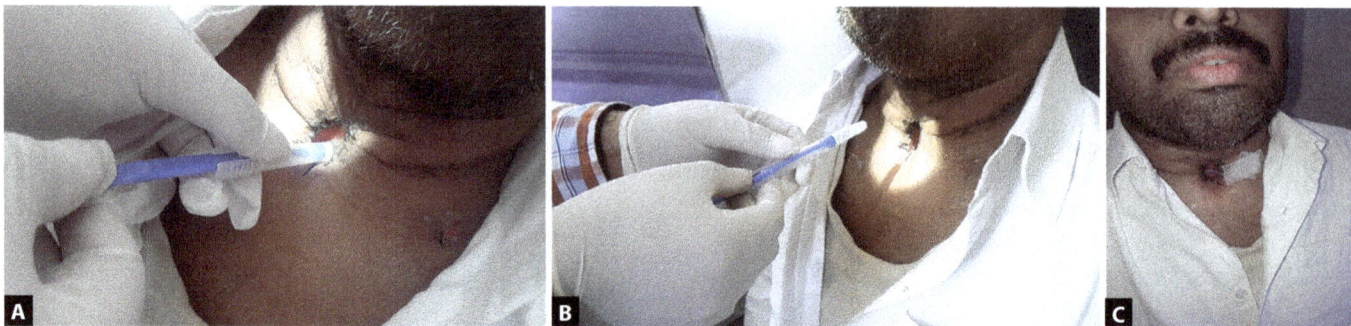

Figs 4A to C Transeshophageal puncture (TEP) procedure with Provox prosthesis

SUPERFICIAL VOCAL CORD INJECTION

It means injection of material into superficial subepithelial space using a fine-gauze needle. The material injected includes either collagen or steroids. The subepithelial space is small and only about 0.1–0.2 cc of material can be injected. Steroid injection following phonosurgical procedures to alter the wound healing response is the most common indication. These steroid injections are given serially, i.e. 2–3 injections with a gap of 2 weeks between each injection. Sometimes, it is used to inject collagen-based products, e.g. camera, however, as a lot of precision is required, this is better done under general anesthesia.[26] This injection can be given either transorally or through the channel of fiberoptic laryngoscope.

BOTOX INJECTION

Conventionally Botox injection is done under electromyographic (EMG) guidance either through percutaneous cricothyroid route or thyrohyoid membrane route. The injection is done into the thyroarytenoid muscle for adductor spasmodic dysphonia.

In certain rare cases, injection may be done into false cord and interarytenoid area. This is done for a small number of adductor spasmodic dysphonia patients who have not improved with injection into thyroarytenoid muscle and patients with essential tremor where maximum tremor is in the supraglottis area.[27] This injection into the false cord can either be done through transoral approach or endoscopic approach. Injection into interarytenoid muscle is more challenging and needs a combination of endoscopic and percutaneous approach. An EMG needle is passed percutaneously below the thyroid cartilage and once it enters the laryngeal lumen the visualization is shifted to endoscopic view and needle is directed to the posterior commissure and injection done in the interarytenoid muscle under EMG guidance.

TRANSNASAL ESOPHAGOSCOPY

This has become another addition in the armamentarium of laryngologists in the recent years. This has improved diagnosis and treatment for swallow disorders, dysphagia, reflux, and head neck cancer. Esophagoscopy as described by Jackson C[28] has undergone a lot of changes in the recent years. The latest technology including distal chip cameras, thinner caliber esophagoscopes are responsible for this.[29,30] Topical nasal anesthesia with decongestion is done and TNE can be performed as an office-based procedure with no sedation. The entire tract from nose to gastroesophageal junction is visualized and small procedures like biopsy can also be done. The scope needs to be passed very carefully through the upper esophageal sphincter. As normally esophagus is collapsed at rest insufflation with air, swallowing by patient or drinking water helps to improve the visualization.

Indications for TNE include patients with:[31,32]
- Dysphagia
- Laryngopharyngeal reflux where symptoms persist despite antireflux treatment
- Painful swallowing
- Corrosive ingestion
- Biopsy of suspicious lesions
- Monitoring of esophageal varices
- Chronic cough
- Part of panendoscopy for head and neck cancer patients
- Globus patients
- Balloon dilatation of strictures
- Secondary or revision trachea esophageal puncture
- Flexible laser fiber application
- Injection of Botox for dysphagia in postlaryngectomy patients.

Expertise is required in doing the patients with Zenker's diverticulum. TNE provides a big advantage over conventional upper gastrointestinal (GI) endoscopies as it is done without sedation. In upper GI endoscopy majority of complications are related to cardiopulmonary issues[33] which is avoided in TNE. It is a very safe procedure. In literature with so many large series of TNE only one case of perforation[34] has been reported. Rates of self-limiting epistaxis were reported around 1–2% while vasovagal events were reported around 0.3%.[31,35] There have been many studies comparing TNE to upper GI endoscopy and results are equal while patients prefer TNE to more elaborate conventional upper GI endoscopies.[36-38]

Office-based diagnosis and treatment has immensely improved patient management and we are moving forward with new procedures or interventions which can be carried out with under local anesthesia, without sedation and at lowered cost and less complications. However, it must be kept in mind that there are certain procedures and intervention where general anesthesia is required.

REFERENCES

1. Rosen CA, Amin MR, Sulica L, et al. Advances in office based diagnosis and treatment in laryngology. Laryngoscope. 2009;119:S18-212.
2. Hogikyan ND. Transnasal endoscopic examination of the subglottis and trachea using topical anesthesia in the otolaryngological clinic. Laryngoscope. 1999;109(7):1170-3.
3. Milstein CF, Charbel S, Hicks DM, et al. Prevalence of laryngeal irritation signs associated with reflux in asymptomatic volunteers: impact of endoscopic technique (rigid vs flexible laryngoscope). Laryngoscope. 2005;11:2256-61.
4. Carretta A, Melloni G, Ciriaco P, et al. Preoperative assessment of patients with post intubation tracheal stenosis: rigid and flexible bronchoscopy versus spiral CT scan with multiplanar reconstructions. Surg Endos. 2006;20:905-8.
5. Bogdasarian RS, Olson NR. Posterior glottis laryngeal stenosis. Otolaryngol Head Neck Surg. 1980;88:765-72.
6. Sataloff RT, Bough ID Jr, Spiegel JR. Arytenoid dislocation diagnosis and treatment. Laryngoscope. 1994;104(1):1353-61.
7. Murry T, Tabaee A, Owczarzak V. Respiratory training therapy and management of laryngopharyngeal reflux in the treatment of patients with cough and paradoxical vocal fold movement disorder. Ann Otol Rhinol Laryngol. 2006;115:754-8.
8. Sulivan MD, Heywood BM, Beukelmann DR. A treatment for vocal cord dysfunction in female athletes: an outcome study. Laryngoscope. 2001;111:1751-5.
9. Whited RE. A prospective study of laryngotracheal sequelae in long term intubation. Laryngoscope. 1984;94:367-77.
10. Cummings CW. Cummings Otolaryngology head and neck surgery, 4th Edition. Philadelphia: Elsevier Mosby; 2005.
11. Gaissert HA, Burns J. The compromise airway: tumors, strictures and tracheomalacia. Surg Clin North Am. 2010;90:467-72.
12. Belafsky PC, Kuhn MA. Office airway surgery. Otolaryngol Clin N Am. 2013;46:63-74.
13. Lee KH, Ko GY, Song HY, et al. Benign tracheobronchial stenosis: long term clinical experience with balloon dilatation. J Vasc Interv Radiol. 2002;13:909-14.
14. Rees CJ. In office unsedated transnasal balloon dilatation of the oesophagus and trachea. Curr Opin Otolaryngol Head Neck Surg. 2007;15:401-4.
15. Knott DP, Lorenz RR, Eliachar I, et al. Reconstruction of a tracheobronchial tree disruption with bovine pericardium. Interact cardiovasc Thorac Surg. 2004;3:554-6.
16. Rees CJ, Halum SL, Wijewickrama RC, et al. Patient tolerance of in office-pulsed dye laser treatments to the upper aerodigestive tract. Otolaryngol Head and Neck Surg. 2006;134:1023-7.
17. Andrews BT, Graham SM, Ross AF, et al. Technique, utility and safety of awake tracheoplasty using combined laser and balloon dilatation. Laryngoscope. 2007;117:2159-62.
18. Leventhal DD, Krebs E, Rosen MR. Flexible laser bronchoscopy for subglottic stenosis in the awake patient. Arch Otolaryngol Head Neck Surg. 2009;135:467-71.
19. Rees CJ, Postma GM, Koufman JA. Cost savings of unsedated office based laser surgery for laryngeal papillomas. Ann Otol Rhinol Laryngol. 2007;116:45-8.
20. Chheda NN, Rosen CA, Belfsky PC, et al. Revision laryngeal surgery for the suboptimal injection of Calcium hydroxyapatite. Laryngoscope. 2008;118:2260-3.
21. Carroll TL, Rosen CA. Trial vocal cord injection. J Voice. 2010;24(4):494-8.
22. Mathison CC, Vilari CR, Klein AM, et al. Comparison of outcomes and complications between awake and sleep injection laryngoplasty. a case control study. Laryngoscope. 2009;119:1417-23.
23. Amin MR. Transthyroid approach for vocal cord augumentation. Ann Otol Rhinol Laryngol. 2006;115:699-702.
24. Postma GN, Bach KK, Belafsky PC, et al. The role of transnasal oesophagoscopy in head and neck oncology. Laryngoscope. 2002;112:2242-3.
25. Bastian RW, Coliins SL, Kaniff T. Indirect videolaryngoscopy versus direct endoscopy for larynx and pharynx cancer staging. Towards elimination of preliminary direct laryngoscopy. Ann Otol Rhinol Laryngol. 1989;98:693-8.
26. Superficial vocal cord injection. In: Rosen CA, Simpson CB (Eds). Operative techniques in laryngology. Heidelberg, Germany: Springer; 2008.
27. Simpson CB, Amin MR. Office-based procedures for the voice. Ear Nose Throat J. 2004;83(7):6-9.
28. Jackson C. The life of Chevalier Jackson: An autobiography. New York, NY: Macmilan; 1938.
29. Aviv JE, Takoudes TG, Ma G, et al. Office-based oesophagoscopy: a preliminary report. Otolaryngol Head Neck Surg. 2001;125:170-5.
30. Belafsky PC, Postma GN, Daniel E, et al. Transnasal oesophagoscopy. Otolaryngol Head Neck Surg. 2001;25:588-9.
31. Postma GN, Cohen JT, Belafsky PC, et al. Transnasal oesophagoscopy: revisited (over 700 consecutive cases). Laryngoscope. 2005;115:321-3.
32. Amin MR, Postma GN, Setzen M, et al. Transnasal oesophagoscopy: a position statement from the American Bronchoesophagological Association (ABEA). Otolaryngol Head Neck Surg. 2008;138:411-4.
33. Sharma VK, Nguyen CC, Crowell MD, et al. A national study of cardiopulmonary unplanned events after upper GI endoscopy. Gastrointest Endosc. 2007;66:27-34.

34. Zaman A, Hahn M, Hapke R, et al. A randomized trial of per oral versus transnasal unsedated endoscopy using an ultrathin videoendoscope. Gastrointest Endosc. 1999;49(3): 279-84.

35. Dumortier J, Napolean B, Hedelius F, et al. Unsedated transnasal EGD in daily practice: results with 1100 consecutive patients. Gastrointest Endosc. 2003;57:198-204.

36. Birkner B, Fritz N, Schatke W, et al. A prospective randomized comparison of unsedated ultrathin versus standard esophagogastroendoscopy in routine patient gastroenterology practice: does it work better through the nose? Endoscopy. 2003;35:647-51.

37. Sorbi D, Gostout CJ, Henry J. Unsedated small caliber esophagogastroduodenoscopy (EGD) versus conventional EGD a comparative study. Gastroentrology. 1999;117:1301-7.

38. Thota PN, Zuccaro G jr, Vargo JJ 2nd, et al. A randomized prospective trial comparing unsedated esophagoscopy via transnasal and transoral routes using a 4 mm video endoscope with conventional endoscopy with sedation. Endoscopy. 2005;37:559-65.

Recurrent Respiratory Papillomatosis

KK Handa, Anup Singh Yadav

INTRODUCTION

Recurrent respiratory papillomatosis (RRP) is the most common benign neoplasm affecting pediatrics larynx. With an unpredictably predictable course, the disease has a notorious tendency to recur and spread throughout the upper aerodigestive tract of children and adults, taking a huge emotional turmoil on the family of the effected and economic burden on society.

The huge amount of literature available to date agrees on unreliability of long-term eradication of RRP lesions; however, currently available therapeutic modalities provide some promise in reducing the number and frequency of the operative procedures requiring general anesthesia and its attendant risks.

EPIDEMIOLOGY

Recurrent respiratory papillomatosis is a disease of viral etiology, caused by human papillomavirus (HPV) type 6 and 11. Although rare, the disease remains the most common benign neoplasm among children and second most common cause of childhood hoarseness.

True incidence and prevalence of the disease remains unknown; however in 1995, based on a survey of otolaryngologists in the United States, the Task Force on RRP reported a projected total of 3,623 new cases and 9,015 active cases of adult RRP, and a projected total of 2,354 new cases and 5,970 active cases of pediatric RRP. The Task Force data were extrapolated to estimate an RRP prevalence of 4.3 per 100,000 children and 1.8 per 100,000 adults in the United States.[1] The National Registry of children with RRP, composed of the clinical practices at 22 pediatric otolaryngology sites, calculated a mean number of procedures at 19.7 per child with an average of 4.4 procedures per year.[2]

Recurrent respiratory papillomatosis can affect people of any age, the youngest patient documented at 1 day of life and the eldest recognized at 84 years of age.[1] Two clinically distinct forms of RRP can be recognized as:[3]

1. Juvenile-onset RRP (JORRP).
2. Adult-onset RRP (AORRP).

Juvenile-onset RRP is diagnosed most commonly between 2 years and 4 years of age, 75% diagnosed before 5th birthday.[3] It is equally common between girls and boys and is more aggressive than AORRP. Within the subgroup, JORRP tends to be more aggressive the younger the patient is. Children diagnosed with RRP before age of 3 years have been found to be 3.56 times more likely to undergo more than four surgeries, and at twice the risk for having more than two anatomic sites involved with lesions, when compared with children diagnosed with JORRP after 3 years of age.[4] AORRP is less common than JORRP, most commonly diagnosed between 20 years and 40 years of age, has a slight male predilection and tends to be less aggressive than JORRP in general.[3] In adolescence, incidence of RRP nadirs and it is distinctly uncommon for onset of RRP to be in this age group and arbitrarily all the patients diagnosed before adolescence are categorized as JORRP.[1]

ETIOLOGY

Recurrent respiratory papillomatosis is a disease of viral etiology, HPV types 6 and 11 being the proven culprits. HPV belongs to family Papovaviridae. It is a small, nonenveloped, icosahedral capsid virus with 7,900 base pair long double-stranded circular deoxyribonucleic acid (DNA) containing genome. HPV is epitheliotropic, meaning thereby that they preferentially infect epithelial cells. Nearly 100 different types of HPV have been identified, being grouped on the basis of shared genetic code homology, with viruses that share less than 90% identity in specific regions of the virus being defined as separate types. Papillomaviruses exhibit absolute species specificity, however within a host species, epithelial specificity is less absolute.[5]

The most common types of HPV affecting the airway are types 6 and 11, and these are the types most often implicated in genital condylomata. Viral subtype seems to predict severity of disease to some extent and children infected with HPV-11 appear to be having more sinister disease prognosis leading to more aggressive airway obstruction and more frequent need of tracheostomy.[6] HPV 16,18,31, and 33 have also been implicated in RRP, albeit rarely.[7]

Another important aspect of HPV infection of airway is that apart from the lesion itself, the virus has been consistently demonstrated in the adjacent normal appearing tissue, which accounts for the recurrence of disease despite apparent surgical eradication of the lesion.[8] Smith et al.[9] have demonstrated the presence of HPV DNA in macroscopically normal sites in RRP patients at a rate of 61%.

Biology of Human Papillomavirus Infection

Human papillomavirus genomes have all open reading frames (ORFs) located on one of the two viral DNA strands, and only this strand is transcribed. The HPV genome (Fig. 1) has three distinctive parts: a noncoding upstream regulatory region, designated long control region (LCR) and two coding ORFs named according to the phase of infection they are expressed in early (E) and late (L) regions. The E region expresses a total of 6 (E1-2 and 4-7) and L region expresses 2 proteins (L1 and 2) in that temporal sequence.

The replication cycle of HPV is tightly linked to the differentiation of the epithelium it infects and it has a preferential tropism for the stem cells in the basal layer of epithelium. After infection of the basal cells, the virus can either stay as latent infection in grossly and histologically normal mucosa or it can express actively to lead to proliferative papillomatous lesions.

Viral genome integration into the host DNA heralds the active expression of viral transcription and replication which begins with expression of E1 and E2 proteins in basal cell layer. The E1 and E2 proteins regulate viral replication and expression of the other early viral genes. As the infected cell migrates toward the superficial layers of the squamous epithelium, the E6 and E7 oncogenes are expressed and modify the cell cycle to retain the differentiating host

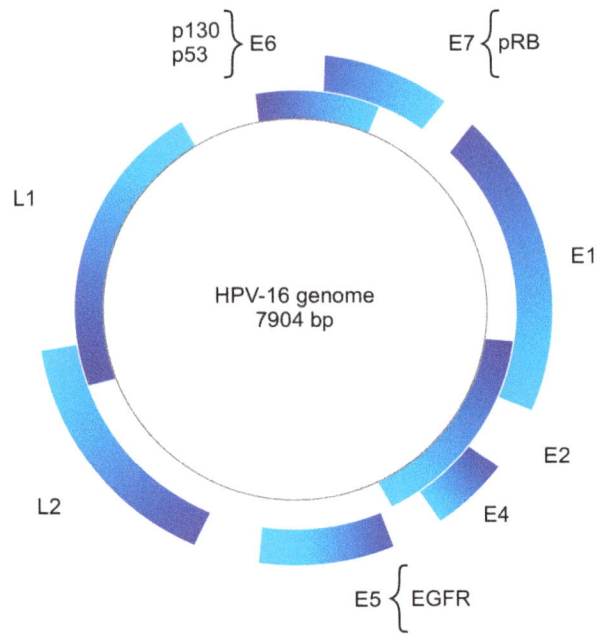

Fig. 1 Human papillomavirus-16 genome. The circular HPV-16 genome is 7,904 base pairs and encodes 6E and 2L major proteins. The primary cellular targets of these proteins are indicated on the genome diagram: E6 ubiquitinates p53, E7 competes for binding with E2F to the hypophosphorylated active form of retinoblastoma tumor suppressor gene product (pRB), and E5 upregulates estimated glomerular filtration rate (EGFR) *Source:* Adapted from reference 10

keratinocyte in a state that is favorable for amplification of the viral genome. The E6 oncoprotein ubiquitinates p53, thereby flagging it for proteosomal degradation via the ubiquitin-proteasome pathway. The E7 protein competes for binding with E2F to the hypophosphorylated active form of the retinoblastoma tumor suppressor gene product, pRB, thus releasing the transcription factor E2F to bind and activate its targets to facilitate cell cycle progression. The binding affinity of E6 and E7 to p53 and pRB, respectively, differentiates the low and high risk types of HPV, which is based on the risk of the infected cell progressing to malignant transformation.[10]

Expression of late proteins, L1 and L2 occurs in granular epithelial layer and lead to formation of major and minor capsid proteins, respectively. L1 spontaneously forms pentamers that assemble with the L2 protein to form the viral capsule.[10]

PATHOPHYSIOLOGY

Grossly the papillomata have a fleshy wart-like appearance and can present as superficial spreading "velvety" appearance or as exophytic "cauliflower" projections. The lesions are pinkish to white in appearance and can be sessile or pedunculated.

The dotted-appearance corresponding to fibrovascular core can be appreciated on microlaryngoscopy.

Recurrent respiratory papillomatosis has a predilection for squamocolumnar junctional zones in respiratory tract and in general, papillomas occur most commonly on the limen vestibuli, the nasopharyngeal surface of the soft palate, the midzone of the laryngeal surface of the epiglottis, the upper and lower margins of the ventricle, the under surface of the vocal folds, the carina, and at bronchial spurs.[11]

Histologically the lesions appear as "fronds" of nonkeratinized stratified squamous epithelium overlying a fibrovascular core. The basal epithelium can be normal to hyperplastic with characteristic koilocytosis (vacuolated cells with clear cytoplasmic inclusions). The delayed maturation of epithelium in signaled by dyskeratosis, parakeratosis and significantly thickened basement membrane.

The virus cannot bind to live tissue; instead, it infects epithelial tissues through microabrasions or other epithelial trauma that exposes segments of the basement membrane. The infected basal cells do not divide at rapid rates but it is the disproportionate increase in the number of dividing infected basal cells which leads to rapid expansion of RRP tissue mass.[12]

The virus is not cytolytic but spreads to adjacent areas by degeneration of desquamated epithelial cells and it is the latent infection in apparently healthy mucosa that has to be eliminated to affect a "cure" for the disease.

MODE OF TRANSMISSION AND RISK FACTORS OF DISEASE

The association between genital HPV infection and RRP incidence is well-established. Different series have noted 50–70% of patients of RRP cohort being born to mothers who had genital warts during pregnancy or childbirth.[13,14] As noted by Kashima et al.[15] 72% of JORRP patients versus 36% of patients with AORRP had the clinical triad of:

- Being the firstborn (longer 2nd stage of labor in primigravidae)
- Being delivered vaginally (direct viral exposure in the birth canal), and
- Being born to a teenage mother (newly acquired genital HPV infection especially low socioeconomic status).

In the same review, AORRP patients were found to have more numbers of lifetime sexual partners and higher frequency of oral sex.

The presence of HPV in the genital tract of women of child-bearing age is believed to be at least 25% worldwide;[16] clinical infection of pregnant women in the United States is between 1.5% and 5%.[17] Despite this large number of infected patients and close association between maternal condyloma and RRP, only a small proportion of children born to mothers with active genital condylomata at the time of vaginal delivery go on to develop RRP, estimated risk[18,19] being only approximately 1 in 231–400. What deters the remaining 230–399 from catching the disease, remains unknown. Apart from the vertical mode of transmission, the reports of neonatal papillomatosis suggest possibility of *in utero* transmission.[20]

An increased frequency of HLA-DRB1*0102 has been noted in white patients with RRP pointing towards genetic susceptibility.[21] Occurrence of RRP in immunosuppressed children and adults is documented; however, a strong correlation cannot be made out.[1]

PRESENTING SYMPTOMATOLOGY

Involvement of vocal cord as the first site leads to appearance of first symptom as *hoarseness*, which because of its subtle nature in children tends to go unnoticed till *Stridor*, initially inspiratory and later biphasic, appears as the next alarming feature. However, in infants with an already precarious airway, acute respiratory distress may be the presenting symptom, occurring with an otherwise common cold. Other symptoms secondary to involvement of upper aerodigestive tract can appear, including:

- Chronic cough
- Dyspnea
- Recurrent upper respiratory tract infection (URTIs)
- Recurrent pneumonia
- Failure to thrive
- Dysphagia.[3]

This wide array of possible symptomatology tends to conceal the real underlying pathology and child may be misdiagnosed as:

- Asthma
- Croup
- Allergies
- Bronchitis
- Vocal nodule.

The low index of suspicion of this rare disease with the subtle presenting features leads to a delay in diagnosis of up to a year after initial symptomatology.

Course of disease is highly unpredictable with a waxing and waning course of remission and exacerbation being a common one, however the disease may undergo spontaneous remission or may present in an extremely aggressive manner, needing surgical debridement every few days to weeks. Many a times, however, a certain pattern may roughly be anticipated after observing initial few episodes on which to base the further follow-up of the patient. Fatalities in disease course are usually ascribed to airway complications related to frequent surgical intervention or to distal spread and attendant obstructive sequelae.

TRACHEOSTOMY IN RECURRENT RESPIRATORY PAPILLOMATOSIS

Tracheostomy is an obvious need in a significant number of cases, given the unpredictable presentation of disease, and comes as a life saving measure without doubt. However, there are attendant real risks associated with the procedure, with a potential to complicate future disease course. Similar sequelae can be attributed to use of endotracheal tube in these patients.

Shapiro et al.[22] noted that children who need tracheostomy tends to present at a younger age with more severe disease and frequently with distal airway spread before tracheostomy. However, there are others who suggest that tracheostomy can itself contribute in spreading the disease further in the airway. The possible explanation includes creation of de novo squamocolumnar junction at the site of tracheostomy and direct implantation or chronic irritation of respiratory epithelium leading to metaplastic changes. Cole et al.[23] reported that distal spread of disease with tracheal papilloma occurred in half of their patients who underwent tracheostomy. More specifically, prolonged tracheostomy and presence of subglottic papillomas at the time of tracheostomy has been associated with a higher risk of distal spread (Fig. 2).

The general consensus is that tracheostomy should be avoided until absolutely necessary. If it has to be done, decannulation should be considered as soon as possible after surgical debridement of papillomas and securing airway (Fig. 3).

EXTRALARYNGEAL SPREAD

Extralaryngeal spread of RRP has been noted to occur in up to 30% of children and 16% of adults. Most commonly affected sites are oral cavity, trachea, bronchi, and esophagus in that order.[1,11]

Distal spread to trachea occurs in up to 5% and lung involvement occurs in up to 1% of cases (Fig. 4). Pulmonary involvement occurs twice as commonly in males than in females and heralds a grave prognosis leading to progressive obstructive and infective sequelae with destruction of lung parenchyma and in more aggressive cases leading to malignant transformation which has been reported in 1.6% of cases by Dedo and Yu.[24] Risk of malignancy mandates radiological monitoring and adequate biopsy of the lesion in progressive cases. These pulmonary neoplasms display a moderate to well-differentiated histology and appear on imaging as solid or cystic areas with central liquefactive necrosis. Appearing initially as noncalcified peripheral nodules, these lesions ultimately progress to engulf the functioning lung parenchyma terminating invariably fatal. The extralaryngeal spread and malignant transformation appear to be more

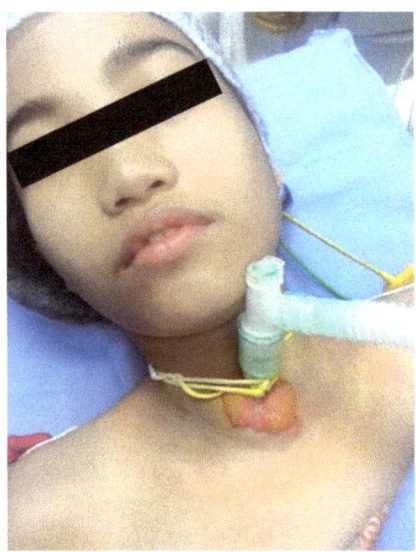

Fig. 2 Extensive tracheal papillomatosis coming out of stoma

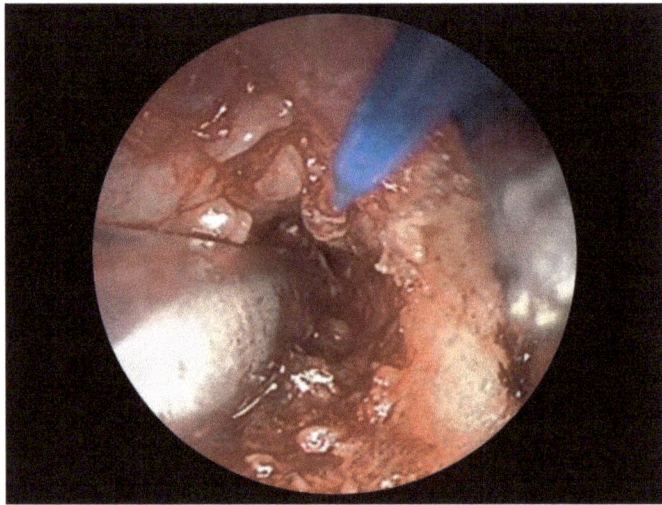

Fig. 3 Extensive tracheal papillomatosis. Use of fiber laser

commonly associated with HPV-11 conferring it a moderate risk category between type 6 on benign end and 16 and 18 on high risk end of the spectrum.[25,26]

PATIENT EVALUATION

Ask about:
- Age of onset and rate of progression
- Concomitant infection
- History of trauma or surgery
- Previous critical cardiorespiratory adverse events
- Significant perinatal event (including maternal condyloma acuminata)

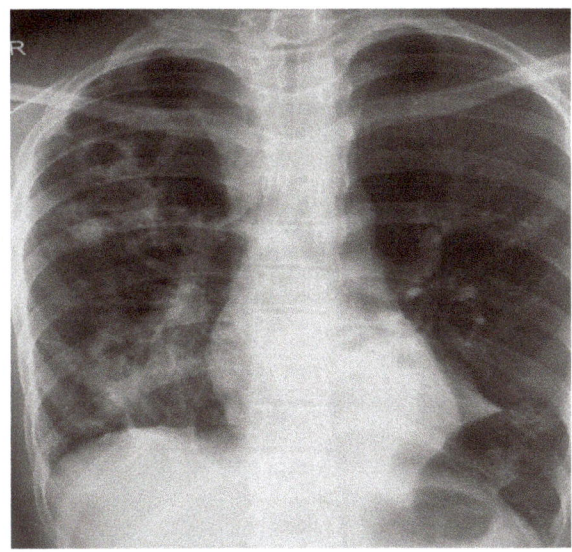

Fig. 4 Lung involvement in a patient with extensive laryngeal papillomatosis

Look for:
- Respiratory distress—Alae nasi, accessory muscles, cyanosis, tachypnea, respiratory fatigue.
- Obvious skin lesions so an alternate or concomitant congenital pathology.

Listen to:
- Voice or cry
- Stridor—Over nose, mouth, neck and chest
  - Phase of respiration and character of stridor
  - Positional variation of characteristics.

In a stable situation, further examination of patient's airway should proceed with flexible nasopharyngoscopy to have a direct look at endolarynx to confirm the diagnosis, assess the glottic chink and stage the lesion. However, if the signs of respiratory distress or fatigue are apparent, the patient should immediately be shifted to operation theater with all the basic amenities to secure airway under controlled condition being handy.

Once lesion is visualized with fiberoptic laryngoscopy, it should be:
- Photographed
- Staged and
- Biopsied—with optional HPV typing

Education and counseling of the family of an RRP patient is crucial to make them understand about the social and economic implications associated.

Staging severity: It is highly relevant to develop a standardized staging system to:
- Track the disease progression
- Treat the patient in a protocol format
- Physician-to-physician communication and
- To assess and compare the results of various interventions in a meaningful way.

Figure 5[27,28] shows the staging assessment sheet and pictorial representation of sites to be scored using the current standard staging system, developed using software designed at University of Washington and licensed to the American Society of Pediatric Otolaryngology (ASPO), computerized and available online.

Genetic and Immunological Aspects

The rarity of number of children with RRP as opposed to the large scale HPV exposure has not yet been fully explained. Recently some light has been shed on the host immunity playing some role in this aspect.

It has been shown that although humoral immunity remains intact in RRP patients, the mucosal cellular immunity fails to mount appropriate response and a significant relationship has been found between low CD4/CD8 counts and JORRP.[29] Additionally, CD28 coexpression in tumor infiltrating lymphocytes from papillomata of RRP patients has been shown to be deficient in severe RRP cases.[30] HPV-11 E6-induced dendritic cell dysfunction has been shown to skew IL-10 and interferon (IFN) gamma expression towards increased IL-10 expression in RRP patients.[31] Further evidences suggest that HPV may evade immune recognition by decreasing major histocompatibility complex (MHC-1) surface expression via downregulation of transporter associated with antigen presentation (TAP-1) on dendritic cells and TAP-1 protein expression is inversely proportional to frequency of disease recurrence.[32]

A strong correlation has been shown between specific human leukocyte antigen (HLA) alleles and HPV infection and its severity, with simultaneous expression of certain alleles conferring a greater risk of developing severe RRP.[33,34]

MANAGEMENT

Surgical Treatment

Surgery remains the current standard of care with adjuvant pharmacotherapy being considered for severe cases. With the currently available therapeutic modalities, curative intent cannot be expected. Hence the realistic goals of surgery include reducing the tumor burden, achieving a patent airway, decrease the spread of the disease and at the same time, to avoid the sequelae of overzealous extirpative treatment resulting in excessive scarring, webbing, and stenosis with suboptimal voice outcomes.

The surgery should be performed in a "hair-cutting" or "lawn mowing" fashion, debulking the obstructive papillomas

Staging assessment for recurrent laryngeal papillomatosis

Patient initials: _____   Date of surgery: _____   Surgeon: _____

Patient ID #: _____   Institution: _____

1. How long since the last papilloma surgery? ____days, ____weeks, ____ months, ____years.
    ____do not know, ____1st surgery
2. Counting today's surgery, how many papiloma surgeries in the past 12 months?____
3. Describe the patient's voice today: ____aphonic, ____abnormal ____normal, ____ other
4. Describe the patient's stridor today: ___absent, _____present with activity, ___present at rest,
    ____do not know
5. Describe the urgency of today's intervention: ____scheduled, ____urgent, ____emergent

For each site, score as: 0 = None, 1 = Surface lesion, 2 = Raised lesion, 3 = Bulky lesion

Larynx:
Epiglottis

Lingual surface _____ Laryngeal surface _____
Aryepiglottic folds: Right ____   Left ____
False vocal cords: Right ____   Left ____
True vocal cords: Right ____   Left ____
Arytenoids: Right ____   Left ____
Anterior commissure ____ Posterior commissure _____
Subglottis ____

Trachea:
Upper one-third ____
Middle one-third ____
Lower one-third ____
Bronchi: Right _____   Left ____
Tracheotomy stoma ____

Other:
Nose_____
Palate____
Pharynx___
Esophagus____
Lungs_____
Other_____

Total score all sites: _____

Fig. 5 Staging assessment

down to the level of grossly normal appearing adjacent mucosa and not disturbing the submucosa and deeper structures which do not harbor the virus. Omnipresent cryptic infection of apparently healthy adjacent mucosa cannot be removed surgically and should not be attempted.

Recurrent respiratory papillomatosis is a "chronic disease" and even with the use of combined modalities, patient has to undergo multiple surgeries with an average of 4.1–4.4 surgeries needed in the first year of diagnosis alone.[1] It is not rare or exceptional for the patients to undergo hundreds of surgeries during the lifetime, however, it is impossible to predict the future course and prognostication of the disease based on initial picture of presentation. A more practical strategy is to thoroughly examine the larynx at monthly intervals for the first few months to establish a rough pattern of disease progression behavior rather than waiting for the symptoms to appear and undertake an emergency surgery with its greater attendant risks including need for tracheostomy.

Anesthetic Considerations

A variety of anesthetic techniques have been used as listed in the Table 1.[1]

Regardless of the technique of anesthesia, one must be mindful of:

- Risk of losing an already jeopardized airway at induction, conferred by the muscle relaxants
- Risk of mucosal microtraumas and distal implantation of disease.

Although seemingly intimidating, intubation through the papilloma is usually successful, avoiding the need of tracheostomy. The use of intravenous medications,

Table 1 Variety of anesthetic techniques	
Anesthesia techniques	Recurrent respiratory papillomatosis (RRP) task force data
• Laser safe endotracheal tube	46.00%
• Jet ventilation	26.00%
• Apneic technique	16.00%
• Spontaneous ventilation	12.00%

typically propofol and remifentanil, achieves the objective of suppressing arousal while maintaining spontaneous respiration.

Surgical Techniques

Surgical options have undergone significant advancement from the days of debulking with cup forceps with hand-held laryngoscope under direct naked vision, to microlaryngoscopy under suspension, using laser ablation to the use of laryngeal microdebrider for disease removal.

Surgical options currently available include:
- Cold steel instrumentation
- Laser ablation (CO_2 laser and angiolytic lasers)
- Laryngeal microdebrider
- Coblator wand-assisted debridement.

After anesthesia, larynx is carefully examined under microscopic vision and a graphic documentation and staging of disease is undertaken. Biopsies are next taken from appropriate sites before the surgeon moves on to debulk the disease.

Cold Steel

Before 1970s, when the laser was introduced for laryngeal applications, cold instruments using laryngeal forceps and scissors have been the mainstay of surgical removal of papillomas. The technique of cold instrumentation has undergone impressive refinements. The principle of submucosal excision, hydrodissection, and microflap techniques offer great control in high risk areas like the anterior and posterior commissures, however, the amount of papillomas that can be removed this way is modest at best, and bleeding can be intimidating and frustrating given the limited speed at which precise removal of disease with functional preservation has to be achieved.

Carbon Dioxide Laser Excision

From 1970s until 2000, CO_2 was the most commonly used modality for removal of respiratory papillomas. With a wavelength of 10,600 nm, it falls in far infrared spectrum and principally converts light into thermal energy which is absorbed by water present in the cells and causes water vaporization and surface tissue cauterization.

The essential benefits with CO_2 laser are the precision of surgery and excellent hemostasis. After mounting CO_2 laser and micromanipulator over the microscope, endolarynx is visualized via the rigid wide field laryngoscope placed in suspension. It can be used at defocused mode to cauterize the tissue in a broad front fashion to deal with the bulky central papillomas in the initial stage of surgery and later on be shifted to a sharp focus mode as a cutting tool for handling the disease precisely in critical areas like commissures, free edge of true folds and conus.[35] The usual power setting of 2–7 Watts (W) suffices with a repeat mode being used to allow for thermal relaxation. One of the effective techniques described for RRP is the "laser brush technique"[36] which uses lowest wattage setting of 2–3W with an exposure time of 1 second and spot size diameter of 300 microns. It is a layered approach with microhemostasis. The laser is applied in "brush strokes" in an anterior to posterior direction in a broad front over the velvety papillomatous surface resulting in superficial vaporization and carbonization which can be brushed away with a saline-soaked patty and suction. Such multiple brush strokes are applied with microscopic visualization until submucosa can be identified which is the surgical endpoint. The use of a laryngeal spreader makes the removal of subglottic disease easier. Involvement of distal airway can be addressed with the use of flexible fiber-based CO_2 or thulium laser under bronchoscopic ventilation.

Needless to say, laser can be a two-edged sword, and universal laser precautions are of paramount importance. Other hazards specific to surgery for RRP can be:
- Exposure of the operating team to the potentially infective laser "plume" containing active viral DNA,[37,38]
- Collateral thermal damage to deeper tissue leading to glottic edema with airway compromise and delayed effects of scarring,[35]
- Inadvertent damage to surrounding healthy mucosa leading to possibility of creation of a new squamocolumnar junction and increased susceptibility to viral implantation.[35]

Angiolytic Lasers

The two issues of surface cauterization leading to creation of raw surfaces and thermal conductivity with CO_2 laser can be overcome with the angiolytic lasers including 585 nm pulsed-dye laser (PDL) and 532 nm pulsed potassium-titanyl-phosphate (KTP) laser.

The chromophore for these lasers is oxyhemoglobin which selectively absorbs the energy from laser light and results in photoablation of vessels in the central fibrovascular area of the papilloma, leading to extravasation of oxyhemoglobin from microvasculature into the papilloma core resulting in dark purpura, which signals the endpoint with laser treatment. This selective photo vascular ablation achieves the objective of devitalizing the papillomas without creation of raw epithelial surfaces vulnerable to metaplasia, viral implantation and scarring and can be carried out at power settings much lower than that causing collateral thermal damage to deeper tissues.[39,40]

These lasers are best suited to treat the delicate, risky areas like commissures and vocal fold edges, after the bulky lesions have been debrided with other suitable tools. Another extra edge that PDL or KTP lasers offer is the office-based treatment that can be undertaken under local anesthesia with fiberoptic-based flexible instruments obviating the recurring need of general anesthesia and attendant cost and safety issues.[39,40] This ease of delivery to remote areas makes it suitable for delivery to distal tracheobronchial lesions also.

Microdebrider

Since the time, the microdebrider was first used in laryngologic practice in 1999 by Myer and colleagues,[41] this instrument has become the preferred way to debulk the RRP papillomas. In 2004, a web-based survey of APSO members suggested that 53% (compared to 42% for CO_2 laser) of the respondents preferred the use of laryngeal microdebrider for removing the papillomas.

The laryngeal blades are thinner and longer than sinus blades and are available in skimmer configuration. Their length vary from 18 cm to 45 cm and diameters available are 2.9, 3.5, and 4.0 mm depending on patient age and anatomy. The debrider is set at 1,500 rpm in oscillation mode without irrigation and under microscopic or telescopic guidance; bulk of the papillomas is debrided, followed by finer "trimming" of the delicate areas like anterior commissure and vocal fold edges. To remove the papillomas in ventricle, the skimmer is placed over the floor of ventricle and the papillomas can be sucked and cut by the blade, progressing from posterior to anterior direction, the area in advance of the tip being protected by round and smooth tip of the laryngeal blade. For the medial aspect of true vocal fold, the papillomatous velvet should be sucked gently into the microdebrider for cutting rather than pushing the blade against the cord and risking deeper bites.[42] In the area of anterior commissure, it is wiser to either do subtotal disease clearance or opt for a staged removal of papillomas to avoid risking web formation.

Microdebrider provides a rapid debulking of bulky exophytic papillomatosis and at the same time avoids the risks associated with laser use to the operating staff and the risk of thermal tissue damage and airway fire to the patient. However, the disadvantages include the lack of concurrent hemostasis offered by the use of laser, and the danger of extending the depth of excision to underlying submucosa and musculature. A more prudent way to achieve best obtainable outcome may be to rapidly debride the central bulk of papillomas with microdebrider followed by repeated laser brushing of the peripheral deeper epithelial layers.

ADJUVANT TREATMENT MODALITIES

Although surgical treatment remains the mainstay of RRP management, ultimately up to 10–20% patients will lend up needing adjuvant treatment.

The most widely accepted criteria cited in literature for the use of adjuvant therapy are:[3,43]
- Need of undergoing surgery at a frequency of more than 4 times a year.
- Rapidly regrowing papillomas causing airway compromise
- Distal tracheobronchial spread of papillomas.

Historically, alpha-IFN has been the most common adjuvant therapy, however, with its introduction in late 1990s, the use of intralesional cidofovir has become quite popular. Other promising therapies in use are indole-3-carbinol (I3C) and photodynamic therapy (PDT). Acyclovir, ribavirin, methotrexate, celecoxib, isotretinoin, and mumps vaccine have also been used in past, however, have failed to gain popularity for this indication.

Cidofovir

Cidofovir [(S)-1-(3-hydroxy-2-phosphonylmethoxypropyl) cytosine] is a cytosine analog, with *in vitro* activity against a broad spectrum of viruses including cytomegalovirus, herpes simplex virus types 1 and 2, varicella-zoster virus, Epstein–Barr virus, human herpesvirus-6, human herpesvirus-8, polyomaviruses, adenovirus, and HPV.[44] It has been approved by the US Food and Drug Administration (FDA) for use in cytomegalovirus retinitis in acquired immunodeficiency syndrome (AIDS) patients.[45] In this setting, it is used intravenously and adverse effects include nephrotoxicity, myelosuppression, hepatic dysfunction and ocular toxicity. Teratogenic potential too, has been demonstrated. Topical use, even though not FDA approved, has been popular in various cutaneous conditions.[45] Subcutaneously injected cidofovir has been shown to cause mammary adenocarcinoma in rodents,[46] in humans, however, the histological studies have found no evidence to support the carcinogenicity attributable to cidofovir topical application.[47-49]

The mechanism of action of cidofovir largely remains unknown, however, it acts to induce apoptosis and improve immune response.[50] It has been shown to reduce expression of E6 and E7 proteins with increase in active p53 in an *in vitro* model of HPV-associated tumors.[51]

The use of cidofovir to treat papillomas was described first by Van Cutsem et al.[52] in 1995, who treated a 69-years-old patient's hypopharyngeal and esophageal papillomas by direct intralesional cidofovir injection. Since then numerous case series and reports of cidofovir use in RRP, with and without surgical debridement, have been published with encouraging results.[53-58] The first attempt at conducting a placebo-controlled, double-blinded, randomized controlled trials was attempted by The *National Institute of Allergy and Infectious Diseases* (NIAID) collaborative study group in late 1990s, but the study was stopped prematurely because of poor patient accrual. The only patient with whom the treating investigator found encouraging results, ultimately turned out to be in the control, placebo arm.[59]

To date, the only prospective, randomized, double-blind, placebo-controlled trial for use of cidofovir in RRP conducted by McMurray et al.[60] in 2008, showed significant improvement in Derkey severity score in both the cidofovir and placebo group at the end of 12 months, without significant difference between the two arms, suggesting that the encouraging results of the earlier nonrandomized studies might as well have been spuriously favoring the use of cidofovir in the absence of control arm. The study was limited by a small sample size (n = 19) and a change in the cidofovir concentration midway through the trial, from 0.3 mg/mL in children and 0.75 mg/mL in adults, to 5 mg/mL in both adults and children.

Recently, eighteen statements were approved by the RRP Task Force after discussion of the survey results in RRP task force meeting held in April 2012, with the salient points about the use of intralesional cidofovir being as follows:[61]

- *Indication*: Initiated for patients requiring six or more surgeries per year, or for whom the interval between surgeries is decreasing, or in children with extralaryngeal or excessively bulky papilloma disease.
- *Dosing:* Recommended in concentrations in the range of 2.5–7.5 mg/mL. Based upon the literature, doses should not exceed 3 mg/kg.
- *Volume*: An endolaryngeal injection volume less than 4 mL is typical in adults and adolescents, and 2 mL in children so as not to obstruct the airway.
- *Dosing schedule:* Typically up to 5 doses at interval of 2–6 weeks.
- Routine biopsies for adults (and preferably in children too) with RRP should be obtained at the time of each direct laryngoscopy.
- Informed consent process should include mention of the risk of acute kidney injury in children.

Alpha Interferon

Interferons are biological response modifying proteins produced by human leucocytes in response to a variety of stimuli including viral infection and they act on cellular receptors to inhibit viral protein translation and tilt the balance of cellular metabolism towards an antiproliferative, antiviral and immunoprotective state.[62]

For use in RRP IFN alpha is used in two forms—IFN alpha-2a and-2b, the two of them differing by two amino acid sequences. Initially obtained from pooled blood products, currently it is synthesized in much purer form using recombinant technology.[62,63] Conventional IFNs have been taken off the market and replaced now with the "pegylated" form. This modification stabilizes the IFNs in the presence of degrading host enzymes and increases its half-life needing only weekly subcutaneous injections as opposed to daily injections in case of conventional IFNs.

Use of alpha interferon in RRP was first reported in 1981 by Haglund et al.[62] Thereafter, multiple uncontrolled as well as controlled studies have shown the beneficial effects of INF therapy in RRP.[63-66] A popular regimen as proposed by levanthal et al.[67] includes escalating the dose rapidly to a dose of 5 million units/m^2/day given subcutaneously for 1 month and thereafter continuing the same dose 3 times/week for next 6 months. The initial benefits with its use, however, have not found to be sustained and a rebound phenomenon with accelerated papilloma growth has been observed on discontinuation of therapy. Formerly the most popular adjuvant therapy, the use of IFN alpha has been supplanted by more recently added more tolerable adjuvant like cidofovir, in view of associated toxicity with the use of the former, both early, as well as late. Early or the acute side effects include fever with flu-like symptoms, nausea and vomiting, which tends to be mitigated to some extent by night-time dose administration and tolerance usually develops within 2 weeks to these side effects. Late or the chronic side effects include hepatic dysfunction, coagulopathy, leucopenia, thrombocytopenia, alopecia, growth retardation in children, and rarely but significantly spastic diplegia and seizure disorder have been reported.

As suggested by Gerein et al.[68] an enhanced response may exist for HPV-6 than type 11. Recently, Peg-IFN alpha-2a has been combined with granulocyte macrophage colony stimulating factor (GMCSF), both being potent stimulators of dendritic cells maturation, activation and proliferation, showing promise in RRP treatment. However, the trial was a Descriptive observational study and control group was not included.[69]

Photodynamic Therapy

Photodynamic therapy (PDT) involves the use of photo-sensitizing agent to destroy the rapidly proliferating papillomatous tissue. These agents have been in use since early 1900s for tumor ablative properties. The photosensitizing drug is administered systemically and is concentrated in the papillomata followed by laser activation of the drug resulting in production of reactive oxygen species causing vascular stasis and tumor destruction.[70]

The traditionally used agent di-hematoporphyrin ether (DHE, Photofrin-II) is injected intravenously in a dose of 4.25 mg/kg, which has been found superior to lower doses, 48–72 hours before exposure to 630 nm argon pumped-dye laser delivering energy density of 50 J/cm^2.[71] This results in singlet oxygen production and induction of cellular apoptosis. Photosensitivity, however, remains a significant side effect lasting for up to 6–9 months, with skin erythema, blistering and ocular discomfort even with indoor fluorescent light.

To overcome this limitation, search of alternative photosensitizer led to development of meso-tetra-hydroxyphenyl-chlorin (m-THPC or Foscan). This agent is a second generation photosensitizer and has a better efficacy and side effect profile, with photosensitivity lasting only for 2–3 weeks. PDT has uniquely been shown to provide additional immune benefits in case of RRP treatment.[72,73] The study with Foscan, showed a transient initial worsening of the disease activity followed by delayed beneficial response.[72] This pattern was explained by the authors to be because of a rapid increase in amount of antigen presented to the immature antigen presenting cells (APCs) resulting in a shift of HPV-specific immune response from low-HPV level T-cell ignorance or tolerance to high antigen load associated T-cell suppression or energy state leading to initial disease worsening. Later on with the maturation of APCs function, however, ability of immune system to respond to viral antigens improved, leading to a beneficial response. 3–5 years follow-up of the patients showed disease recurrence, albeit at low level.[72] Notably, however, viral DNA is not eliminated from tissue with either of the agents.

Use of PDT may be more desirable in handling endobronchial lesions. Further large scale studies are needed to evaluate the comparative benefits with these two agents and to better elucidate the mechanism of action of these drugs.

Indole-3-Carbinol

Indole-3-carbinol is a phytochemical found in cruciferous vegetables like broccoli, brussels, cabbage, and cauliflower. It gets activated only after being macerated. I3C acts as a potent-inducer of CYP-450 mediated metabolism of estrogen causing preferential induction of 2 hydroxylation relative to 16 alpha hydroxylation of estrogen (higher 2-OHE1: 16α-OHE1 ratio). As opposed to 16 alpha hydroxyestrone (16α-OHE1), 2 hydroxyestrone (2-OHE1) is devoid of peripheral estrogenic activities and rather has a weak antiestrogenic nature translating into a lower cellular proliferative potential conferred by the action of I3C on respiratory papillomata.[74]

Indole-3-carbinol, though available naturally in crucifer vegetables, its absorption from eating vegetables is highly nonuniform. It is available over the counter as tablet formulation, the doses for adults being 200–400 mg daily and for children weighing less than 25 kg, 100–200 mg daily. It has a very good safety profile, but at higher doses it can cause dizziness and gastric discomfort.[75]

In an open label prospective study taking 33 patients, with a mean duration of 57.6 months of follow-up, Rosen et al.[76] showed that 33% had complete response, 30% had partial response and 36% had no response to I3C therapy. Children, overall, had a poorer response than adults in their study.

Another compound Di-indolyl-methane (DIM) is an active dimer of I3C, forming naturally in acidic medium, and having better absorbability and shelf life than I3C. Used at a typical dose of 4 mg/kg/day, it has no significant side effects reported.

Hence, I3C or DIM are natural products, easily administered with low side effect profile with moderate efficacy and their use needs to be investigated in further controlled studies.

Heat-shock Protein E7: Therapeutic Vaccination

Heat-shock protein E7 (HspE7) is an immunotherapeutic recombinant protein with 638 amino acids, covalently linking C terminus of Hsp65 derived from mycobacterium bovis Bacille Calmette–Guérin and E7 protein of HPV-16. The HspE7 protein is produced in *Escherichia coli* expression strain BLR (DE3). The fusion protein has been shown to possess antiviral activity *in vivo* and *in vitro* against HPV-16 and also cross reactivity against other strains, however, individual components of the combination, given separately or as mixture, show no clinical activity.

In an open-label, single arm interventional study conducted by Derkey et al.[77] in 8 university-affiliated medical centers, 27 patients aged 2–18 years were injected subcutaneously with HspE7 at monthly intervals for 3 doses after baseline surgical debridement. The study revealed significant decrease in posttreatment intersurgical interval as well as postintervention Derkey scoring, which was sustained over time. Therapy was well-tolerated, with only mild injection site reactions.

HspE7 therapy appears promising and needs further randomized large scale studies to establish comparative efficacy.

Mumps Vaccine

Use of mumps vaccine injection in RRP lesions is an intriguing hypothesis and has been tested in nonrandomized studies to offer benefits with a remission rate of around 80% with follow-up of up to 2 years with minimal, if any, side effects.[78,79] Although a pattern is reflected in these case series, specific attribution of benefits needs controlled trials.

ANTIREFLUX THERAPY IN RECURRENT RESPIRATORY PAPILLOMATOSIS

Antireflux treatment appears to be a rational therapy based on following effects:

- Preventing laryngeal mucosal damage
- Specific immunomodulatory effects of certain class of antacids.

Theoretically, mucosal damage and potential metaplastic changes caused by laryngopharyngeal reflux (LPR) can provide a milieu for viral implantation and propagation and also add onto the ongoing vocal deterioration already in effect by the established primary disease. Moreover, H_2 antihistaminic agents (ranitidine/cimetidine) have been shown to have immunomodulatory properties,[80] which can be expected to provide benefits against a number of viral affections, including RRP. Cimetidine at high doses (30–40 mg/kg) has been shown to shift the balance of helper T-cells in favor of TH1 response, increasing the TH1:TH2 ratio. Currently available case series and nonrandomized studies suggest that control of LPR can result in significant control of disease activity,[81,82] including in previously resistant cases[83] and possibly complete remission. Even though randomized controlled studies are still awaited for objectification, presently available literature supports the routine use of antireflux therapy as an adjunct to surgical treatment.

Retinoids

Retinoids are vitamin A analogs and have ability to alter *in vitro* differentiation of human laryngeal keratinocytes into ciliated, nonkeratinized epithelium and hence make the tissue microenvironment less conducive to viral affection. Deficiency of vitamin A has been shown to promote squamous differentiation in the upper aerodigestive tract while its excess can channel the differentiation toward mucous hyperplasia. Retinoids, however, are a class of proteins and different agents may have opposite effects on epithelial differentiation.[84]

With this background, 13 cis-retinoic acid (accutane) or isotretinoin, has been tried in cases affected with RRP in a dose of 1–2 mg/kg for up to 6 months or till the subject develops significant side effects.[85] The side effects with retinoids include skin peeling, cheilitis, photosensitivity and arthralgia. Liver function tests, blood counts with peripheral smear, urinalysis should be obtained prior to starting treatment and at 2 monthly intervals thereafter. In view of its teratogenic side effects, it should be used with extreme caution in women of childbearing age group.

Despite some case report favoring the use of accutane in RRP,[86,87] better designed studies have failed to reproduce the results and the double-blind placebo-controlled trial by Bell and colleagues[85] was halted prematurely because of severe side effects in all the subjects in the treatment arm, without appreciable effects on RRP disease activity. Another study has suggested a possible synergistic role of 13-cis retinoic acid with IFN in case of distal tracheobronchial spread of the disease.[88]

Cyclooxygenase-2 Inhibitors

The enzyme cyclooxygenase-2 (COX-2) has been shown to be over expressed in RRPs, mediated via epidermal growth factor, and to promote papillomata growth.[89] Celecoxib (celebrex) is a selective COX-2 inhibitor and has documented antipapilloma activity in rabbits. Based on the pilot data, a US National Institute of Health (NIH) funded multi-institutional, double-blinded, randomized controlled trial taking adults and children over 2 years of age is underway.

Acyclovir

Acyclovir is an antiviral agent which needs activation by the viral enzyme thymidine kinase. Despite the absence of this activating enzyme in HPV, it is interesting that effectiveness of this agent has been documented in several case series.[90-92] This antipapillomatous activity of acyclovir is probably because of its effect on coinfectors like Herpes simplex virus-1, cytomegalovirus and Epstein-Barr virus. Such coinfections have been observed in both children[93] and adults.[94] Adults with coinfection in RRP seem to run a more aggressive disease course.[95] Use of acyclovir in RRP has been shown to be largely free from adverse effects in the three case series reported till date. However, lack of controlled studies makes it difficult to reach any evidence-based conclusion.

Ribavirin

Ribavirin is an antiviral agent used most commonly for respiratory syncytial virus pneumonia in pediatric age group. Individual case report[95] and series[96,97] have shown some benefit with its use in RRP. Ribavirin is used at a dose of 23 mg/kg/day, divided in 4 daily doses, after an intravenous loading dose. Side effects of ribavirin therapy include moderate to severe anemia with reticulosis, headache and fatigue. A small randomized control trial by Ostrow and colleagues[98] showed an increase in post-treatment intersurgical interval. However, larger randomized studies are needed before the efficacy of its use can be established.

Zinc has been proposed as being useful in curtailing RRP in a single case report in a child with RRP with documented zinc deficiency. However, there are no other trials or evidence base to its use.[99]

Prophylactic Vaccination

There is huge amount of interest in research regarding prophylactic vaccination for HPV-associated diseases.

Currently two vaccines are approved for general use, working by way of induction of humoral immunity:

- *Cervarix*: a European-approved product of Glaxo-Smith-Kline is a bivalent vaccine composed of L1 epitopes of HPV 16 and 18. It has been shown to have efficacy for cervical cancer prevention.[100] However, being devoid of HPV 6 and 11 epitopes, it cannot be expected to provide protection against RRP or genital warts.[101]

- *Gardasil*, a product of Merck, was approved by the US FDA on June 8, 2006, following the recommendations of Advisory Committee on Immunization Practices (ACIP), based on phase III future II trial[102] and several well-designed phase II studies. It contains recombinant virus-like particles designed from L1 protein of HPV type 6, 11, 16 and 18. Hence in addition to being beneficial for cancer prevention, it can protect against benign lesions like warts and, by corollary, lesions like RRP. The ACIP recommendation state it to be administered to all girls aged 11–12 years, and as young as 9 years, as deemed necessary, with catch up vaccination for previously unvaccinated females aged 13–26 years.[103]

The neonatal transmission of HPV infection, and hence RRP affliction may theoretically be hampered via two mechanisms:

1. Direct humoral immunity transfer to the neonate from maternal antibody pool, and
2. Direct booster immunization of neonates "at risk", as in case of hepatitis B vaccination,[104] which needs further trials to assess the level and durability of neonatal immunization.

Immunization in conjunction with cesarean delivery before rupture of amnion may provide added benefits for protection at individual level.

Another aspect of HPV immunization is male vaccination,[105] which is already being implemented in Australia,[106] where the quadrivalent vaccine is registered for use in boys aged 9–15 years in addition to girl's vaccination, even though the infection is usually asymptomatic in males.[107] The idea is based on the legit concept of "Herd immunity" which states that all women and men in a specific age group be vaccinated so that the vaccine-protected individuals outnumber the infected once and with the vaccination of subsequent generation, the immunity is adapted by the community rather than being limited to individual level.

NEW FRONTIERS IN RECURRENT RESPIRATORY PAPILLOMATOSIS

There has been significant development in the field of immunopathogenesis and molecular targeting in the treatment of RRP lately, with ongoing research unfolding the basic pathophysiology of the disease, development of preventive and therapeutic vaccination being one of the impressive milestones. Some of the research areas are highlighted below.

The role of apoptosis dysregulation was explored by Poetker and colleagues,[108] who studied a host of apoptotic and antiapoptotic factors in relation to RRP pathophysiology. One of the peculiar proteins *survivin*, which is an antiapoptotic factor, expressed normally during developmental fetal stages as well as in certain preneoplastic and neoplastic conditions, was shown to be raised significantly, up to fivefold as compared to normal laryngeal epithelium. This antiapoptotic factor may be a potential future target for novel therapeutic strategies.

Another important molecular target in research has been the vascular endothelial growth factor-A (VEGF-A), involved in angiogenesis and also over expressed in certain neoplasms. This molecule has been retrospectively studied by Rahbar et al.[109] in 12 formalin-fixed laryngeal papilloma specimen and comparing them with 5 normal laryngeal autopsy samples, they showed that VEGF-A mRNA was strongly expressed in papilloma specimen and VEGF receptors 1 and 2 mRNA was seen to be expressed strongly in endothelium of vascular core of papillomas, compared to normal laryngeal epithelium where no such activity was seen. More specifically, HPV-16 E6 and E7 proteins can upregulate VEGF expression[110,111] and E5 increases VEGF expression via the EGFR pathway.[112] Recently a case report on use of bevacizumab, an anti-VEGF monoclonal antibody, was published by Nagel et al.[113] showing significant regression of intraparenchymal, pulmonary, nonmalignant lesions of RRP in an adult male in whom no other adjuvant therapy seemed to be promising. Thereafter, one retrospective chart review[114] and two prospective nonrandomized studies[115,116] have shown beneficial effect of combined photoangiolytic laser with sublesional bevacizumab injection in doses of up to 50 mg in single shot, without any appreciable local or systemic side effects. Future use for RRP may be promising and awaits randomized controlled trials.

Epidermal growth factor receptor (EGFR) is commonly over expressed in many head and neck carcinomas and for these cases it has shown promise as an adjuvant treatment. HPV-16 and 18 have been implicated in oropharyngeal cancers and in particular, HPV-16 viral protein E5 has been shown to enhance EGFR pathway activation.[117] EGFR over expression is also well documented in laryngeal papillomas[118] which are caused by the HPV types 6 and 11. Based on this background, EGFR inhibitors, like cituximab, have been used in case reports[119-121] and recently in a case series by Moldan et al.[122] taking four severely affected patients with RRP, resulting in improvement in Derkey score in all four of them and increased intersurgical interval in three out of four patients. However, no direct correlation has been proposed between level of EGFR expression and response of papillomas to EGFR inhibitor therapy. Moreover, in head and neck cancers, EGFR expression is greater in tobacco-associated cancers than HPV-related cases, and over expression of EGFR has been correlated with poor prognostication and a poor response to EGFR inhibitor therapy. Use of these agents in RRP needs a lot of research work before their use can be mainstreamed for this purpose.

The lifecycle of HPV is restricted to epithelium. There is no viremic phase during viral infection and propagation. The individuals with RRP seem to be unable to mount an adequate local immune response to HPV infection rather than being in a state of systemic immunodeficiency. This local immune defect is thought to be a reduced number of local dendritic cell population needed as an epithelial adaptive defense. Based on this idea, the concept of "*Dendritic cell vaccination*" is being developed by Dr Owain R Hughes.[123] The CD14+ve monocytes are harvested from peripheral blood and cultured over 5 days in presence of interleukin-4 (IL-4) and GMCSF to yield a population of immature dendritic cells. These immature cells are then primed to HPV 6 or 11 E6 epitopes for 24 hours and then transformed to a mature form by incubating in the presence of prostaglandin E2 (*PGE2) and tumor necrosis factor-alpha* (TNF-alpha). These mature dendritic cells can, and then act as antigen presenting cells to the T-cells causing a clonal expansion of cellular population active against RRP cells. Certain fatty acids, like conjugated linoleic acid (CLA) and eicosapentaenoic acid (EPA) are being proposed for concomitant therapy in RRP for their immunomodulatory properties, to restore the down regulated TH1 response in this disease.[124,125]

Finally, the largest area of active research is being undertaken by Buchinsky[126] and colleague as a multicenter initiative, recruiting 400 patients from 21 institutions, to explore the critical genes governing the susceptibility to RRP, of the few affected by this disease, despite hundreds of the neonates exposed to active infection during vaginal delivery.

RECURRENT RESPIRATORY PAPILLOMATOSIS RESOURCES

Accomplishments of RRP Task Force, initiated in 1994 following a survey of members of ASPO, the American Broncho-Esophagological Association (ABEA) and the American Academy of Otolaryngology–Head and Neck Surgery (AAO-HNS), need no introduction. Headed by Daniel Craig Derkay, MD (Eastern Virginia Medical School), huge amount of work in establishing a US nationwide registry with analysis of demographics, currently available treatments and the continued research activities with dissemination of knowledge regarding RRP is a big leap forward to fight RRP.

The RRP foundation is an internet-based community (www.rrpf.org), established in 1992. Directed by Bill Stern, it comprises of RRP patient's families, researchers and medical care providers and, provides invaluable information on the subject and a common platform to share them their experiences with the disease. The biannual newsletter serves to flash over the psychosocial aspects and new advancements and trials being run in the field of RRP. Another web-based resource community is active at website (www.rrpwebsite. org).

SUMMARY

Recurrent respiratory papillomatosis is a chronic unpredictably predictable disease affecting millions all over the world costing heavily on the health care system. It is caused by HPV type 6 and 11, with demonstrable biological differences between the two. It is unlikely to be diagnosed in the initial stages, unless kept in the mind with a high-index of suspicion. The treatment is surgical with some benefits of adjuvant therapy in certain cases, none of them being effective as stand-alone treatment. At present, even though it remains incurable, with the arrival of preventive and therapeutic vaccination, there are high hopes that future will unfold in favorable ways leading to RRP being a disease of past to be mentioned in books.

REFERENCES

1. Derkay CS. Task force on recurrent respiratory papillomatosis: a preliminary report. Arch Otolaryngol Head Neck Surg. 1995;121(12):1386-91.
2. Armstrong LR, Derkay CS, Reeves WC. Initial results from the national registry for juvenile-onset recurrent respiratory papillomatosis. RRP Task Force. Arch Otolaryngol Head Neck Surg. 1999;125:743.
3. Derkay CS. Recurrent respiratory papillomatosis. Laryngoscope. 2001;111(1):57-69.
4. Reeves WC, Ruparelia SS, Swanson KI, et al. National registry for juvenile-onset recurrent respiratory papillomatosis. Arch Otolaryngol Head Neck Surg. 2003;129(9):976-82.
5. Auborn KJ, Steinberg BM. In: Pfister H (Ed). Papillomaviruses and Human Cancer. Boca Raton, Florida: CRC Press; 1990.
6. Wiatrek BJ, Wiatrek DW, Broker TR, et al. Recurrent respiratory papillomatosis: a longitudinal study comparing severity associated with human papilloma viral types 6 and 11 and other risk factors in a large pediatric population. Laryngoscope. 2004;114:1-23.
7. Derkay CS, Darrow DH. Recurrent respiratory papillomatosis. Ann Otol Rhinol Laryngol. 2006;115(1):1-11.
8. Rihkaren H, Aaltonen LM, Syranen SM. Human papillomavirus in laryngeal papillomas and in adjacent normal epithelium. Clin Otolaryngol. 1993;18:470-4.
9. Smith EM, Pignatari SS, Gray SD, et al. Human papillomavirus infection in papillomas and nondiseased respiratory sites of

patients with recurrent respiratory papillomatosis using the polymerase chain reaction. Arch Otolaryngol Head Neck Surg. 1993;119(5):554-7.

10. Best SR, Niparko KJ, Pai SI. Biology of human papillomavirus infection and immune therapy for HPV-related head and neck cancers. Otolaryngol Clin North Am. 2012;45:807-22.

11. Kashima H, Mounts P, Leventhal B, et al. Sites of predilection in recurrent respiratory papillomatosis. Ann Otol Rhinol Laryngol. 1993;102:580-3.

12. Steinberg BM, DiLorenzo TP. A possible role for human papillomaviruses in head and neck cancer. Cancer Metastasis Rev. 1996;15:91.

13. Quick CA, Kryzek RA, Watt SL, et al. Relationship between condylomata and laryngeal papillomata clinical and molecular virological evidence. Ann Otol Rhinol Laryngol. 1980;89:467-71.

14. Hallden C, Majmudar B. The relationship between juvenile laryngeal papillomatosis and maternal condylomata acuminata. J Reprod Med. 1986;31:804-7.

15. Kashima HK, Shah F, Lyles A, et al. A comparison of risk factors in juvenile-onset and adult-onset recurrent respiratory papillomatosis. Laryngoscope. 1992;102:9-13.

16. Ho GY, Bierman R, Beardsley L, et al. Natural history of cervicovaginal papillomavirus infection in young women. N Engl J Med. 1998;338:423.

17. Bennett RS, Powell KR: Human papillomaviruses: associations between laryngeal papillomas and genital warts. Pediatr Infect Dis J. 1987; 6:229.

18. Silverberg MJ, Thorsen P, Lindeberg H, et al. Condyloma in pregnancy is strongly predictive of juvenile-onset recurrent respiratory papillomatosis. Obstet Gynecol. 2003;101:645.

19. Shah KV, Stern WF, Shah FK, et al. Risk factors for juvenile onset recurrent respiratory papillomatosis. Pediatr Infect Dis J. 1998;17:372.

20. Kosko JR, Derkay CS. Role of cesarean section in prevention of recurrent respiratory papillomatosis—is there one? Int J Pediatr Otorhinolaryngol. 1996;35:31.

21. Bonagura VR, Vambutas A, DeVoti JA, et al. HLA alleles, IFN-gamma responses to HPV-11 E6, and disease severity in patients with recurrent respiratory papillomatosis. Hum Immunol. 2004;65:773-82.

22. Shapiro AM, Rimell FL, Shoemaker D, et al. Tracheotomy in children with juvenile-onset recurrent respiratory papillomatosis: the Children's Hospital of Pittsburgh experience. Ann Otol Rhinol Laryngol. 1996;105:1.

23. Cole RR, Myer CM, Cotton RT. Tracheotomy in children with recurrent respiratory papillomatosis. Head Neck. 1989;11:226.

24. Dedo HH, Yu KC. CO2 laser treatment in 244 patients with respiratory papillomas. Laryngoscope. 2001;111:1639.

25. Katsenos S, Becker HD. Recurrent respiratory papillomatosis: a rare chronic disease, difficult to treat, with potential to lung cancer transformation: apropos of two cases and a brief literature review. Case Rep Oncol. 2011; 4(1):162-71.

26. Cook JR, Hill DA, Humphrey PA, et al. Squamous cell carcinoma arising in recurrent respiratory papillomatosis with pulmonary involvement: emerging common pattern of clinical features and human papillomavirus serotype association. Mod Pathol. 2000;13(8):914-8.

27. Derkay CS, Malis DJ, Zalzal G, et al. A staging system for assessing severity of disease and response to therapy in recurrent respiratory papillomatosis. Laryngoscope. 1998;108:935-7.

28. Hester RP, Derkay CS, Burke BL, et al. Reliability of a staging assessment system for recurrent respiratory papillomatosis. Int J Pediatr Otorhinolaryngol. 2003;67:505-9.

29. Stern AY. Felipovich. RT, Segal CK. Immunocompetency in children with recurrent respiratory papillomatosis: prospective study, Ann. Otol. Rhinol. Laryngol. 2007;116(3):169-71.

30. Bonagura VR, Hatam L, DeVoti J, et al. Recurrent respiratory papillomatosis: altered CD8(+) T-cell subsets and T(H)1/T(H)2 cytokine imbalance. Clin. Immunol. 1999;93(3):302-11.

31. DeVoti JA, Steinberg BM, Rosenthal DW, et al. Failure of gamma interferon but not interleukin-10 expression in response to human papillomavirus type 11 E6 protein in respiratory papillomatosis. Clin Diagn Lab Immunol. 2004;11(3):538-47.

32. Vambutas A, Bonagura VR, Steinberg BM. Altered expression of TAP-1 and major histocompatibility complex class I in laryngeal papillomatosis: correlation of TAP-1 with disease. Clin Diagn Lab Immunol. 2000;7(1):79-85.

33. Bonagura VR, Du Z, Ashouri E, et al. Activating killer cell immunoglobulin-like receptors 3DS1 and 2DS1 protect against developing the severe form of recurrent respiratory papillomatosis. Hum. Immunol. 2010;71(2):212-9.

34. Gelder CM, Williams OM, Hart KW, et al. HLA class II polymorphisms and susceptibility to recurrent respiratory papillomatosis. J Virol. 2003;77(3):1927-39.

35. Derkay CS, Darrow DH. Recurrent respiratory papillomatosis of the larynx: current diagnosis and treatment. Otolaryngol Clin North Am. 2000;33(5):1127-41.

36. Andrus GJ, Shapshay SM. Contemporary management of laryngeal papilloma in adults and children. Otolarygol Clin N Am. 2006;39:135-58.

37. Hallmo P, Naess O. Laryngeal papillomatosis with human papillomavirus DNA contracted by a laser surgeon. Eur Arch Otorhinolaryngol. 1991;248:425.

38. Kashima HK, Kessis T, Mounts P, et al. Polymerase chain reaction identification of human papillomavirus DNA in CO_2 laser plume from recurrent respiratory papillomatosis. Otolaryngol Head Neck Surg. 1991;104:191.

39. Valdez TA, McMillan K, Shapshay SM. A new laser treatment for vocal cord papilloma 585-nm pulsed dye. Otolaryngol Head Neck Surg. 2001;124:421-5.

40. Franco RA Jr, Zeitels SM, Farinelli WA, et al. 585-nm pulsed dye laser treatment of glottal papillomatosis. Ann Otol Rhinol Laryngol. 2002;111:486-92.

41. Myer CM, Willging JP, McMurray S, et al. Use of a laryngeal micro resector system. Laryngoscope. 1999;109(7):1165-6.

42. Hoff SR, Koltai PJ. Operative management of juvenile-onset recurrent respiratory papillomatosis. Oper Tech Otolaryngol. 2012;23:117-123.

43. Schraff S, Derkay CS, Burke B, et al. American Society of Pediatric Otolaryngology members' experience with recurrent respiratory papillomatosis and the use of adjuvant therapy. Arch Otolaryngol Head Neck Surg. 2004;130(9):1039-042.

44. Kimberlin DW. Acyclovir derivatives and other new antiviral agents. Semin Pediatr Infect Dis. 2001;12:224-34.

45. Safrin S, Cherrington J, Jaffe H. Cidofovir: review of current and potential clinical uses. Antiviral Chemo. 1999;5:111-20.

46. Derkay C. Cidofovir for recurrent respiratory papillomatosis (RRP): a re-assessment of risks. Int J Pediatr Otorhinolaryngol. 2005;69(11):1465-7.

47. Lindsay F, Bloom D, Pransky S, et al. Histologic review of cidofovir-treated recurrent respiratory papillomatosis. Ann Otol Rhinol Laryngol. 2008;117:113-7.

48. Sajan JA, Kerschner JE, Merati AL, et al. Prevalence of dysplasia in juvenile-onset recurrent respiratory papillomatosis. Arch Otolaryngol Head Neck Surg. 2010;136:7-11.

49. Blumin JH, Handler EB, Simpson CB, et al. Dysplasia in adults with recurrent respiratory papillomatosis: incidence and risk factors. Ann Otol Rhinol Laryngol. 2009;118:481-5.

50. Shehab N, Sweet BV, Hogikyan ND. Cidofovir for the treatment of recurrent respiratory papillomatosis: a review of the literature. Pharmacotherapy. 2005; 25(7):977-89.

51. Abdulkarim B, Sabri S, Deutsch E, et al. Antiviral agent cidofivir restores p53 function and enhances the radiosensitivity in HPV-associated cancers. Oncogene. 2002;21:2334-46.

52. Van Cutsem E, Snoeck R, Van Ranst M, et al. Successful treatment of a squamous papilloma of the hypopharynx-esophagus by local injections of (S)-1-(3-hydroxy-2-phosphonylmethoxypropyl) cytosine. J Med Virol. 1995;45:230-5.

53. Snoeck R, Wellens W, Desloovere C, et al. Treatment of severe laryngeal papillomatosis with intralesional injections of cidofovir [(S)-1-(3-hydroxy-2 phosphonylmethoxypropyl) cytosine]. J Med Virol. 1998;54(3):219-25.

54. Pransky SM, Magit AE, Kearns DB, et al. Intralesional cidofovir for recurrent respiratory papillomatosis in children. Arch Otolaryngol Head Neck Surg. 1999;125(10):1143-8.

55. Pransky SM, Brewster DF, Magit AE, et al. Clinical update on 10 children treated with intralesional cidofovir injections for severe recurrent respiratory papillomatosis. Arch Otolaryngol Head Neck Surg. 2000;126(10):1239-43.

56. Wilson WR, Hashemiyoon R, Hawrych A. Intralesional cidofovir for recurrent laryngeal papillomas: preliminary report. Ear Nose Throat J. 2000;79(4):236-8, 240.

57. Chhetri DK, Blumin JH, Shapiro NL, et al. Office-based treatment of laryngeal papillomatosis with percutaneous injection of cidofovir. Otolaryngol Head Neck Surg. 2002;126(6):642-8.

58. Naiman AN, Abedipour D, Ayari S, et al. Natural history of adult onset laryngeal papillomatosis following multiple cidofovir injections. Ann Otol Rhinol Laryngol. 2006;115(3):175-81.

59. Kimberlin DW. Current status of antiviral therapy for juvenile-onset recurrent respiratory papillomatosis. Antiviral Res. 2004;63(3):141-51.

60. McMurray JS, Connor N, Ford CN. Cidofovir efficacy in recurrent respiratory papillomatosis: a randomized, double-blind, placebo-controlled study. Ann Otol Rhinol Laryngol. 2008;117:477-483.

61. Derkay CS, Volsky PG, Rosen CA, et al. Current use of intralesional cidofovir for recurrent respiratory papillomatosis. Larygoscope. 2012;123(3):705-12.

62. Haglund S, Lundquist P, Cantell K, et al. Interferon therapy in juvenile laryngeal papillomatosis. Arch Otolaryngol Head Neck Surg. 1981;107:327-32.

63. McCabe BF, Clark KF. Interferon and laryngeal papillomatosis. The Iowa experience. Ann Otol Rhinol Laryngol. 1983;92(1): 2-7.

64. Lusk RB, McCabe BF, Mixon JH. Three year-experience of treating recurrent respiratory papilloma with interferon. Ann Otol Rhinol Laryngol. 1987;96:158-62.

65. Kashima H, Levethal B, Dedo H, et al. Interferon alfa-n1 (Wellferon) in juvenile onset recurrent respiratory papillomatosis: results of a randomized study in twelve collaborative institutions. Laryngoscope. 1988;98:334-40.

66. Healy GB, Gelber RD, Trowbridge AL, et al. Treatment of recurrent respiratory papillomatosis with human leukocyte interferon: results of a multicenter randomized clinical trial. N Engl J Med. 1988;319(7):401-7.

67. Leventhal BG, Kashima HK, Mounts P, et al. Long-term response of recurrent respiratory papillomatosis to treatment with lymphoblastoid interferon alfa-N1. Papilloma Study Group. N Engl J Med. 1991;325(9):613-7.

68. Gerein V, Rastorguev E, Gerein J, et al. Use of interferon-alpha in recurrent respiratory papillomatosis: 20-year follow-up. Ann Otol Rhinol Laryngol. 2005;114(6):463-71.

69. Suter-Montano T, Montano E, Martinez C, et al. Adult recurrent respirator papillomatosis: a new therapeutic approach with pegylated interferon alpha 2a (Peg-IFNα-2a) and GM-CSF. Otolaryngol Head Neck Surg. 2013;148(2):253-60.

70. Dougherty TJ, Gomer CJ, Henderson BW, et al. Photodynamic therapy. J Natl Cancer Inst. 1998;90:889-905.

71. Abramson AL, Shikowitz MJ, Mullooly VM, et al. Variable light-dose effect on photodynamic therapy for laryngeal papillomas. Arch Otolaryngol Head Neck Surg. 1994;120:852-5.

72. Shikowitz MJ, Abramson AL, Steinberg BM, et al. Clinical trial of photodynamic therapy with meso-tetra (hydroxyphenyl) chlorin for respiratory papillomatosis. Arch Otolaryngol Head Neck Surg. 2005;131(2):99-105.

73. Lee RG, Vecchiotti MA, Heaphy J, et al. Photodynamic therapy of cottontail rabbit papillomavirus-induced papillomas in a severe combined immunodeficient mouse xenograft system. Laryngoscope. 2010;120(3):618-24.

74. Newfield KM, Goldsmith A, Bradlow HL, et al. Estrogen metabolism and human papillomavirus- induced tumors of the larynx: chemoprophylaxis with indole-3-carbinol. Anticancer Res. 1993;13:337-42.

75. Rosen CA, Woodson GE, Thompson JW, et al. Preliminary result of the use of indole-3-carbinol for recurrent respiratory papillomatosis. Otolaryngol Head Neck Surg. 1998;118: 810-5.

76. Rosen CA, Bryson PC. Indole-3-carbinol for recurrent respiratory papillomatosis: long-term results. J Voice. 2004;18(2):248-53.

77. Derkay CS, Smith RJH, McClay J, et al. HspE7 treatment of pediatric recurrent respiratory papillomatosis: final results of an open-label trial. Ann Otol Rhinol Laryngol. 2005;114(9):730-7.

78. Pashley NR. Can mumps vaccine induce remission in recurrent respiratory papilloma? Arch Otolaryngol Head Neck Surg. 2002;128(7):783-6.

79. Lieu JE, Molter DW. Another potential adjuvant therapy for recurrent respiratory papillomatosis. Arch Otolaryngol Head Neck Surg. 2002;128(7):787-8.

80. Brockmeyer NH, Kreuzfelder E, Chalabi N, et al. The immunomodulatory potency of cimetidine in healthy volunteers. Int J Clin Pharmacol Ther Toxicol. 1989;27:458-62.

81. Borkowski G, Sommer P, Stark T, et al. Recurrent respiratory papillomatosis associated with gastroesophageal reflux disease in children. Eur Arch Otorhinolaryngol. 1999;256(7):370-2.

82. Harcourt JP, Worley G, Leighton SE. Cimetidine treatment for recurrent respiratory papillomatosis. Int J Pediatr Otorhinolaryngol. 1999;51(2):109-13.

83. McKenna M, Brodsky L. Extraesophageal acid reflux and recurrent respiratory papilloma in children. Int J Pediatr Otorhinolaryngol. 2005; 69:597.

84. Lotan R. Effects of vitamin A and its analogs (retinoids) on normal and neoplastic cells. Biochim Biophys Acta. 1980;605:33.

85. Bell R, Hong WK, Itri LM, et al. The use of cisretinoic acid in recurrent respiratory papillomatosis of the larynx: a randomized pilot study. Am J Otolaryngol. 1988;9:161-4.

86. Eicher S, Taylor-Cooley L, Donovan D. Isoretinoin therapy for recurrent respiratory papillomatosis. Arch Otolaryngol Head Neck Surg. 1994;120:405-9.

87. Osborne C, LeBoeuf H, Jones D. Isotretinoin in respiratory papillomatosis. Ann Intern Med. 2000;132:1007.

88. Lindeberg H, Elbrond O. Laryngeal papillomas: The epidemiology in a Danish subpopulation 1965-1984. Clinical Otolaryngol. 1991;l5(2):125-31.

89. Wu R, Coniglio SJ, Chan A, et al. Up-regulation of Rac1 by epidermal growth factor mediates COX-2 expression in recurrent respiratory papillomas. Mol Med. 2007;13:143.

90. Kiroglu M, Cetik F, Soylu L, et al. Acyclovir in the treatment of recurrent respiratory papillomatosis: a preliminary report. Am J Otolaryngol. 1994;15(3):212-4.

91. Endres DR, Bauman NM, Burke D, et al. Acyclovir in the treatment of recurrent respiratory papillomatosis. A pilot study. Ann Otol Rhinol Laryngol. 1994;103(4):301-5.

92. Lopez AD, Perez PB, Betancor L, et al. Acyclovir in the treatment of laryngeal papillomatosis. Int J Pediatr Otorhinolaryngol. 1991;21(3):269-74.

93. Rimmell F, Shoemaker D, Pu A, et al. Pediatric respiratory papillomatosis: prognostic role of viral typing and cofactors. Laryngoscope. 1997;107:915-8.

94. Pou A, Rimmell F, Jordan J, et al. Adult respiratory papillomatosis: human papillomavirus type and viral coinfections as predictors of prognosis. Ann Otol Rhinol Laryngol. 1995;104:758-62.

95. Balauff A, Sira J, Pearman K, et al. Successful ribavirin therapy for life-threatening laryngeal papillomatosis post liver transplantation. Pediatr Transplant. 2001;5(2):142-4.

96. McGlennen RC, Adams GL, Lewis CM, et al. Pilot trial of ribavirin for the treatment of laryngeal papillomatosis. Head Neck. 1993;15(6):504-12.

97. Morrison GA, Kotecha B, Evans JN. Ribavirin treatment for juvenile respiratory papillomatosis. J Laryngol Otol. 1993;107(5):423-6.

98. Ostrow M. Proceedings of 17th International Papillomavirus Conference. Charleston, SC, 1999.

99. Bitar M, Baz R, Fuleihan N, et al. Can zinc be an adjuvant therapy for juvenile onset recurrent respiratory papillomatosis? Int J Pediatr Otorhinolaryngol. 2007;71:1163-73.

100. Paavonen J, Jenkins D, Bosch FX, et al. Efficacy of a prophylactic adjuvanted bivalent L1 virus-like particle vaccine against infection with HPV types 16 and 18 in young women: an interim analysis of a phase II double-blind, randomized controlled trial. Lancet. 2007;369:2161-70.

101. Pederson C, Petaja T, Strauss G, et al. Immunization of early adolescent females with HPV type 16 and 18 L1 virus-like particle vaccine containing ASO4 adjuvant. J Adolesc Health. 2007;40:564-71.

102. Villa LL, Costa RL, Petta CA, et al. Prophylactic quadrivalent HPV (types 6,11, 16 and 18) L1 virus-like particle vaccine in young women: a randomized double-blind placebo-controlled multi-centre phase II efficacy trial. Lancet Oncol. 2005;6: 271-8.

103. Markowitz LE, Dunne EF, Saraiya M, et al. Quadrivalent HPV: recommendations of the ACIP. MMWR Recomm Reports. 2007;56(2):1-24.

104. Schaffer A, Brotherton J, Booy R. Do human papillomavirus vaccines have any role in newborns and the prevention of recurrent respiratory papillomatosis in children? J Paediatr Child Health. 2007;43(9):579-80.

105. Block SL, Nolan T, Sattler C, et al. Comparison of the immunogenicity and reactogenecity of a prophylactic quadrivalent human papillomavirus (types 6,11, 16 and 18) L1 virus-like particle vaccine in male and female adolescents and young adult women. Pediatrics. 2006;118:2135-45.

106. May J. HPV vaccination-a paradigm shift in public health. Aust Fam Physician. 2007;36(3):106-11.

107. Gallagher TQ, Derkay CS. Recurrent respiratory papillomatosis: update 2008. Curr Opin Otolaryngol Head Neck Surg. 2008;16(6):536-42.

108. Poetker DM, Sankler AD, Scott CL, et al. Survivin expression in juvenile-onset recurrent respiratory papillomatosis. Ann Otol Rhinol Laryngol. 2002;111:957-61.

109. Rahbar R, Vargas SO, Folkman J, et al. Role of vascular endothelial growth factor-A in recurrent respiratory papillomatosis. Ann Otol Rhinol Laryngol. 2005;114:289-95.

110. Lopez-Ocejo O, Viloria-Petit A, Bequet-Romero M, et al. Oncogenes and tumor angiogenesis: the HPV-16 E6 oncoprotein activates the vascular endothelial growth factor (VEGF) gene promoter in a p53 independent manner. Oncogene. 2000; 19(40):4611-20.

111. Walker J, Smiley LC, Ingram D, et al. Expression of human papillomavirus type 16 E7 is sufficient to significantly increase expression of angiogenic factors but is not sufficient to induce endothelial cell migration. Virology. 2011;410(2):283-90.

112. Kim SH, Juhnn YS, Kang S, et al. Human papillomavirus 16 E5 up-regulates the expression of vascular endothelial growth factor through the activation of epidermal growth factor receptor, MEK/ ERK1,2 and PI3K/Akt. Cell Mol Life Sci. 2006; 63(7–8):930-8.

113. Nagel S, Busch C, Blankenburg T, et al. Behandlung der respiratorischen Papillomatose--Kasuistik zur systemischen Therapie mit Bevacizumab [Treatment of respiratory papillomatosis—a case report on systemic treatment with bevacizumab]. Pneumologie. 2009;63(7):387-9.

114. Zeitels SM, Lopez-Guerra G, Burns JA, et al. Microlaryngoscopic and office-based injection of bevacizumab (Avastin) to enhance 532-nm pulsed KTP laser treatment of glottal papillomatosis. Ann Otol Rhinol Laryngol Suppl. 2009;201: 1-13.

115. Rogers DJ, Ojha S, Maurer R, et al. Use of adjuvant intralesional bevacizumab for aggressive respiratory papillomatosis in children. JAMA Otolaryngol Head Neck Surg. 2013;139(5):496-501.

116. Zeitels SM, Lopez-Guerra G, Burns JA, et al. Local injection of bevacizumab (Avastin) and angiolytic KTP laser

treatment of recurrent respiratory papillomatosis of the vocal folds: a prospective study. Ann Otol Rhinol Laryngol. 2011;120(10):627-34.

117. Pim D, Collins M, Banks L. Human papillomavirus type 16 E5 gene stimulates the transforming activity of the epidermal growth factor receptor. Oncogene. 1992;7(1):27-32.

118. Johnston D, Hall H, Di Lorenzo TP, et al. Elevation of the epidermal growth factor receptor and dependent signaling in human papillomavirus-infected laryngeal papillomas. Cancer Res. 1999;59(4):968-74.

119. Bostrom B, Sidman J, Marker S, et al. Gefitinib therapy for Life-threatening Laryngeal Papillomatosis. Arch Otolaryngol Head Neck Surg. 2005;131(1): 64-7.

120. Limsukon A, Susanto I, Soo Hoo GW, et al. Regression of Recurrent Respiratory Papillomatosis with Celecoxib and Erlotinib Combination Therapy. Chest. 2009;136(3): 924-6.

121. Loyo M, Pai SI, Netto GJ, et al. Aggressive recurrent respiratory papillomatosis in a neonate. Int J Pediatr Otorhinolaryngol. 2008;72(6):917-20.

122. Moldan MM, Bostrom BC, Tibesar RJ, et al. Epidermal growth factor receptor inhibitor therapy for recurrent respiratory papillomatosis. F1000Research. 2013;2:202.

123. HughesOR. Toward prevention or cure for recurrent respiratory papillomatosis. Laryngoscope. 2012;122(4):S63-4.

124. Louw L, Seedat R, Claassen A. HPV-induced recurrent laryngeal papillomatosis: fatty acid role-players. Asia Pac J Clin Nutr. 2008;17:208-11.

125. Louw L. Effects of conjugated linoleic acid and high oleic acid safflower oil in the treatment of children with HPV-induced laryngeal papillomatosis: a randomized, double-blinded and crossover preliminary study. Lipids Health Dis. 2012;11:136.

126. Buchinsky FJ, Derkay CS, Leal SM, et al. Multicenter initiative seeking critical genes in respiratory papillomatosis. Laryngoscope. 2004;114(2):349-57.

Lasers in Phonosurgery and Laryngology

KK Handa

INTRODUCTION

Laser is another technologically advanced tool in the armamentarium of ENT (ear, nose, and throat) surgeons in general and laryngologists in particular. The types of lasers used in laryngology include carbon dioxide (CO_2) laser, Nd:YAG (neodymium: yttrium-aluminum-garnet), diode and KTP (potassium-titanyl-phosphate) laser. CO_2 laser is rod delivery laser while the rest are fiber lasers. However, recently, even CO_2 laser has come in a fiber mode, e.g. omniguide and waveguide.

Carbon dioxide laser is the best accepted international standard for precise work in the larynx. The laser scores over the cold instrumentation in precision, better healing, hemostasis and less scarring. The CO_2 laser induces very little collateral thermal tissue interaction when compared with other wavelengths used in the medical field, e.g. Nd:YAG laser, argon laser, or KTP laser. The CO_2 thermal penetration ranges in microns, whereas that of other wavelengths ranges in millimeters.[1] These features make the CO_2 laser the surgical workhorse when tissue incision or vaporization with minimum concomitant collateral damage is required.[1] The wavelength of CO_2 laser (10.6 μm) lies outside the visible spectrum and therefore an aiming beam of helium neon/diode is required. The latest generation CO_2 laser is equipped with the robotic scanner and AcuBlade. The AcuBlade is a scanner software which allows the beam to travel across the target as a straight or curved line. Various lengths 0.5–3.5 mm and various depths 0.2–2.0 mm are programmable.

Before starting a laser program in laryngology with CO_2 laser it is important that the surgeon checks the compatibility of the microscope, micromanipulator, and the laser machine (Fig. 1).

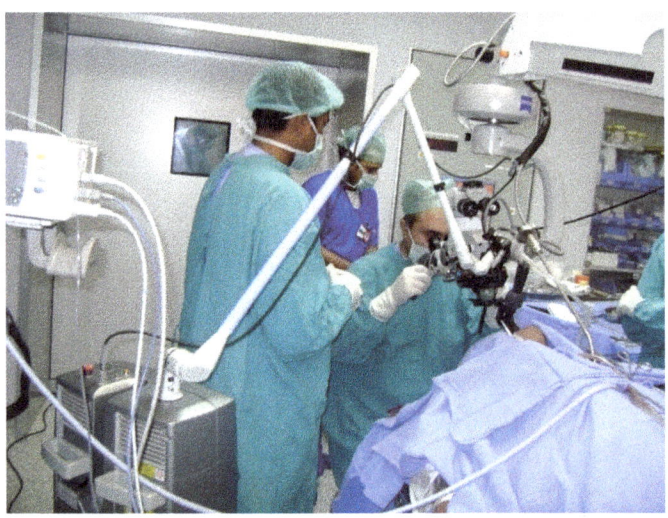

Fig. 1 Use of carbon dioxide Lumenis system with micromanipulator and robotic scanner

Also required are certain specific instruments including jet black laryngoscopes to prevent reflection and having a smoke evacuator (Fig. 2).

LASER SAFETY PROTOCOL

Before any laser surgery, an exhaustive laser safety protocol needs to be followed and includes:
- Wearing of protective eyewear for the surgeon, personnel around, and the patient
- Avoidance of inflammable gases like nitrous oxide. Air-oxygen mixture is preferred and fraction of inspired oxygen (FiO_2) needs to be less than 30

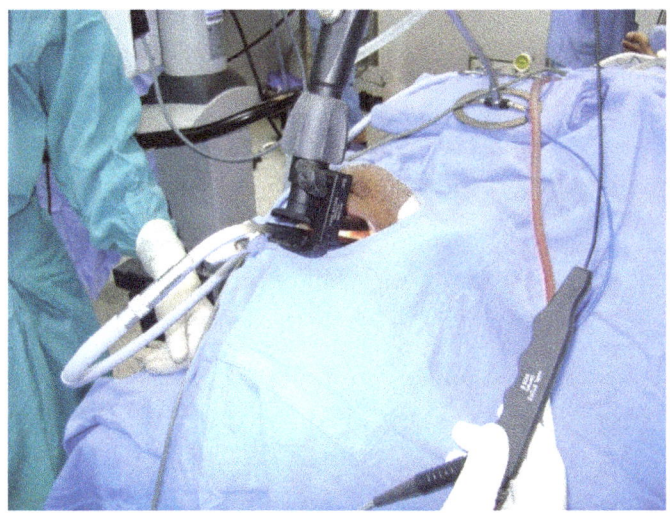

Fig. 2 Use of Steiner adjustable flange laryngoscope with a smoke evacuator

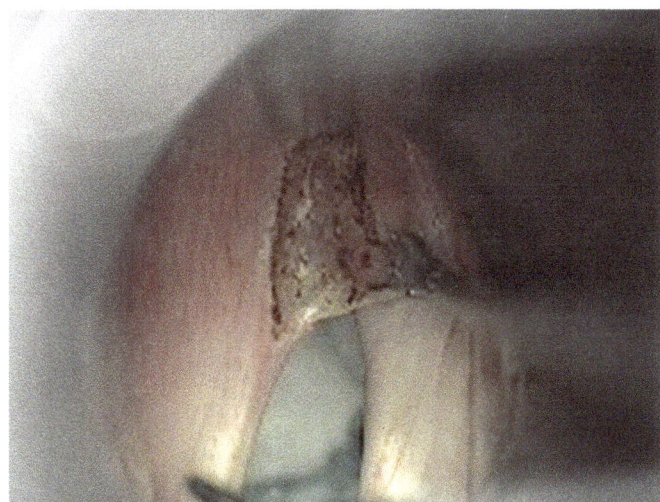

Fig. 3 Raising of a microflap with carbon dioxide laser

- Any combustible materials like charred tissue, gauze, etc. must be away from the beam
- It is preferable to use laser protective endotracheal tubes.
- Display of warning board outside the operation theater.

VOCAL CORD CYSTS AND POLYPS

Carbon dioxide laser can be used very successfully for intracordal cysts using the mini microflap technique (Fig. 3). The vocal cord cysts are of two types: mucus retention cyst and the epidermoid cysts. The vocal cord cysts lie very close to the vocal ligament; hence high degree of precision is required in dealing with them. The use should only be in expert hands and a beginner should use phonomicrosurgical techniques. An epithelial cordotomy 1 mm lateral to the cyst is done and the cyst is grasped with Bouchayer forcep and separated medially from the epithelium and laterally from the vocal ligament. In case the cyst ruptures care must be taken to remove the entire epithelium. The epithelium needs to be redraped. CO_2 laser gives the right amount of precision required in dealing with a lesion as delicate as an epidermoid cyst. The AcuBlade system has been shown to be a better alternative in this setting.[2]

Carbon dioxide laser is also useful for removing benign lesions like polyps and is especially useful for hemorrhagic or telangiectatic polyps (Fig. 4).

ABDUCTOR CORD PARALYSIS

Carbon dioxide laser is a very effective tool for the management of bilateral abductor cord paralysis. Posterior transverse laser cordotomy (PTLC) was first described by Dennis and Kashima[3] as a technique for providing an airway at the posterior glottis without preoperative tracheotomy; they

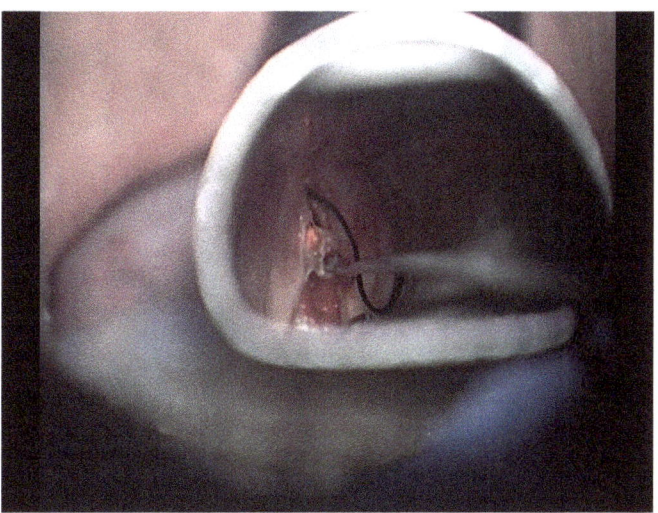

Fig. 4 Carbon dioxide laser for a laryngeal polyp

reported it as a successful method with satisfactory functional results. The other procedures include posterior cordectomy with or without partial arytenoidectomy, suture lateralization with longitudinal laser cordotomy.

LEUKOPLAKIA AND KERATOSIS

Carbon dioxide laser is a very effective tool for dealing with leukoplakia and keratotic lesions of the vocal cords (Fig. 5).

RECURRENT RESPIRATORY PAPILLOMATOSIS

Recurrent respiratory papillomatosis is another suitable condition for microsurgery using CO_2 laser. The laser may be used alone or along with a soft-tissue shaver (microdebrider). The soft-tissue shaver is used to debulk the papillomas and CO_2 laser is used for fine work. The use of CO_2 laser is likely to produce very little damage to the vocal cords. This is a very important aspect as these patients need to undergo repeat surgeries because of the biological behavior of the papillomas and once vocal cords are scarred cannot be corrected.

EARLY LARYNGEAL CANCER

Transoral laser surgery for early laryngeal cancer is an accepted modality today. The benefits are of short treatment duration, lower costs, oncological control similar to radiotherapy and possibility of successive treatments. The argument of better

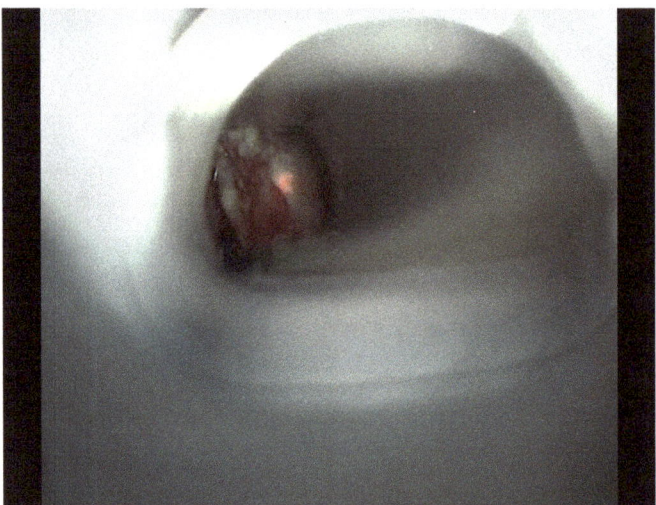

Fig. 5 Keratosis of vocal cords; carbon dioxide laser being used in an ablative mode

voice results with radiotherapy may not be entirely true today. Endoscopic laser surgery offers overall voice quality equivalent to that of radiotherapy for patients with T1a midcord glottic carcinoma. In lesions beyond T1a, the voice improves with speech therapy or primary or secondary vocal cord reconstruction can be done with autologous fat or other materials.

A retrospective cohort study[4] was conducted of all individuals who received either radiation therapy (RT) or transoral laser microsurgery (TLM) for the treatment of Tis or T1a glottis squamous cell carcinoma (SCC) between 2004 and 2009 at the London Regional Cancer Program.[5] The primary outcome measure was voice-related quality of life (V-RQOL), as assessed by the V-RQOL questionnaire. Secondary outcomes included local control, overall survival, and laryngectomy-free survival. 57 patients were eligible for this study; 34 received RT and 23 received TLM. 40 (70.2%) of the 57 patients completed the V-RQOL. No statistically significant difference in total V-RQOL score was observed between the RT and TLM cohorts (p = 0.228). There was, however, a trend toward higher scores (i.e. less voice disability) in the physical function domain of the V-RQOL for the RT group (90.0%) as compared to the TLM group (80.2%) (p = 0.05). No significant differences were observed in recurrence or overall survival between the two groups. The study concluded that both oncologic outcomes and self-rated V-RQOL are similar in patients treated with RT and TLM for early-glottic carcinoma.

Another study by Peretti et al.[6,7] did a cost analysis, comparison of voice results and the curative results between external beam radiation and laser surgery for early cancer larynx (Figs 6A and B). The study concluded that cure rates are equal; voice results are comparable and the total cost of external radiotherapy significantly higher as compared to the laser surgery for early cancer larynx and the author

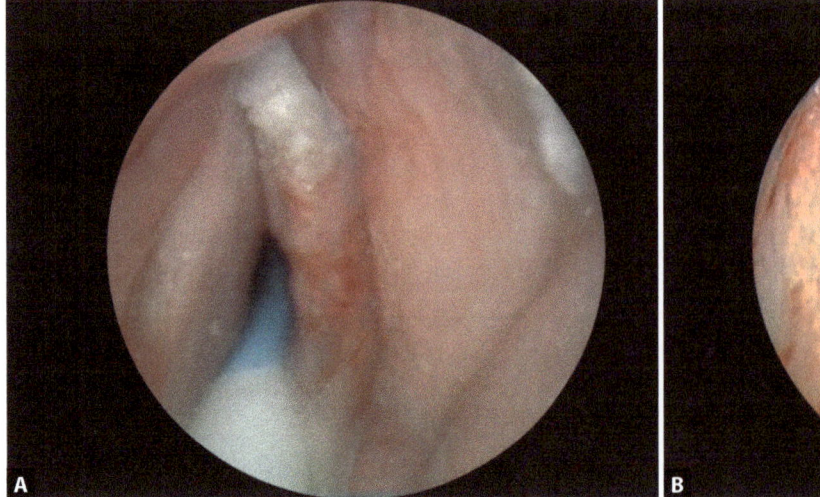
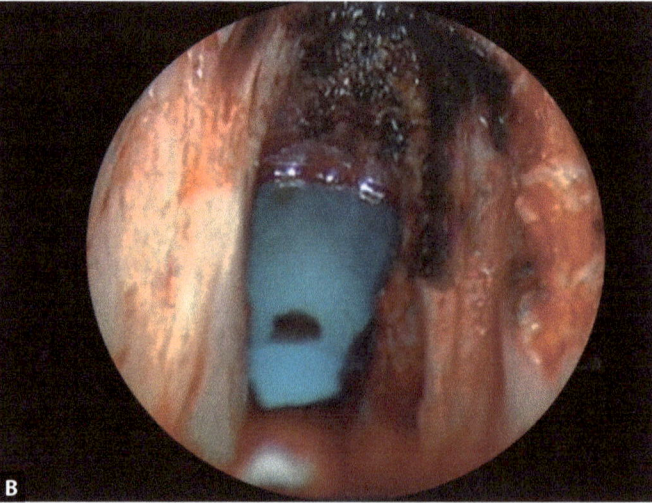

Figs 6A and B Laser excision of early cancer larynx confined to one cord: Intraoperative picture

recommended laser surgery over external beam radiotherapy. Peretti et al.[7,8] also confirmed good surgical outcomes for T1, Tis and selected T2 and T3 glottic tumors with laser. They also achieved high rates (65%) of rescue endoscopic retreatment in case of early detected local failure, achieving an ultimate local control with laser alone of 93.4%, 95%, 85.6%, and 71.6% for Tis, T1, T2, and T3, respectively. Another study[8] from the same center concluded that selected recurrences after primary RT for T1 and T2 glottic carcinoma are eligible for endoscopic salvage surgery with oncologic results comparable to those with open neck procedures but with a lower complication rate and a favorable functional outcome.

VOCAL CORD POLYPS

Carbon dioxide laser has been advocated for the treatment of benign vocal fold lesions since Benninger's 2000 randomized trial[9] demonstrated the absence of difference in outcomes on blinded comparisons of stroboscopy, voice quality or recovery between cold instruments and laser in the treatment of benign superficial vocal fold lesions. With improvement introduction of the AcuBlade system the results are getting better.

Laser is of benefit in vascular polyps where it scores over conventional instruments in terms of hemostasis and precision.

VASCULAR LESIONS

Vascular lesions, like hemangiomas of larynx, subglottic hemangioma in children, are very suitably dealt with the CO_2 laser.

LARYNGOTRACHEAL STENOSIS

Most commonly used in the airway for laryngotracheal stenosis are CO_2, Nd:YAG and the KTP laser. The CO_2 laser has been the mainstay in the management of most airway lesions because of surgeon's familiarity and its precise cutting properties. Its main drawback is difficulty with delivery of the beam through the subglottiscope or bronchoscope. The development of microsubglottoscopy with specially designed scopes and more sophisticated micromanipulators has overcome this problem to a large degree. The Nd:YAG laser has the advantage of transmission through flexible fibers and delivery by either contact or noncontact mode. This greatly facilitates its use via the bronchoscope when addressing tracheal stenosis. Nd:YAG laser also offers good hemostatic properties, but its heat diffusion characteristics may cause surrounding thermal damage. KTP is a better hemostat because of it preferential absorption by hemoglobin.[9]

Laser is useful for limited stenosis of larynx and trachea. Stenosis of the supraglottic and glottic larynx may be approached with standard suspension microlaryngoscopy while exposing stenosis of the subglottis or upper trachea may require the rigid bronchoscope or specially designed subglottiscopes.[10] As described by Ossoff et al.,[11] the subglottiscope modification of the Dedo laryngoscope provides access to the subglottis with a port for jet ventilation, while still allowing the use of the microscope and the CO_2 laser aiming system. Laser is also useful for managing postoperative granulations and webs in the glottis.

Laryngomalacia

It is normally a self-limiting condition in children and here CO_2 laser can be very effectively used if the condition does not improve.

Sleep Surgery

With surgery for sleep disorders and snoring gaining more acceptance lasers are being commonly used for palate procedures, such as LAUP (laser-assisted uvulopalatoplasty), uvulopalatal flap, tonsillectomies and for base of tongue reduction.

Office-based Laser Surgery

Kaufmann et al.[12] have described good results with unsedated office-based laser surgery (UOLS) of the larynx and trachea for laryngotracheal pathology including recurrent respiratory papillomas, granulomas, leukoplakia, and polypoid degeneration. UOLS delivered by flexible endoscopes has dramatically impacted office-based surgery by reducing the time, costs, and morbidity of surgery. Of the 443 cases, 406 were performed with the pulsed-dye laser, 10 with the CO_2 laser, and 27 with the thulium: yttrium-aluminum-garnet laser. There were no significant complications in this series. Use of office-based laser procedure is gaining popularity, especially in USA because of avoidance of general anesthesia, shorter duration, and cost advantage.

Laser Use with Robotic Systems

Now with the popularization of transoral robotic surgery lasers using Da Vinci robots laser systems, which are compatible with the robotic arms, are being developed as laser cutting is more precise and heals with less scarring than commonly used diathermy-based cutting or coagulation instruments. Thulium and CO_2 fibers have been used in some centers with good success.[13]

CONCLUSION

Laser is a useful tool which scores over conventional instrumentation in terms of better precision, better hemostasis, and less surrounding tissue damage resulting in less postoperative scarring. However, a proper case selection, proper laser safety precautions, and surgeons and personnel properly trained are a prelude to running a proper laser program.

REFERENCES

1. Remacle M, Hassan F, Cohen D, et al. New computer-guided scanner for improving CO_2 laser-assisted microincision. Eur Arch Otorhinolaryngol Head Neck. 2005;262(2):113-9.
2. Matar N, Amoussa K, Verduyckt I, et al. CO_2 laser-assisted microsurgery for intracordal cysts: technique and results of 49 patients. Eur Arch Otorhinolaryngol. 2010;267(12):1905-9.
3. Dursun G, Gökcan MK. Aerodynamic, acoustic and functional results of posterior transverse laser cordotomy for bilateral abductor vocal fold paralysis. J Laryngol Otol. 2006;120(4):282-8.
4. Sjögren EV, van Rossum MA, Langeveld TP, et al. Voice outcome in T1a midcord glottic carcinoma: laser surgery vs radiotherapy. Arch Otolaryngol Head Neck Surg. 2008;134(9):965-72.
5. Osborn HA, Hu A, Venkatesan V, et al. Comparison of endoscopic laser resection versus radiation therapy for the treatment of early glottic carcinoma. J Otolaryngol Head Neck Surg. 2011;40(3):200-4.
6. Brandenburg JH. Laser cordotomy versus radiotherapy: an objective cost analysis. Ann Otol Rhinol Laryngol. 2001;110(4);312-8.
7. Peretti G, Piazza C, Cocco D, et al. Transoral CO_2 laser treatment for T(is)-T(3) glottic cancer: the University of Brescia experience on 595 patients. Head Neck. 2010;32(8):977-83.
8. Puxeddu R, Piazza C, Mensi MC, et al. Carbon dioxide laser salvage surgery after radiotherapy failure in T1 and T2 glottic carcinoma. Otolaryngol Head Neck Surg. 2004;130(1):84-8.
9. Benninger MS. Microdissection or microspot CO_2 laser for limited vocal fold benign lesions: a prospective randomized trial. Laryngoscope. 2000;110(2 Pt 2 Suppl 92):1-17.
10. Bhattacharya N, Fried MP. Operative techniques in otolaryngology. Head Neck Surg. 1999;10(4):290-3.
11. Ossoff RH, Duncavage JA, Dere H. Microsubglottoscopy: An expansion of operative microlaryngoscopy. Otolaryngol Head Neck Surg. 1991;104:842-8.
12. Koufman JA, Rees CJ, Frazier WD, et al. Office-based laryngeal laser surgery: a review of 443 cases using three wavelengths. Otolaryngol Head Neck Surg. 2007;137(1):146-51.
13. Handa KK. Lasers in laryngology: Current status. Int J Phonosurg Laryngol. 2011. pp. 6-8.

Adult Laryngotracheal Stenosis

KK Handa, Dhananjay Kumar

INTRODUCTION

Laryngotracheal stenosis (LTS) is characterized by abnormal narrowing of the central airway from glottis inlet to carina.[1] It is a life-threatening, extrathoracic restriction of pulmonary ventilation in which luminal compromise can occurs at the level of the larynx, subglottis or trachea.[2] LTS causes flow-dependent ventilatory insufficiency that clinically manifests as exertional dyspnea, effort intolerance and stridor.[3,4]

It is caused by various benign and malignant conditions. Historically, external injury and infection to the airway were the main causes of LTS but currently the sequelae of intubation have become the primary causative factor.[5]

Stenosis of the subglottis and trachea are well-recognized complications of prolonged intubation and tracheostomy.[6,7] Nearly 10% of intubated patients will subsequently develop stenosis.[8] Incidence of LTS following laryngotracheal intubation and tracheostomy ranges from 6% to 21% and 0.6% to 21%, respectively.[9,10]

Laryngotracheal stenosis is generally considered as a structural entity and defined on the basis of percent stenosis, distance from vocal folds, overall length, but it has heterogeneous pathophysiology.[2] It results from the proliferation of granulation tissue and fibrous tissue into the laryngotracheal lumen.

Laryngotracheal stenosis has multiple etiologies. Mostly involved sites are subglottis and tracheal area followed by glottic area. Supraglottic stenosis is comparatively rare condition.

The risk of airway stenosis appears to rise with prolonged intubation, particularly the subglottic injury can occur within hours of intubation.[11,12] Post-tracheostomy airway stenosis, benign and malignant neoplasms, radiation, and collagen-vascular diseases are other causes of LTS.[5] Many studies suggest that laryngopharyngeal reflux may be the primary etiology in some cases and may be associated with subglottic stenosis (SGS) regardless of the cause.[13] Rarely few patients develop idiopathic LTS.

Thus, there is a variety of patients that is at risk of developing LTS with different etiological factors. Adult LTS remains a challenge for ear, nose, and throat (ENT) surgeons regarding its management.

ETIOLOGY

Laryngotracheal stenosis is a relatively rare disease with multiple etiologies. It can be divided in two types:[14]
1. *Primary stenosis*: When the wall of larynx or trachea involved by disease.
2. *Secondary stenosis*: Where compression of pathological process at surroundings causes airway narrowing.

Causes of Primary Stenosis

Causes of primary stenosis include:
- Iatrogenic
- Post-traumatic
- *Postinfective:* Tuberculosis (TB), syphilis, scleroma, and diphtheria
- *Connective tissue disorder:* Wegener granulomatosis and relapsing polychondritis
- Pemphigoid cicarticans
- Epidermolysis bullosa
- Amyloidosis or sarcoidosis.

Causes of Secondary Stenosis

Causes of secondary stenosis include:
- Thyroid diseases
- Hypertrophic thymus
- Tumor or cysts of the neck or mediastinum
- Retrotracheal abscess or cold abscess.

Causes of Adult Laryngotracheal Stenosis[2,15-17]

Causes of adult laryngotracheal stenosis are listed as:
- Trauma:
  - External laryngotracheal trauma
    - Blunt neck trauma
    - Penetrating wound of larynx
    - Radiation therapy
    - Endotracheal burn (thermal or chemical)
  - Internal laryngotracheal injury
  - Prolonged endotracheal intubation
  - Tracheostomy
  - Surgical procedures
- Chronic inflammatory disease:
  - Diphtheria/syphilis/TB/leprosy/sarcoidosis/scleroma/fungal histoplasmosis
- Benign neoplasms:
  - *Intrinsic:* Papilloma/chondroma/minor salivary gland neoplasm/neural neoplasms
  - *Extrinsic:* Thyroid or thymus lesion
- Malignant neoplasms:
  - *Intrinsic:* Squamous cell carcinoma/sarcomas/lymphoma/salivary gland tumor
  - *Extrinsic:* Thyroid lesion
- Collagen vascular disorders:
  - Wegener granulomatosis
  - Relapsing polychondritis
- Idiopathic
  - Stenosis with unknown etiology.

Gelbard et al.[2] reported in their study the incidence of common etiologies as follows:
- *Iatrogenic:* 54.5%
- *Autoimmune:* 18.5%
- *Idiopathic:* 18.5%
- *Traumatic:* 8%.

Intubation as Etiological Factor

The incidence of LTS after prolonged or repeated intubation has been estimated to range from 3% to 8% in both adults and children. Nordin and Lindholm[18] correlated the grade of damage with duration of intubation and cuff characteristics and concluded that the cuff over the tracheal surface is more important than the length of intubation. The microcirculation of the laryngeal mucosa stops at a presence of 30 mm Hg. The low volume with high pressure cuffs is more likely to cause ischemic injury than high volume with low pressure cuff.

Whited et al.[19] found that patients intubated for 2–5 days had 0–2% incidence of chronic stenosis, those intubated for 5–10 days had 4–5% incidence, and those with an indwelling tube for more than 10 days had 12–14% incidence. But tracheal stenosis can be caused by intubation lasting as short as 24 hours only.[20]

CLASSIFICATION OF LARYNGOTRACHEAL STENOSIS

There are various grading systems available.

Myer-Cotton Staging[21]

This staging is for mature, firm, and circumferential stenosis, confined to the subglottis. It describes the stenosis based on the percent relative reduction in cross-sectional area of the subglottis.

It is determined by the different sizes of endotracheal tubes. There are four grades of stenosis:

Grade I: Lesions have less than 50% obstruction

Grade II: 51–70% obstruction

Grade II: 71–99% obstruction

Grade IV: Lesions have no detectable lumen or complete stenosis.

Lano Classification[22]

Described in 1998 and is based on number of subsites involved in the stenosis. Subsites include the glottis, subglottis, and trachea. It does not take into account length or diameter of stenosis.

Grade I: One subsite involved

Grade II: Two subsites involved

Grade III: Three subsites involved.

McCaffrey Classification[23]

This grading system was described by McCaffery in 1992. This system was based on subsites and length of stenosis but not on lumen diameter.

Grade I: Confined to the subglottis or trachea and less than 1 cm

Grade II: Isolated to the subglottis and greater than 1 cm

Grade III: Subglottic and tracheal lesions not involving the glottis

Grade IV: With glottis involvement.

Cohen Grading System[24]

Cohen proposed the classification of anterior glottic web or stenosis.

Type I: Involvement of 35% or less of the glottis with little or no subglottic involvement.

Type II: Involvement of 35–50% of the glottis with minimal subglottic involvement.

Type III: Involvement of 50–75% of the glottis extending to the lower border of cricoids.

Type IV: Thick web covering the 75–90% of the glottis and extending to the lower border of the cricoid.

Bogdasarian and Oslon Classification[25]

They classified the posterior glottic web or stenosis.

Type I: Vocal process adhesion.

Type II: Posterior commissure stenosis with scarring in the interarytenoid plane and the surface of the posterior cricoid lamina.

Type III: Posterior commissure stenosis with unilateral cricoarytenoid joint ankylosis.

Type IV: Posterior commissure stenosis with bilateral cricoarytenoid joint ankylosis.

For Isolated Tracheal Stenosis[26]

Anand et al. apply a grading system for surgical consideration in tracheal stenosis. It was based on length or severity or location of the tracheal stenosis which was described as follows:
- *Length:* Less than 1 cm or 1–3 cm or more than 3 cm
- *Severity:* Mild or moderate or severe
- *Location:* Glottic or cervical or thoracic.

Freitag et al.[27] proposed a classification system for tracheobronchial stenosis which divides the stenosis into structural and dynamic types and classify by degree of stenosis, location, and transition zone.

DIAGNOSIS

Clinical Assessment

The proper history and complete physical examination of patients is important. Most of the cases of LTS are related with laryngotracheal trauma or intubation history so the duration of injury and history of any previous airway evaluation or repair procedure should be recorded. Patient may present with complaints of breathing difficulty or stridor in severe cases, hoarseness, swallowing difficulty, and difficulty in clearing secretions. Majority of the cases present with airway symptoms. Reports from recent studies also shows that significant subjective and objective changes in the voice of such patients.

Diagnostic Procedures

Office-based flexible fiberoptic laryngoscopy is necessary for evaluating the vocal cord mobility as well as site and grading of stenosis. Rigid video laryngoscopy with 90° or 70° telescope also provides insight including the cord mobility. A retrograde examination may be done in tracheostomized patients in the outpatient department with 30° telescope of 4 mm diameter and this will add information about subglottis and suprastomal trachea.

Direct laryngoscopic and tracheoscopic examination under general anesthesia aided by various rigid telescopes helps to define the extent and severity of the stenosis and also to monitor the success of treatment. It is important to define the site, circumferential involvement, length and number of tracheal rings involved, distance from free edge of vocal cord, status of cartilages, and mobility of vocal cords during reversal. Biopsy may be mandated in patients suspected of having any specific lesion, e.g. Wegener's or tuberculosis.

Noninvasive methods are also available and have a promising future but their clinical role still remains unclear. Nouraei et al. developed a method that is based on flow-volume loops and used to quantify the mechanical extent and clinical impact of LTS.[28]

Imaging

- X-ray soft tissue neck anteroposterior and lateral view. It is considered as base line imaging to see the evidence of narrowing of airway or any stenosis. Small area of calcification may be seen in previous injury cases. Barium swallow may be helpful in evaluating hypopharynx and esophagus.
- Computed tomography (CT) is considered as the standard imaging technique to evaluate the cartilaginous framework and cricoarytenoid joint. Spiral CT with 3D reconstruction allows evaluation of the extent, shape, and site of the stenosis.
- Magnetic resonance imaging is occasionally useful for soft tissue delineation.
- Ultrasonography has become a very useful bedside tool to quickly identify the lumen diameter and length of stenosis. However, ultrasound is very operator dependent.

In 2006, Carretta et al.[29] compared the preoperative CT imaging with intraoperative rigid endoscopy findings and found that endoscopy is better diagnostic procedure and can be considered as gold standard.

Other Evaluations

There are tests that can be done where specific causes of stenosis are suspected. Immunologic or rheumatologic workup can be helpful in patients with suspicion of having Wegener's granulomatosis or other autoimmune disorder. Reflux laryngitis should be kept in mind during preoperative evaluation and also in postoperative management. In 1991, Koufman[30] showed that 73% of patients with SGS had abnormal pH probe results. Maronian et al.[13] show that 5 of the 7 patients (71%) with idiopathic SGS tested had positive pH probe studies (pH below 4 in the pharyngeal probe).

MANAGEMENT

Due to multiple and variety of etiologies, adult LTS remains a challenging disease for the otolaryngologists to diagnose and treat.

The goal of any treatment modality[31] is:
- Airway patency
- Glottic competence for airway protection against aspiration
- Acceptable voice quality.

Decannulation and closure of preliminary tracheostomy, if any, is another goal of modern therapy addressing airway stenosis.[32] Determining the proper management of adult LTS is challenging for otolaryngologists even in modern medical history. There is no single reconstructive technique that applies to all of the LTS cases. The choice of the surgical procedure depends on the severity, location, and length of the stenosis, as well as on the preference of the surgical team.

Management of LTS is a challenging problem that demands a multidisciplinary approach. The length, location, and severity of stenosis all are considered in the treatment of LTS. There are various treatment options for LTS such as endoscopic dilatations, laser surgery, laryngotracheal reconstruction (LTR) with or without stenting, resection end-to-end anastomosis, cricotracheal resection (CTR), and anastomosis, etc. The procedure should be according to patient characteristics (degree and consistency of stenosis, patient age and general condition of patient). Mild LTS can be managed with endoscopic techniques including CO_2 laser, dilatation, steroid injections, and antineoplastic agents applications. These are safe and well tolerated but are associated with recurrence and may need to repeat the procedures.[33]

Open surgical procedures provides long-term decannulation rate but associated with risks of morbidity and mortality.[33] If immediate repair is not being feasible then securing the airway is necessary. Tracheostomy with smallest tube is advisable. It will cause less injury to tracheal mucosa and also helps in preservation of voice. Definitive procedure for LTS is considered after the securing airway. The best chance for the good result after procedure lies in the initial operation.

The different modalities of management of LTS are as following:
- Endoscopic methods
- Open surgical methods.

Endoscopic Management

Endoscopic Dilatation

Endoscopic dilatation with dilators (rigid/balloon) is effective and useful method in early stages of stenosis (Grade 1 and Grade 2). Rigid dilators having the risk of shearing of airway mucosa. New dilators like balloon dilators are better than rigid dilators. Endoscopic dilatation is useful in immature, soft and minimally thick scar and in stenosis with Wegener's granulomatosis.

In recent time, the balloon dilatation became popular and can also be used in high-grade stenosis as a primary procedure. In a systemic review of dilatation as primary procedure, Chueng et al.[34] reported 50% success rate with balloon dilatation and 50–78% success rate as balloon dilatation combined with adjuvant therapy. Balloon dilatation (Fig. 1) needs more repetitive interventions than LTR with a higher restenosis rate 63.2% versus 31.3%.[35]

Herrington et al.[15] in 2006 showed that 70% of patients undergoing dilatation needed repeated procedures. He also recommended that dilatation is useful in grade I or II stenosis before considering open procedures.

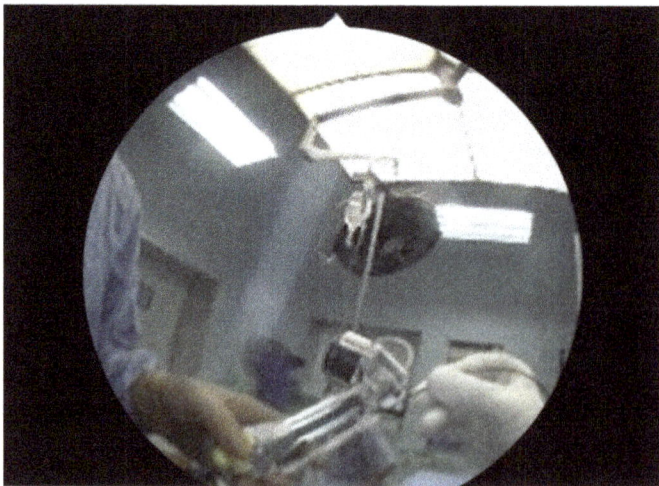

Fig. 1 Balloon dilator for use in early stage laryngotracheal stenosis

Dilatation is useful to avoid a tracheostomy in immature stenosis. It also widened the lumen before stenting.[36] When the open surgical procedure is not feasible (i.e. poor general condition of the patient), dilatation can be helpful.

As per literature, approximately three-fourths of patients treated with dilatation as primary procedure requires a subsequent intervention.[15,37] So, possible recurrence and need of repeated dilatation is disadvantage of this method.

Laser-assisted Procedure

Strong and Jako[38] started doing laser microsurgery with the CO_2 laser. Laser surgery (Fig. 2) has advantages of hemostasis and a fair visual field. Experimental data suggests that wound after laser use show early re-epithelialization, slow fibroblast proliferation and collagen formation. Anterior and posterior glottic webs or stenosis can be addressed with the use of the CO_2 laser to perform a micro-trapdoor technique maximally to preserve mucosa.[39,40] Laser ablation of cotton grade I or II stenosis is shown to be effective in lesions which are noncircumferential and less than 1 cm in length. A staged quadrant by quadrant method may be used at 6 week intervals.[41] The major complications are restenosis, thermal damage, and secondary scarring.

Supraglottic stenosis is mainly managed by laser excision or release of stenosis. Endoscopic surgical treatment with CO_2 laser in operative room is a viable method. Office-based procedure with a pulsed potassium titanyl phosphate (KTP) laser is also described and reported as effective and safe.

Ossoff et al.[42] introduced the laser radial incisions with dilatation. Roediger FC[43] reported that endoscopic laser radial incisions with mitomycin–C (MMC) application (ELRM) are the effective methods of managing SGS with idiopathic causes. They also mentioned that ELRM reduces the airway

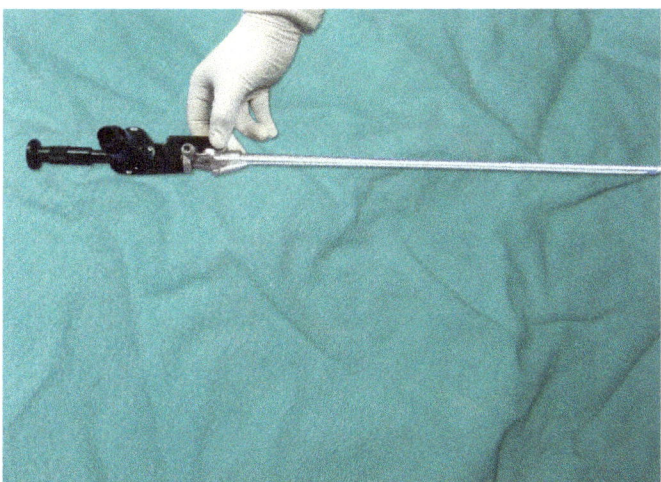

Fig. 2 Bronchoscopic attachment to the rigid rod laser system for laser delivery to trachea

symptoms and decreases the need for tracheostomy in patients with Wegener's granulomatosis-related stenosis.

Thin anterior web can be treated by microsurgical knife or CO_2 laser release and placement of keel. Stent or keel is required to prevent restenosis.[44] The web can be divided at anterior one-third of free edge of true vocal cord into superficial and deep laterally based flaps and flaps covered the exposed area of vocal cords and so keel can be avoided by this technique. Posterior glottic stenosis is a major challenge because the voice is generally normal. The preferred method for posterior glottic stenosis is excision of scar through a micro-trapdoor flap method (an inferiorly based interarytenoid area flap). Flap elevation can be done by laser or microsurgical instruments. In this procedure the submucosal scar is removed and reposition of flap should be done. This procedure was described by Dedo et al.[45] Yilmaz et al. reported micro-trapdoor flap technique.[46]

In restenosis cases and advanced cases with cricoarytenoid joint fixation, an endoscopic arytenoidectomy is performed with laser microsurgery. Open laryngofissure approach with posterior cricoid split and grafting is another method of repair. In 2002, Inglis et al.[47] introduced the endoscopic posterior cricoid split as an alternative to managing isolated posterior glottic stenosis.

Endoscopic Microdebrider Use

The microdebrider has been successfully used in the adult or pediatric airway to remove suprastomal and peristomal granulation tissue.[48] Airway obstruction following LTR is often caused by granulation tissue formation and the microdebrider has been used for management of this problem.

Limitations of Endoscopic Procedures

Simpson et al.[49] described the factors which are predictive of poor results or failure with endoscopic management of LTS.
- Circumferential scarring with cicatrical contracture
- Scarring longer than 1 cm in vertical direction
- Tracheomalacia and loss of cartilage
- History of severe bacterial infection associated with tracheostomy
- Posterior laryngeal inlet scarring with arytenoid fixation.

Galluccio et al.[50] analyze the results of their large series including 21 cases of SGS and concluded that the endoscopic treatment of complex SGS is generally contraindicated.

Open Surgical Methods

The requirements for successful LTS surgery are adequate exposure, normal tissue preservation, and recurrence prevention by promoting primary healing. There are two general open surgical strategies.

1. First approach involves full resection of stenosis segment of trachea with or without cricoid ring and primary anastomosis.
2. Second approach is laryngotracheoplasty or LTR which describes surgical removal of the lumen stenosis and scar, along with reconstruction without segmental tracheal resection. Tracheal or CTR with primary anastomosis gives excellent long-term success rates and high rates of decannulation.

For supraglottic stenosis, the open surgical method described in literature is transcervical supraglottic laryngectomy with preservation of recurrent laryngeal nerves, hyoid bone, and soft tissue adjacent to scarred area.[51]

Anterior glottic stenosis develops from the result of external laryngeal trauma, after endoscopic vocal cord surgery or surgical laryngeal procedure (in malignancy). In recurrent cases with thick scar or stenosis and in web thicker than 1 cm involving the subglottis or combined with posterior glottis stenosis, the open procedure should be in consideration. Laryngofissure approach with placement of an umbrella keel is an adequate procedure in these cases. Keel should be kept in place for 2–4 weeks and removal can be done when anterior one-third of vocal cord becomes epithelized.

Loss of the anterior segment of the thyroid cartilage as a result of trauma or oncologic surgery requires reconstruction of the cartilaginous support. The preferred method for such reconstruction is epiglottopexy laryngoplasty described by Kambic et al.[52]

Posterior glottic stenosis occurs mostly due to prolonged endotracheal intubation or trauma. Due to interarytenoid scarring success of surgery depends upon the degree and depth of scarring. Cricoarytenoid joints mobility should also be considered.

Complete glottic stenosis is difficult to manage. Incising the scar in an anteroposterior line. With posterior cartilage grafting and stenting may be tried. Open procedures for SGS are different laryngotracheal reconstruction procedures and CTR with anastomosis. For pure tracheal stenosis, preferred technique is tracheal resection and anastomosis.

VARIOUS OPERATIVE TECHNIQUES FOR LARYNGOTRACHEAL STENOSIS

External Expansion Surgeries

This includes anterior laryngofissure with cartilage grafting, anterior or posterior cricoid split or both with or without graft or stenting.

Anterior laryngofissure or cricoid split is mainly for anterior wall stenosis or collapse of anterior cartilaginous wall. The cartilage graft should be in such shape that it could not be prolapsed in the lumen. Boat-shaped cartilage graft with outer flange is an option. The perichondrium of the graft is placed towards the inner lumen of airway so that it helps in re-epithelization. A sternocleidomastoid myoperiosteal flap is also described as an alternate for augmentation of anterior cricoid and cervical trachea (Friedman et al.) in SGS cases.[53]

Posterior cricoid split and grafting is require in more severe cases of stenosis, i.e. in posterior glottis or SGS, circumferential stenosis. Laryngofissure is required to expose the posterior cricoid area. Many times stenting is required in these procedures to maintain the cartilage in place and lumen patency.

These LTR procedure (Figs 3A and B) can be done in single stage procedure (SS-LTR) or double stage procedure (DS-LTR). In SS-LTR, patients are decannulated in immediate

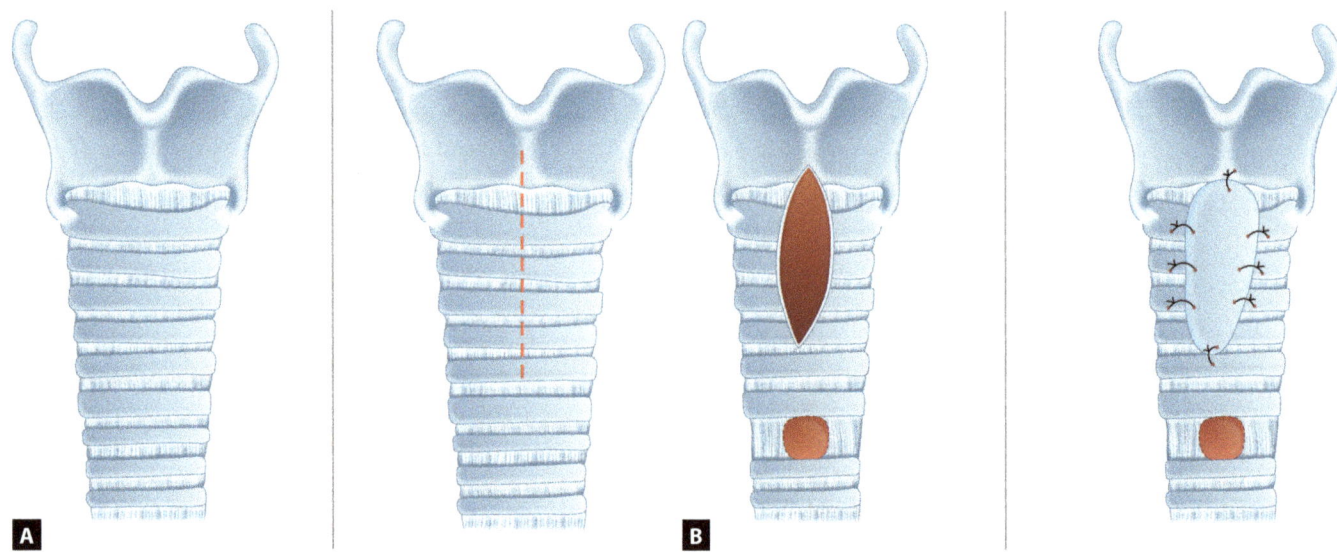

A **B**

Figs 3A and B Steps of laryngotracheal reconstruction. (A) Laryngotracheal fissure; (B) Use of costal cartilage to expand the cricoid and the rest of laryngotracheal framework

postoperative period and left intubated for 1 week with intensive care unit (ICU) stay. In DS-LTR, patients are not decannulated and left with stent for months. Isabelle et al.[54] reported good decannulation rate with staged LTR.

Serial photos of a patient undergone LTR have been shown in Figures 4A to D.

Cricotracheal Resection and Anastomosis

Cricotracheal resection for the treatment of SGS in an adult was first reported by Conley[55] in 1953. SGS is challenging to manage because it has close relationship of cricoid cartilage with recurrent laryngeal nerve. CTR is recommended for

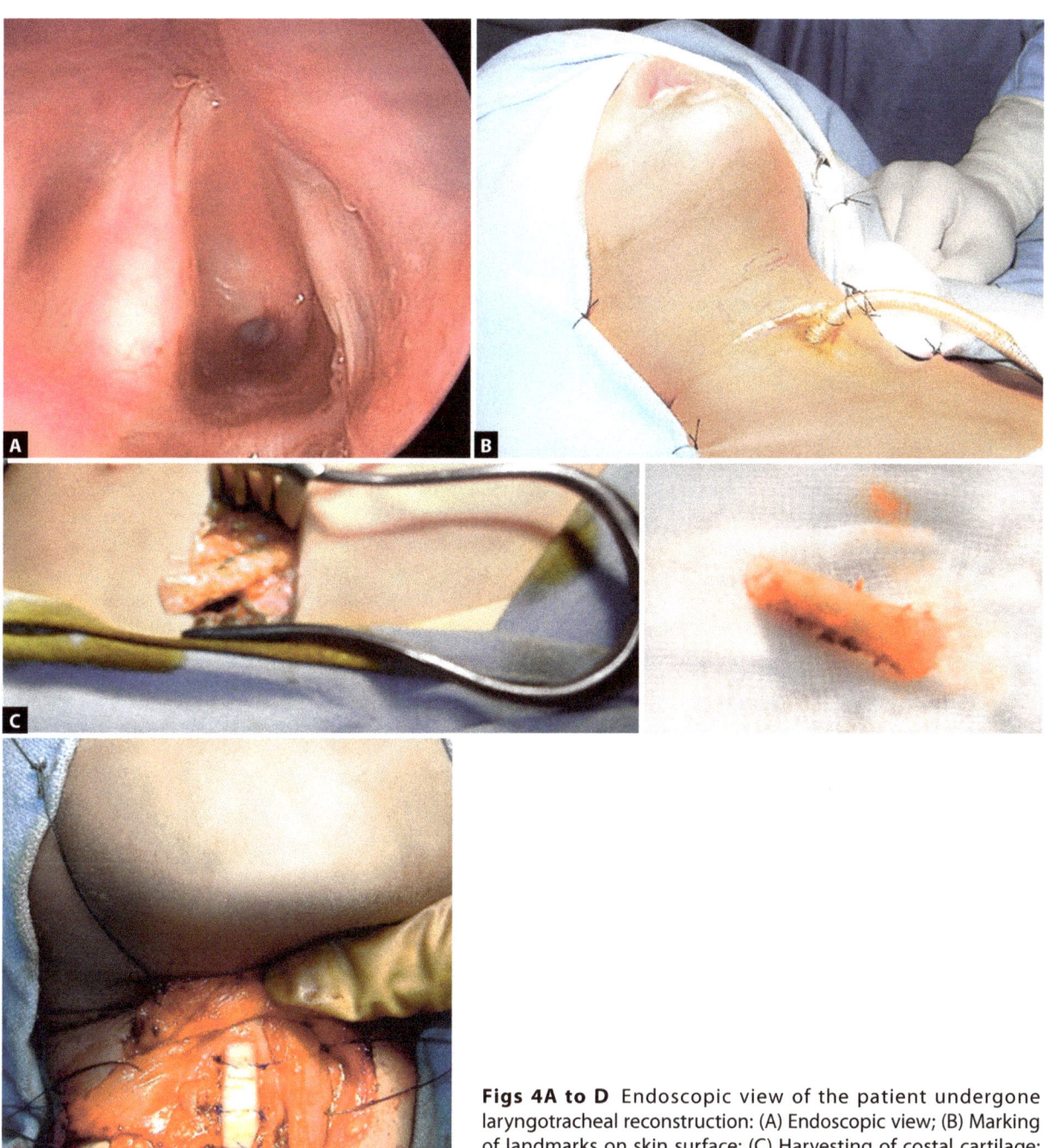

Figs 4A to D Endoscopic view of the patient undergone laryngotracheal reconstruction: (A) Endoscopic view; (B) Marking of landmarks on skin surface; (C) Harvesting of costal cartilage; (D) Cartilage graft used to expand the cricoid cartilage anteriorly

treating patients with high-grade SGS (Cotton grade 3 and 4) and also when there is poor structural integrity of cartilage of affected area. CTR is also indicated as a salvage procedure after failed LTR. Position and length of the stenosis are the deciding factor to do CTR. Patient selection depends on the distance of the stenosis from the vocal cords.

Cricoid ring is the only complete circumferential support of the airway lumen. So, segmental resection of cricoid and primary anastomosis is an accepted technique. The anterior and lateral walls of cricoid are removed and the posterior portion is left. For standard CTR procedure 2–4 mm distance between vocal cords and stenosis is required. If anterior SGS involves the vocal cord then CTR should be avoided. Maddaus et al.[56] described a technique for stenosis which is less than 5 mm of mobile vocal cords. After removal of anterior cricoid arch, the thyroid cartilage incised vertically and affected mucosa is removed by incising the upper limit of the stenosis. The posterior cricoid plate is covered by membranous flap from the distal tracheal stump. If posterior glottis scar is present then posterior cricoid split and cartilage graft with CTR can be done. Couraud[57,58] described a technique for SGS with involvement of glottis, compromised vocal cords or laryngeal cartilage damage by previous procedures. After laryngofissure the cricoid plate is incised and divides in midline. Free cartilage or bone graft can be interposed to enlarge the larynx lumen.

Procedure

Cricotracheal resection can be performed in single stage, i.e. when patient is decannulated intraoperatively or two stage, i.e. with use of suprastomal stent or T-tube (Figs 5A and B).

Technique

Horizontal neck incision made over neck 2 finger above suprasternal notch. Incision can include tracheostoma whenever required. Subplatysmal flap is elevated superiorly up to hyoid bone and inferiorly till sternal notch. Strap muscles are divided in midline and retracted laterally. Thyroid isthmus is divided in midline and thyroid gland retracted laterally. Thyroid cartilage, cricoid cartilage, and tracheal rings are exposed. Anterior tracheal wall should be exposed till sternal notch to allow the mobilization of trachea, if needed. The position of innominate vessels should be kept in mind at inferior level dissection.

An anterior cricoid split is made and extended to visualize the limit of stenotic segment. Superiorly a horizontal incision is made at inferior level of thyroid cartilage and passed laterally just anterior to cricothyroid joints. Lateral exposure of cricoid cartilage is done in subperichondrial plane. Complete resection of anterior cricoid arch from posterior cricoid plate is performed. Removal of anterior cricotracheal complex is performed with extension of this incision. In 1974, Gerwat and Bryce described for the first time an original technique to preserve the posterior cricoid plate and recurrent laryngeal nerves.[59]

Care should be taken at this point to avoid the injury to recurrent laryngeal nerves and vascular supply should be preserved. The incision of the posterior mucosa is made just below the cricoarytenoid joints. The exposure of cricoid plate is completely done.

The membranous trachea then dissected and separated from the anterior wall of the esophagus till the level of cricoid plate. The widening of cricoid plate posteriorly and laterally

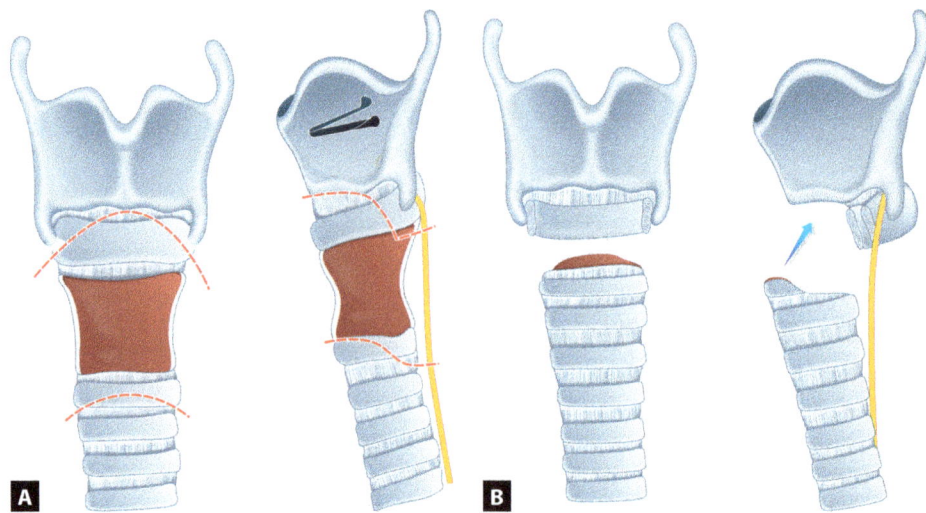

Figs 5A and B Cricotracheal resection steps

with diamond burr is done. Inferior midline thyrotomy is done up to the anterior commissure to widened the subglottic lumen to match the distal tracheal lumen. The cricoid plate is covered with membranous trachea after its upward mobilization.

Anastomosis

Posterior anastomosis is done with interrupted Vicryl suture with knots tied inside the lumen. Fibrin glue can be used to secure the membranous trachea to the cricoid plate. After mucosal closure, the patient is nasotracheally intubated or T-tube or suprastomal stent is placed and secured. Anterior and lateral anastomosis can be done with 3-0 Prolene or Vicryl suture. Anastomosis between first normal tracheal ring and cricoid plate laterally should be in subperichondrial plane to bring mucosa of the subglottis in close contact with mucosa of trachea. Anteriorly the thyrotracheal anastomosis is done by Vicryl or Prolene suture with knots tied outside. The traction sutures placed into the distal trachea earlier may then pass around hyoid bone to reduce the anastomotic tension further.

Contraindications and Cautions of Cricotracheal Resection[60]

- Subglottic stenosis extending into the anterior two-thirds of the vocal cords
- Long segment stenosis (>40–50% of trachea) relative contraindication
- Down syndrome
- Untreated methicillin-resistant *Staphylococcus aureus* (MRSA) colonization
- Uncontrolled gastroesophageal reflux disease (GERD) or eosinophilic esophagitis may compromise surgical outcomes.

Complications of Cricotracheal Resection

- *Laryngeal edema:* Often seen 1–2 weeks after the procedure
- *Restenosis:* In approximately 10% of the patients
- Recurrent laryngeal nerve injury
- *Dehiscence of anastomosis:* This is rare but serious complication.

Tracheal Resection and End-to-end Anastomosis

It is the choice for circumferential pure tracheal stenosis.

Incision and Exposure

A horizontal neck incision is made. Incision should include stoma, if previous tracheostoma was present. Subplatysmal flap is raised superiorly up to hyoid and inferiorly till suprasternal notch. Laterally, the flap should be reaching the anterior border of sternocleidomastoid muscle. Sternohyoid and sternothyroid muscles are divided in the midline. Thyroid isthmus is divided and ligated.[61]

Tracheal Resection

Exposure of trachea is done from thyroid cartilage to suprarenal notch. Dissection should be blunt with a finger along the anterior wall inferiorly as far as possible. It allows mobilization of the inferior tracheal segment. A vertical incision in the anterior trachea is made to determine the length of stenosis.[62,63] Sharp incision is made over trachea above and below the stenosis till the normal tissue. 2-0 silk suture tied in inferior tracheal ring to hold it and to ease for intraoperative manipulation tracheal segment. Care should be taken at this point to avoid any injury to esophageal wall or to recurrent laryngeal nerves. Usually, maximum 4 cm tracheal length or 8 tracheal rings is excised to avoid anastomotic tension. Up to 6.4 cm of tracheal length (Grillo et al.)[64] can be excised by the use of tracheal release maneuvers. Tracheal release maneuvers can be used including suprahyoid release, infrahyoid release or intrathoracic tracheal mobilization (cranial mobilization).

For the patients who do not have posterior tracheal stenosis, it is possible to leave the posterior tracheal wall intact.

End-to-end Anastomosis

Once the resection of involved tracheal segment is done, end-to-end anastomosis is begun. Firstly, posterior wall repair with 4-0 Vicryl is started without tying the sutures which is left to the end. Then all the anterior cartilaginous sutures are placed. 3-0 Prolene or combination of 3-0 Prolene with 3-0 Vicryl sutures can be used for cartilaginous portion of the trachea. Then all sutures are tied one by one in such way that knot of every suture lies externally. Once the tracheal resection is completed, the patient will need to be intubated transorally. Sometimes small tracheostomy below the level of repair can be done specially in morbid obese patients. Wound is closed in layers and suction drain is placed.

Postoperatively a Grillo Stitch can be placed to avoid extension movement of neck but not performed routinely. Use of adhesive tape from mandibular area to sternal area

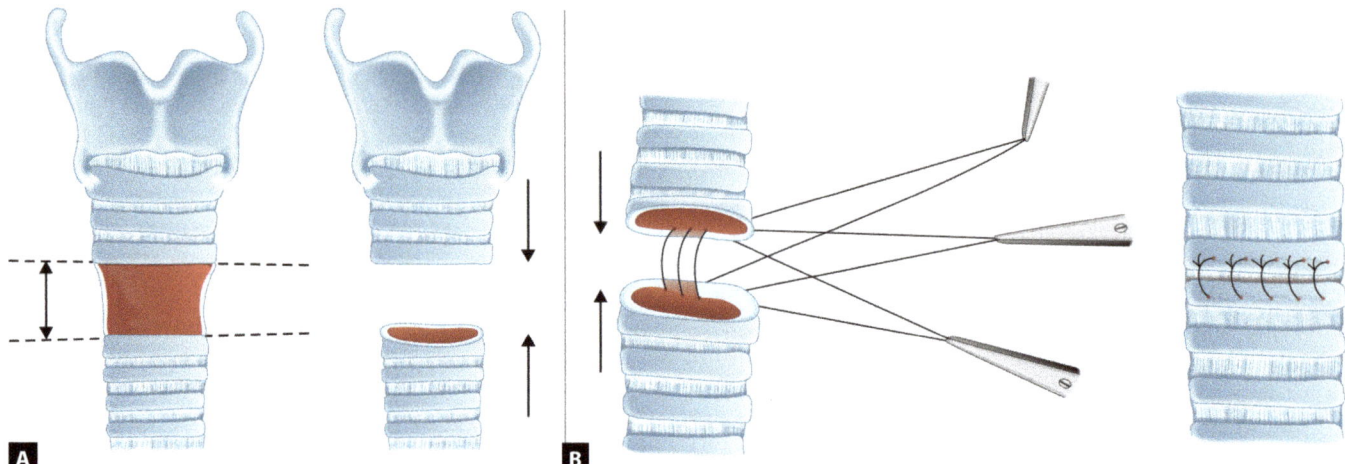

Figs 6A and B Steps of tracheal resection and end-to-end anastomosis

or pillow use and encouragement of patient to keep head in flexed position is feasible and easy (Figs 6A and B).

Complications of Tracheal Resection and Anastomosis

- Granulation tissue formation
- Restenosis
- Wound infection or wound dehiscence
- Laryngeal edema
- Recurrent laryngeal nerve palsy
- Swallowing dysfunction or difficulty.

Stents and Grafts

The first requirement for successful procedure for LTS is establishment of an intact, reasonably shaped skeletal framework to provide a scaffold for the airway.

An ideal cartilage or bone graft does not exist. Rib, iliac crest, hyoid bone, epiglottis, thyroid cartilage, composite auricular cartilage, and nasal septal cartilage are the different sites for grafts. The rib or costal cartilage graft is most commonly used because of its size, strength, and ease of harvesting. Fifth to seventh rib can be used. During the process of rib grafting rare complications are pneumothorax and hematoma formation. Extraperichondrial removal of the rib helps in reducing chances of injury to the pleura.

Stenting may be required to hold the grafts in place. This will improve the success rate of procedure. Montgomery T-tubes and Albouker stents are commonly used. Montgomery T-tube is soft, silicon tube. It is used in subglottic and upper tracheal stenosis. An Aboulker stent is useful in SGS or combined subglottic and laryngeal stenosis. Endotracheal tubes are used as stents in the short-term. For single stage LTR T-tube is mostly used in adult patients.

Stenting is required: (1) to provide support for cartilage and bone grafts or to splint displaced cartilage fragments in the proper position; (2) to allow approximation and immobilization of grafts to a recipient site; (3) to separate opposing raw surfaces during wound healing, and (4) to maintain a lumen in a reconstructed area.

There are different thoughts regarding duration of stenting. Most authors recommend a 6–8 weeks period, but the duration varies from 2 weeks to several months.[65,66] The reported ideal period for stenting ranges from 2 weeks to 10 months. Zalzal et al.[67] showed that when a cartilage graft is inserted, the minimum time necessary for healing is 2 weeks.

Stents can also be used as primary treatment of complicated cases. Patients who have failed multiple attempts at airway reconstruction can be benefited from stent placement.

Complications related with stents are granulation formation at local site and colonization of bacteria. The most common organisms seen are *Staphylococcus aureus* or *Pseudomonas aeruginosa.*

Adjuvant Therapies

Mitomycin C

Mitomycin C can be used as adjuvant therapy following cold knife and laser ablation. It can be used in low-grade stenosis (specially related with autoimmune etiology) and repeated granulation tissue formation. MMC is a naturally occurring antibiotic formed by the *Streptomyces caespitosus*, first isolated in 1956. It is an antimetabolite agent with antineoplastic and antiproliferative properties. MMC can modify wound healing at molecular level and used to interfere with postsurgical scar formation. It was first used in otolaryngologic procedure for tracheal cicatrix after tracheal reconstruction.

Currently 0.4 mg/mL is the recommended concentration at many institutions. It is an alkylating agent that inhibits protein and DNA synthesis. It acts by impeding fibroblast proliferation, thus decreases the probability of restenosis.[68]

Rahbar et al.[69] reported using of topical MMC (at concentration of 0.4 mg/mL for 4 min) as an adjunct to endoscopic laser surgery for LTS. They could successfully decannulate 75% of their patients by this technique.

A prospective randomized double blind placebo controlled trial suggests that, in the endoscopic management of laryngotracheal, two applications of MMC given 3–4 weeks apart after airway surgery (radial incision and dilation) reduces the restenosis rate for 2–3 years after treatment when compared to a single application.[70] MMC use seems cost-effective as it reduces the need of airway dilatation procedure.[71]

Antireflux Therapy

Gastroesophageal or laryngopharyngeal reflux has been suggested as important factor in the development of LTS. Antireflux treatment may be helpful to inhibition of granulation and stenosis formation.

REFERENCES

1. Nouraei SA, Sandhu GS. Outcome of a multimodality approach to the management of idiopathic subglottic stenosis. Laryngoscope. 2013;123(10):2474-84.
2. Gelbard A, Francis DO, Sandulache VC, et al. Causes and consequences of adult laryngotracheal stenosis. Laryngoscope. 2015;125(5):1137-43.
3. Brouns M, Jayaraju ST, Lacor C, et al. Tracheal stenosis: a flow dynamics study. J Appl physiol. 2007;102:1178-84.
4. The American Thoracic Society. Dyspnea, Mechanisms, assessment and management: a consensus statement. Am J Respir Crit Care Med. 1999;159:321-40.
5. Lorenz RR. Adult laryngotracheal stenosis: etiology and surgical management. Curr Opin Otolaryngol Head Neck Surg. 2003;11:467-72.
6. Chew JY, Cantrell RW. Tracheostomy, complications and their management. Arch Otolaryngol. 1973;96:538-45.
7. Keane WM, Denneny JC, Rowe LD, et al. Complications of intubation. Ann Otol Rhinol Laryngol. 1982;91:584-87.
8. Stauffer JL, Olson DE, Petty TL. Complications and consequences of endotracheal intubation and tracheostomy. A prospective study of 150 critically ill adult patients. Am J Med. 1981;70:65-76.
9. Pearson FG, Andrews MJ. Detection and management of tracheal stenosis following cuffed tube tracheostomy. Ann Thorac Surg. 1971;12:359-74.
10. Grillo HC, Donahue DM, Mathisen DJ, et al. Postintubation tracheal stenosis. Treatment and results. J Thorac Cardiovasc Surg. 1995;109:486-92.
11. Klainer AS, Turndorf H, Wu WH, et al. Surface alterations due to endotracheal intubation. Am J Med. 1975;58:674-83.
12. Gould SJ, Young M. Subglottic ulceration and healing following endotracheal intubation in the neonate: a morphometric study. Ann Rhinol Laryngol. 1992;101:815-20.
13. Maronian NC, Azadeh H, Waugh P, et al. Association of laryngopharyngeal reflux disease and subglottic stenosis. Annl otol laryngol rhinol. 2001;110(7):606-12.
14. Szyfter W, Wierzbicka M, Gawecki W, et al. The reasons of laryngo-tracheal stenosis: a review of literature and analysis of 124 patients. Otolaryngol Pol. 2009;63(4):338-42.
15. Herrington HC, Weber SM, Andersen PE. Modern management of laryngotracheal stenosis. Laryngoscope. 2006;116(9):1553-7.
16. Wester JL, Clavburgh DR, Stott WJ, et al. Airway reconstruction in Wegener's granulomatosis associated laryngotracheal stenosis. Laryngoscope. 2011;121(12):2566-71.
17. Parker NP, Bandyopadhyay D, Misono S, et al. Endoscopic cold incision, balloon dilation, mitomycin C application and steroid injection for adult laryngotracheal stenosis. Laryngoscope. 2013;123(1):220-5.
18. Nordin U, Lindholm CE, Wolgast M. Blood flow in the rabbit tracheal mucosa under normal conditions and under the influence of tracheal intubation. Acta Anaesthesiol Scand. 1977;21(2):81-94.
19. Whited RE. Laryngeal dysfunction following prolonged intubation. Ann Otol Rhinol Laryngol. 1979;88:474-8.
20. Yang KL. Tracheal stenosis after a brief intubation. Anesth Analg. 1995;80(3):625-7.
21. Myer CM 3rd, O'Connor DM, Cotton RT. Proposed grading system for subglottic stenosis based on endotracheal tube sizes. Ann Otol Rhinol Laryngol. 1994;103(4):319-23.
22. Lano CF, Duncavage JA, Reinisch L, et al. Laryngotracheal reconstruction in the adult: a ten year experience. Ann Otol Rhinol Laryngol. 1998;107(2):92-7.
23. McCaffrey TV. Classification of laryngotracheal stenosis. Laryngoscope. 1992;102:1335-40.
24. Cohen SR. Congenital glottis webs in children: a retrospective review of 51 patients. Ann Otol Rhinol Laryngol. 1985;121:2-16.
25. Bogdasarian RS, Oslon NR. Posterior glottic laryngeal stenosis. Otolaryngol Head Neck Surg. 1980;88:765-72.
26. Anand VK, Alemar G, Warren ET. Surgical considerations in tracheal stenosis. Laryngoscope. 1992;102:237-43.
27. Freitag L, Ernst A, Unger M, et al. Proposed classification system of central airway stenosis. Eur Respir. 2007;30(1):7-12.
28. Nouraei SM, Patel A, Virk JS, et al. Use of Pressure-volume loops for physiological assessment of adult laryngotracheal stenosis. Laryngoscope. 2013;123:2735-41.
29. Carretta A, Melloni G, Ciriaco P, et al. Preoperative assessment in patients with postintubation tracheal stenosis: Rigid and flexible bronchoscopy versus spiral CT scan with multiplanar reconstructions. Surg Endosc. 2006;20(6):905-8.
30. Koufman JA. The otolaryngologic manifestations of gastroesophageal reflux disease: a clinical investigation of 225 patients using ambulatory 24-hour pH monitoring and an experimental investigation of the role of acid and pepsin in the development of laryngeal injury. Laryngoscope. 1991;101:1-78.
31. Hanna E, Eliachar I. Endoscopically introduced expandable stents in laryngotracheal stenosis: the jury is still out. Otolaryngol Head Neck Surg. 1997;116:97-103.
32. Eliachar I, Goldsher M, Alder O. Combined treatment of concurrent laryngeal and tracheal stenosis. J Laryngol Otol. 1981;9(1):59-66.

33. Parida PK, Gupta AK. Management of laryngotracheal stenosis: our experience. Indian J Otolaryngol Head Neck Surg. 2009;61(4):306-12.

34. Chueng K, Chadha NK. Primary dilatation as a treatment for pediatric laryngotracheal stenosis: a systematic review. Int J Pediatr Otorhinolaryngol. 2013;77(5):623-8.

35. Gunaydin RO, Suslu N, Bajin MD, et al. Endolaryngeal dilatation versus laryngotracheal reconstruction in the primary management of subglottic stenosis. Int J Pediatr Otorhinolaryngol. 2014;78:1332-6.

36. Demello-filho FV, Antonio SM, Carrau RL. Endoscopically placed expandable metal tracheal stents for the management of complicated tracheal stenosis. Am J Otolaryngol. 2003;24:34-40.

37. Clement P, Hans S, de Mones E, et al. Dilatation for assisted ventilation-induced laryngotracheal stenosis. Laryngoscope. 2005;115:1595-8.

38. Strong MS, Jako GJ. Laser surgery in the larynx: early clinical experience with continuous CO_2 laser. Ann Otol Rhinol Laryngol. 1972;81:791-8.

39. Dedo HH, Sooy CD. Endoscopic laser repair of posterior glottis, subglottic and tracheal stenosis by division or microtrapdoor flap. Laryngoscope. 1984;94:445-50.

40. Beste DJ, Toohill RJ. Micro-trapdoor flap repair of laryngeal and tracheal stenosis. Ann Otol Rhinol Laryngol. 1991;100: 420-3.

41. Werkhaven JA, Weed DT, Ossoff RH. CO_2 laser serial microtrapdoor flap excision of subglottic stenosis. Arch Otolaryngol Head Neck Surg. 1993;119(6):676-9.

42. Ossoff RH, Toohill RJ. Carbon dioxide laser management for laryngeal stenosis. Ann Otol Rhinol Laryngol. 1985;94(6): 565-9.

43. Roediger FC, Orloff LA, Courey MS. Adult subglottic stenosis: management with laser incisions and mitomycin-C. Laryngoscope. 2008;118(9):1542-6.

44. Dedo HH. Endoscopic Teflon keel for anterior glottic web. Ann Otol Rhinol Laryngol. 1979;83:467.

45. Langman AW, Dedo HH, Lee KC. The endoscopic Teflon keel for posterior and total glottis stenosis. Laryngoscope. 1989;99:571-7.

46. Yilmaz T, Süslü N, Günaydın RÖ, et al. Microtrapdoor flap technique for treatment of glottis laryngeal stenosis: experience with 34 cases. J Voice. 2016;30(6):751-4.

47. Inglis AF Jr, Perkins JA, Manning SC, et al. Endoscopic posterior cricoid split and rib grafting in 10 children. Laryngoscope. 2003;113(11):2004-9.

48. Rees CJ, Tridico TI, Kirse DJ. Expanding applications for the microdebrider in paediatric endoscopic airway surgery. Otolaryngol Head Neck Surg. 2005;133:509-13.

49. Simpson GT, Strong MS, Healy GB, et al. Predictive Factors of Success or Failure in the Endoscopic Management of Laryngeal and Tracheal stenosis. Ann Otol Rhinol Laryngol. 1982;91(4):384-8.

50. Galluccio G, Lucantoni G, Battistoni P, et al. Interventional endoscopy in the management of benign tracheal stenoses: definitive treatment at long-term follow-up. Eur J Cardiothorac Surg. 2009;35:429-34.

51. Minni A, Gallo A, Croce A, et al. Leroux-Huet Laryngectomy for supraglottic stenosis. Op Tech Otol Head Neck Surg. 1992;3:194-98.

52. Kambic V, Radsel Z, Smid L. Laryngeal reconstruction with epiglottis after vertical hemilaryngectomy. J Laryngol Otol. 1977;9:467-73.

53. Friedman M, Colombo J. Sternocleidomastoid myoperiosteal flap for reconstruction of subglottic larynx and trachea. Op Tech Otol Head Neck Surg. 1992;3:202-5.

54. Liu IY, Mendelsohn AH, Ching H, et al. Staged laryngotracheoplasty in Adult Laryngotracheal stenosis. JAMA otolaryngol Head Neck Surg. 2015;141(3):211-18.

55. Conley JJ. Reconstruction of the subglottic air passage. Ann Otol Rhinol Laryngol. 1953;62:477-95.

56. Maddaus MA, Toth JL, Pearson FG, et al. Subglottic tracheal resection and synchronus laryngeal reconstruction. J Thorac Cardiovasc Surg. 1992;104:1443-50.

57. Couraud L, Jougon JB, Ballester M. Techniquies of management of subglottic stenosis with glottis or supraglotic problems. Chest Surg Clin N. 1996;6:791-809.

58. Couraud L, Martigne C, Houdelette P, et al. Value of cricoid resection in cricotracheal stenosis following intubation. Ann Chir. 1979;33:242-6.

59. Gerwat J, Bryce DP. The management of subglottic laryngeal stenosis by resection and direct anastomosis. Laryngoscope. 1974;84:940-57.

60. White DR, Michael J. Cricotracheal resection and anastomosis. Op Tech Otolaryngol. 2009;20:236-40.

61. Gavilan J, Toledano A, Cerdeira MA, et al. Tracheal resection and anastomosis. Op tech Otolaryngol Head Neck Surg. 1997;8(3):122-9.

62. Mathisen DJ. Subglottic stenosis. Op Tech Thorac Cardiovasc Surg. 1998;3(3):12-53.

63. Grillo HC, Wain JC, Mathisen DJ. Laryngotracheal resection and reconstruction for subglottic stenosis. Ann Thorac Surg. 1992;53(1):54-63.

64. Grillo HC, Mathisen DJ, Ashiku SK, et al. Successful treatment of idiopathic laryngotracheal stenosis by resection and primary stenosis. Ann Otol Rhinol Laryngol. 2003;112(9):798-800.

65. Harris HH, Tobin HA. Acute injuries of the larynx and trachea in 49 patients. Laryngoscope. 1970;80:1376.

66. Schuller DE. Long-term stenting for laryngotracheal stenosis. Ann otol Rhinol Laryngol. 1980;89:515-20.

67. Zalzal GH, Grundfast KM. Broken Aboulker stents in the tracheal lumen. Int J Paediatric Otorhinolaryngol. 1988;16(2):125-30.

68. Perepelitsyn I, Shapshay SM. Endoscopic treatment of laryngeal and tracheal stenosis—Has Mitomycin C Improved the outcome? Otolaryngol Head Neck Surg. 2004;13(1):16-20.

69. Rahbar R, Shapshay SM, Healy GB. Mitomycin: Effects on laryngeal and tracheal stenosis, benefits, and complications. Ann Otol Rhinol Laryngol. 2001;110:1-6.

70. Smith ME, Elstad M. Mitomycin C and endoscopic treatment of laryngotracheal stenosis: are two applications better than one? Laryngoscope. 2009;116:272-83.

71. Ubell ML, Ettema SL, Toohill RJ, et al. Mitomycin C application in airway stenosis surgery: analysis of safety and costs. Otolaryngol Head neck Surg. 2006;134:403-6.

Reconstruction Techniques for the Treatment of Anatomical Upper Respiratory Tract Anomalies in Children

Ravindhra G Elluru

OVERVIEW

Over the past 40 years, there has been a marked evolution in the presentation and management of pediatric laryngeal stenosis. Prior to 1965, this diagnosis indicated the presence of a congenital anterior glottic web or congenital subglottic stenosis (SGS). In many children, congenital SGS could be anticipated to improve with time, even if placement of a temporary tracheotomy tube was required. The advent of prolonged intubation, particularly of the neonate, strikingly changed this situation. Acquired SGS (ASGS) became and currently remains the most frequent cause of laryngeal stenosis. This condition is generally more severe than congenital SGS and does not improve with time. Modern pediatric laryngeal reconstruction was thus born of necessity to manage these otherwise healthy, but tracheotomy-dependent children.

Further improvements in neonatal care, particularly the use of nasopharyngeal continuous positive airway pressure (CPAP), led to a significant decline in the incidence of ASGS in children without other medical problems. The evolution of neonatal care has resulted in the salvage of premature and often medically fragile children whose laryngeal pathology is one component of a myriad of health issues. The overall care of such children is more complex to manage, ideally requiring an interdisciplinary team approach. Additionally, their laryngeal pathology is more severe, with stenosis potentially involving not only the subglottis, but also the supraglottis or glottis.

Both acquired and congenital airway anomalies can occur at various anatomic levels, and their presentation and management are significantly influenced by both the level at which obstruction occurs and the severity of obstruction. To facilitate a discussion of airway reconstruction techniques, it is best to first review the anatomy of the pediatric larynx, and then discuss treatment options for lesions that occur at different levels of the upper airway.

PEDIATRIC VERSUS ADULT UPPER AIRWAY ANATOMY

The three portions of the larynx are (1) supraglottis, (2) glottis, and (3) subglottis (Fig. 1). These laryngeal components are same in adults and children. However, there are some age-related differences that play a role in the development of laryngeal stenosis.[1]

The infant larynx is approximately one-third the size of the adult larynx, but it is proportionally larger than the adult larynx compared with the rest of the tracheobronchial tree. The infant vocal cord is approximately 7–8 mm long, and the adult vocal cord is 14–23 mm long. In the infant, half of the length of the true vocal cord is composed of the vocal process of the arytenoid. In the adult, the vocal process occupies only one-fourth to one-third of the total length of the true vocal cord. Due to the complete ring structure of the cricoid, the subglottis is the narrowest part of the airway. In the infant, the subglottis is approximately 4.5–7 mm in diameter.[2]

The position of the larynx in relation to other structures of the neck is different in infants and adults. In the infant, the superior border of the larynx is located as high as the first cervical vertebra, with the cricoid cartilage positioned at approximately the level of the fourth cervical vertebra.

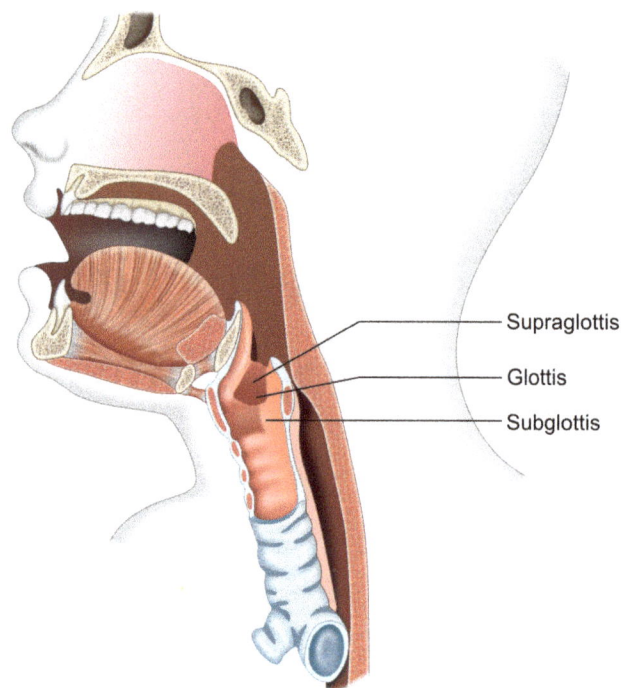

Fig. 1 Sagittal section through the upper respiratory tract demonstrating the areas of the supraglottis, glottis and subglottis

Supraglottis

Glottis

Subglottis

This results in the hyoid overriding the superior larynx in an infant, with the thyroid notch usually being impalpable as a consequence. Because of the superior positioning of the larynx, the epiglottis approximates the dorsal surface of the soft palate. This contributes to the obligate nasal breathing seen in the first months of life. As the child grows into adulthood, the larynx gradually descends, and the cricoid cartilage eventually rests at the level of the sixth cervical vertebra. The infant epiglottis is the structure that demonstrates the most dramatic change in configuration. At birth, the epiglottis, which is shaped like the Greek letter omega (Ω), is narrower and softer than that found in older children and adults. It has a less stable base, and there is a more acute angle between the epiglottis and glottis, allowing the epiglottis to fall into the laryngeal inlet. As the child grows, cartilaginous support of the epiglottis becomes more rigid, the angle of the thyroid cartilage changes from 110° to 120° to an angle of 90° in the adolescent male. In the adult female, this angulation remains more obtuse, as in childhood. Because cartilage, muscle, and submucosal tissues are more pliable and less fibrous in the infant than in the adult and because the airway is narrower at the subglottis, any process that produces edema can cause significant airway obstruction.[2] Circumferential mucosal edema of 1 mm within the larynx of an infant narrows the subglottic space by more than 60%.[3]

LARYNGOMALACIA

Laryngomalacia is the most frequent cause of stridor in the neonate. In most children, symptoms are evident at birth or within the first few days of life. Stridor is generally mild; however, it is exacerbated by feeding, crying, and lying in a supine position. In 50% of children with laryngomalacia, stridor worsens during the first 6 months of life. In virtually all cases, symptoms spontaneously resolve by 1 year of age. In children with severe laryngomalacia (approximately 5%), surgical intervention is required. In such children, symptoms may include apnea, cyanosis, severe retractions, and failure to thrive. Cor pulmonale is seen in very severe cases.[4]

Diagnosis is confirmed by flexible transnasal fiberoptic laryngoscopy.[5] Characteristic findings include short aryepiglottic folds, with prolapse of the cuneiform cartilages. Also, a tightly curled (Ω-shaped) epiglottis is sometimes observed. Owing to the Bernoulli effect, characteristic collapse of the supraglottic structures is observed on inspiration. Additionally, inflammation indicative of reflux laryngitis is often seen. Making the decision as to whether or not to intervene surgically is more so dependent on the severity of symptoms than on the endoscopic appearance of the larynx.

Children with laryngomalacia seldom present with acute airway compromise. In the 5% who require operative management, this may be arranged in a semi-elective fashion within 1–2 weeks of presentation. Preoperative management of gastroesophageal reflux is prudent. Supraglottoplasty (also termed epiglottoplasty) is currently the preferred operative procedure, replacing tracheotomy.[6] It is quick and effective and can be adapted to the infant's specific laryngeal pathology. In general, the cuneiform cartilages are truncated, and the aryepiglottic folds are divided releasing the epiglottis into a more anterior position. Sometimes, the lateral aspects of the epiglottis are trimmed as well.

VOCAL CORD PARALYSIS

Vocal cord paralysis is the second most common cause of neonatal stridor. As with laryngomalacia, the diagnosis is established with awake flexible transnasal fiberoptic laryngoscopy. This condition is subdivided into congenital and acquired paralysis and unilateral and bilateral paralysis. In most cases, bilateral vocal cord paralysis is present at birth, whereas unilateral paralysis is an acquired condition that arises as a result of damage to the recurrent laryngeal nerve. The length and course of the left recurrent nerve in particular places is an increased risk to injury during surgical procedures to the heart, esophagus or thyroid gland.

Although congenital vocal cord paralysis is usually idiopathic, it is also seen with central nervous system pathology such as hydrocephalus and Chiari malformation of the brainstem. In the latter situation, when the underlying cause is successfully treated, vocal cord paralysis is usually reversed. Most children with bilateral paralysis present with significant airway compromise, and an excellent voice. These children usually do not aspirate. Up to 90% of infants with bilateral vocal cord paralysis will ultimately require tracheotomy. By contrast, most children with unilateral vocal cord paralysis have an acceptable airway and a breathy voice. In addition, unlike children with bilateral vocal cord paralysis, those with unilateral vocal cord paralysis are at a higher risk of aspiration.[7,8]

In an infant with stridor and retractions caused by bilateral vocal cord paralysis, placement of a tracheotomy is indicated. The airway can be temporarily stabilized with intubation, CPAP, or high-flow nasal cannula. Since up to 50% of children with congenital idiopathic bilateral vocal cord paralysis have spontaneous resolution of their paralysis by 1 year of age,[8] surgical intervention to achieve decannulation is usually postponed until patients are older than 1 year of age.

Children with acquired bilateral vocal cord paralysis may also experience spontaneous recovery several months after recurrent laryngeal nerve injury if the nerve is still intact.

Most children with unilateral vocal cord paralysis do not require surgical intervention. For those with bilateral paralysis, several surgical options have been used since no particular surgical approach offers a universally acceptable outcome.[9,10] The aim of surgery is twofold: (1) to achieve an adequate decannulated airway while maintaining voice and (2) to prevent aspiration. Surgical options include laser cordotomy, partial or complete arytenoidectomy (endoscopic or open), vocal process lateralization (open or endoscopically-guided) (Fig. 2), and posterior cricoid cartilage grafting.

Acquired bilateral vocal cord paralysis is usually less responsive to treatment than idiopathic cord paralysis, and more than one operative intervention may be required to achieve decannulation. Since some children have an increased risk of aspiration in the immediate postoperative period, swallow function should be evaluated before the child returns to a normal diet.

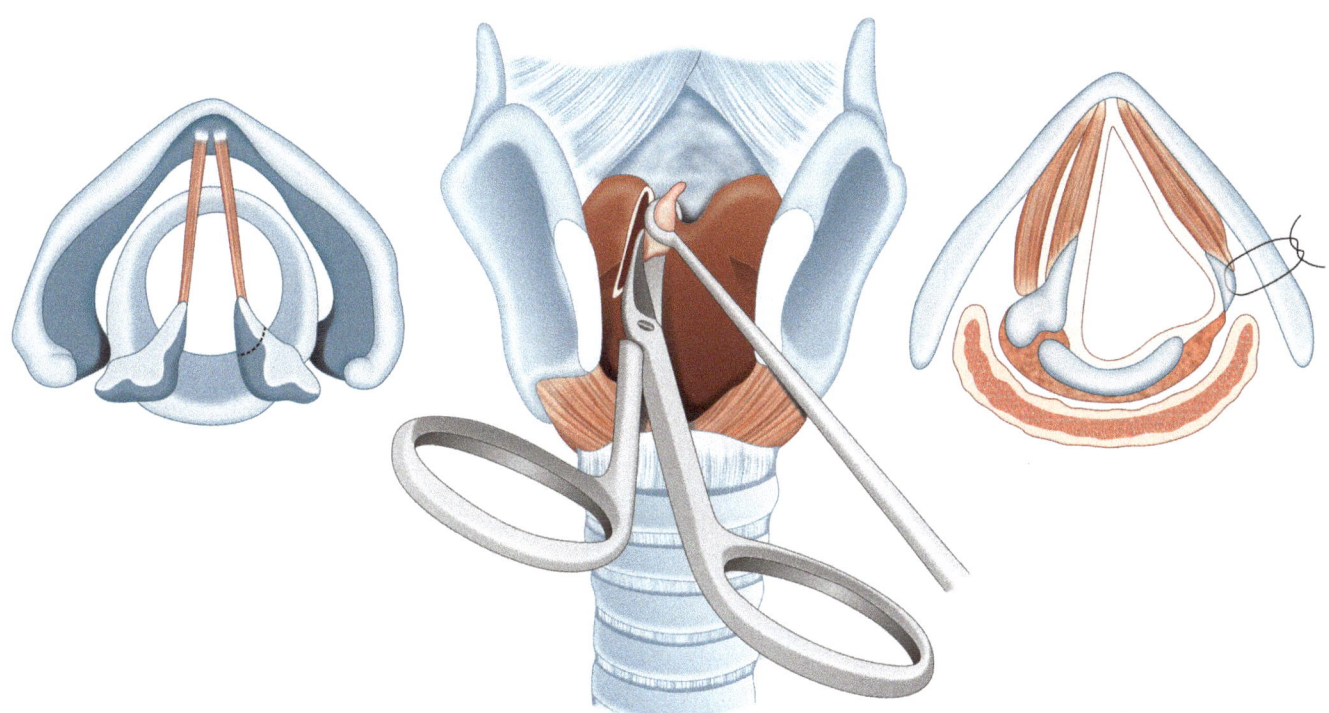

Fig. 2 This schematic represents one of the open operative procedures for widening the glottis airway in a patient with bilateral vocal cord paralysis. In general, the larynx is opened through the neck by dividing the thyroid alae and anterior commissure in the midline. The mucosa over one of the arytenoids is incised and the portion of the arytenoid cartilage that articulates with the cricoid ring is excised. A stitch through the thyroid alae is then used to lasso the vocal process of the arytenoid and lateralize the vocal cord. The larynx is then closed with meticulous attention to approximating the anterior commissure. Vocal cord lateralization without arytenoidectomy can be performed endoscopically

Laryngeal Webs

Laryngeal webs result from a failure of recanalization of the glottic airway in the early weeks of embryogenesis. Recanalization of the larynx occurs in a posterior to anterior manner. In the most severe cases there is a complete failure of recanalization resulting in laryngeal atresia. In less severe cases, a thin anterior glottic web may be the only remnant of the recanalization process. The severity of symptoms, which include dyspnea and voice change, correlates with the size and position of the web. A strong association between anterior glottic webs and velocardiofacial syndrome (VCF) has been identified.[11]

Laryngeal webs are typically thickened anteriorly and thins out towards the posterior edge. Thin webs may elude detection, as neonatal intubation for airway distress may lyse the web. Thick webs require open reconstruction with reconstruction of the anterior commissure and typically temporary placement of a laryngeal keel.[12]

Subglottic Stenosis

Subglottis stenosis is a narrowing of the endolarynx that develops at and below the vocal folds. SGS can results in severe functional impairments, including breathing difficulty and loss of voice. Etiologically, SGS can be congenital or acquired. As many as 92% of SGS cases are of the acquired type with most cases being attributed to intubation injury. Congenital airway anomalies arise from aberrancies in developmental pathways during gestation and include such lesions as laryngeal atresia, stenosis, and webs. Congenital SGS can be associated with other congenital head and neck lesions and syndromes (e.g. a small larynx in a patient with Down's syndrome). In general, the larynx in cases of congenital SGS does grow with time and therefore conservative treatment approaches are sufficient until the size of the subglottic lumen corrects with age and growth.

The incidence of ASGS has been reported to be between 0.4% and 10% of intubated patients. Contributing factors include duration of intubation, size of the endotracheal tube (ETT), history of tracheostomy, reintubation, infection while intubated, and irradiation for oropharyngeal and laryngeal tumors. In general, it is believed that pressure from the ETT causes ischemic injury, leading to ulceration or loss of laryngeal mucosa. When the injury heals inadequately, excessive deposition of scar tissue leads to thickening of the subglottic mucosa tissue, which narrows the airway. The appropriate ETT size is not the largest that will fit, but rather the smallest that allows for adequate ventilation. Ideally, the tube should leak air around it, with subglottic pressures below 25–30 cm of water. Other known cofactors for the development of ASGS include gastroesophageal reflux (GER) and eosinophilic esophagitis (EE).[13-15]

The severity of SGS is typically graded using to the Myer-Cotton grading system.[16] Grade I stenosis corresponds to 0–50%, grade II stenosis corresponds to 51–70%, grade III stenosis corresponds to 71–99%, and grade IV stenosis corresponds to 100% obstruction of the subglottic lumen. Mild SGS may manifest in recurrent upper respiratory infections (often diagnosed as croup) in which minimal subglottic swelling precipitates airway obstruction. Moderate and severe cases of SGS present with symptoms ranging from exercise intolerance, to stridor and dyspnea at rest.

Though not the gold standard for evaluation of the airway, radiological evaluation can offer insight into the anatomy of the airway lesion prior to further other diagnostic evaluations. One of the most helpful diagnostic evaluations is the high-kilovoltage airway film. These films are taken not only to identify the classic "steepling" observed in patients with SGS, but also to identify the extent and length of narrowing, pliability of the airway, and other secondary lesions.

The current gold standard for airway evaluation of SGS, whether congenital or acquired, is airway endoscopy. Airway endoscopy can begin the outpatient setting with a flexible fiberoptic endoscope can provide information about the anatomy of the nasal, nasopharyngeal, oropharyngeal and hypopharyngeal airway. Furthermore, nasopharyngoscopy with the patient awake provides information regarding the static and dynamic anatomy of the larynx and vocal folds. Nasopharyngoscopy can be followed by rigid and possibly flexible endoscopy of the remainder of the airway. In the operating room the airway should be evaluated in an algorithmic manner from the tip of the nose to the bronchi, with photodocumentation for later rereview. Furthermore, during the endoscopy the size of the subglottis should be measured using the Cotton-Myer classification system.

In children with mild symptoms and a minor degree of SGS, conservative management or minimally invasive endoscopic intervention may be sufficient. Endoscopic options include placing chevron incisions in the circumferential scar, followed by balloon dilation. Severe forms of SGS are better managed with open airway reconstruction (Figs 3A and B). Laryngotracheal reconstruction using costal cartilage grafts placed through the split lamina of the cricoid cartilage is reliable and has withstood the test of time.[17]

An open laryngotracheal reconstruction is commenced by isolating the trachea through an anterior cervical incision. A vertical incision is then made through the anterior cricoid lamina and sometimes extended through the midline thyroid alae and anterior commissure. A rib graft is harvested from the same patient through a separate chest incision, contoured to the appropriate dimensions and then sutured in place

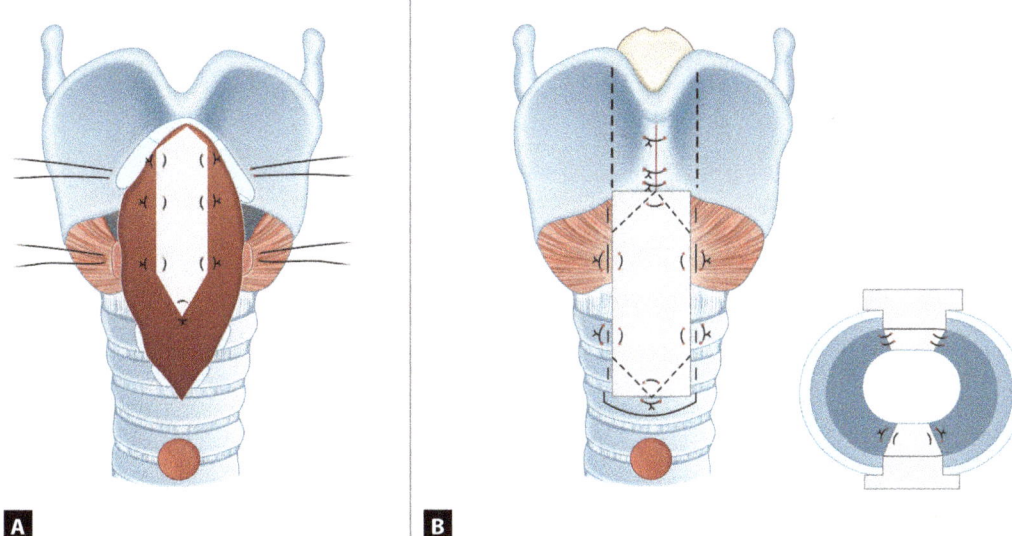

Figs 3A and B (A) This schematic demonstrates the back wall of the subglottis. The back wall of the subglottis has been approached through a vertical incision through the anterior cricoid lamina. A vertical incision has been made in the posterior cricoid lamina as well, and a costal cartilage graft inserted between the edges of the cut posterior cricoid lamina; (B) This schematic demonstrates a costal cartilage graft inserted between the cut edges of the anterior cricoid lamina. Also shown is an axial section through the subglottic ring showing the placement of the anterior and posterior costal cartilage grafts

between the cut edges of the anterior cricoid lamina. In this way, the dimensions of the cricoid ring are augmented, opening up the narrowed subglottic airway. Depending on the degree of stenosis, an anterior graft may be used by itself or in conjunction with a posterior graft placed between the cut edges of a vertical incision in the posterior cricoid lamina.

In cases of grade III and grade IV SGS, a slightly different reconstruction procedure called a cricotracheal resection may be used (Figs 4A and B). This procedure entails removing the anterior half of the cricoid lamina, as well as the mucosa covering the posterior cricoid lamina. In addition, the first several tracheal rings are completely removed. The two cut ends of the airway are then brought back together and closed primarily. The goal of this procedure is to completely remove the stenosed or narrow segment of the airway. Better results have been obtained with cricotracheal resection than with laryngotracheal reconstruction for the management of severe SGS.[18]

Laryngotracheal and cricotracheal reconstruction procedures can be performed as a single- or a double-staged procedure. In a single-staged procedure, the airway is reconstructed and the patient is intubated anywhere from 3 days to –10 days after which he is extubated. Children who undergo a double-staged procedure will have a stent placed at the site of reconstruction, and a tracheotomy below the reconstructed airway. The stents are removed after varying periods of time. The airway is then examined and if deemed adequate, the tracheotomy is removed. Double-staged

procedures are used in cases where prolonged stenting is required and/or the airway contains multiple levels of airway obstruction.[19,20]

The subglottis being anatomically juxtaposed to the vocal folds, stenotic lesions can often extend up to and involve the dorsal aspect of the vocal folds. Therefore, reconstruction procedures frequently involve manipulation of the vocal cord mucosa. The anterior commissure of the vocal folds is sometimes split and reapproximated during the reconstruction procedure which can also lead to altered vocal fold function. Other consequences of airway reconstruction can include scarred and narrow subglottic tissue; fused, off level, webbed, or immobile vocal folds; decreased laryngeal sensitivity, and supraglottic tissue abnormalities.

POSTERIOR LARYNGEAL CLEFTS

Posterior laryngeal clefts result from a fusion failure of the laryngotracheal groove. Although these clefts are generally not obstructive in nature, infants with laryngeal clefts sometimes present with significant aspiration. While gross aspiration may occur with associated apnea, cyanosis, and even pneumonia, often the symptoms are those of microaspiration, with choking episodes, transient cyanosis, and recurrent chest infections. Diagnosis of a laryngeal cleft requires a high-index of suspicion and vigilance during the rigid endoscopy. Laryngeal clefts can be associated with secondary anomalies of the airway including tracheomalacia

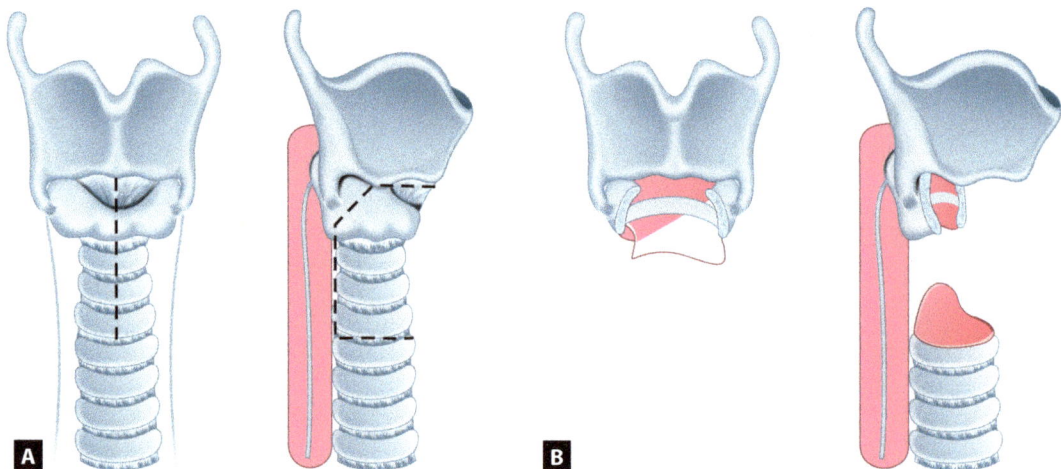

Figs 4A and B This schematic represents a cricotracheal resection. (A) Marks the area of the proximal trachea and anterior cricoid lamina that will be resected; (B) Airway after removing the anterior cricoid lamina and proximal trachea. The two cut edges will be approximated bringing the airway into continuity

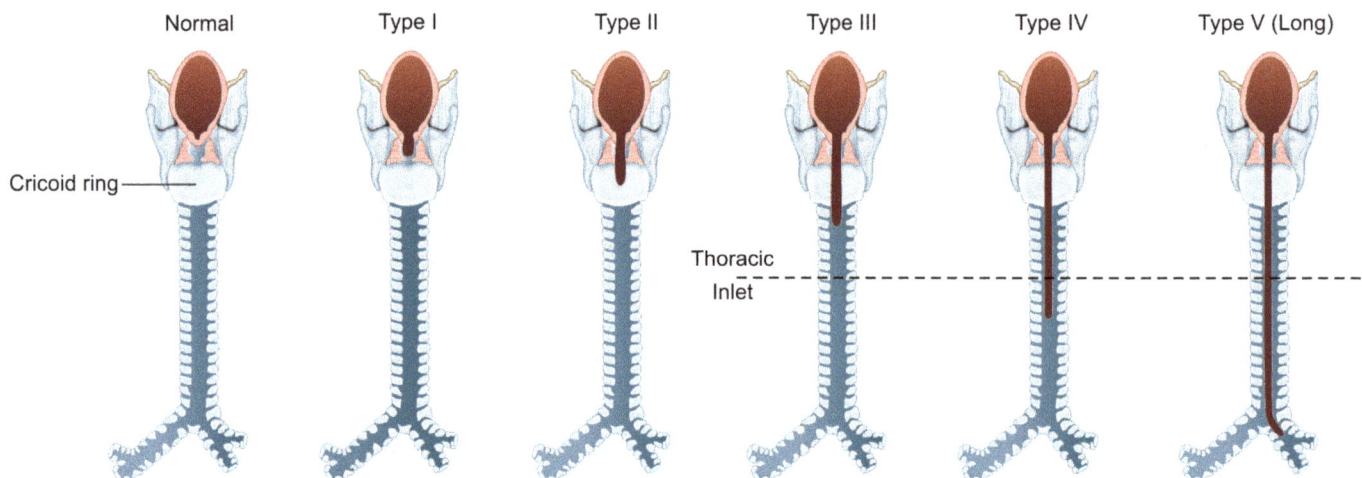

Fig. 5 This schematic represents the types of laryngotracheoesophageal clefts

(>80%) and tracheoesophageal fistula (TEF) (20%) formation. Laryngeal clefts can be associated with other midline defects or syndromes in which midline defects are the hallmark such as Opitz-Frias syndrome (hypertelorism, anogenital anomalies, and posterior laryngeal clefting). Figure 5 shows a modification of the Benjamin and Inglis classification system, with cleft types I to V illustrated.

Management of laryngeal clefts can be challenging and is often multidisciplinary in nature. Prior to repair of the laryngeal cleft, consultation for gastrostomy tube placement or Nissen fundoplication should be considered. Furthermore, if the laryngeal cleft is extensive and an open repair is anticipated or airway symptoms are significant, consideration for placement of a tracheostomy should

be given. The primary and fundamental goal in the management of the child with a laryngeal cleft is to protect the lungs against damage from aspiration. Type I and II laryngeal clefts can often be repaired endoscopically and the chosen approach depends on the comfort level of the surgeon. Longer clefts that extend into the cervical or thoracic trachea, such as type II and type III clefts require open approach. For the open approach, a vertical incision is made in the anterior tracheal wall to assess the posterior tracheal wall to repair the cleft. In general the cleft is repaired in two layers, the esophageal layer and then the posterior tracheal wall. An interposition graft consisting of perichondrium form the clavicle or tibia, or cadaveric dermis can be placed between the trachea and esophagus to help reinforce the repair.

VASCULAR COMPRESSION

Vascular compression of the airway, particularly innominate artery compression, is not uncommon. In most cases, however, it is asymptomatic or minimally symptomatic. Although symptomatic vascular compression of the trachea or bronchi is rare, it is associated with marked symptoms, including biphasic stridor, retractions, a honking cough, and "dying spells." Symptoms tend to exacerbate when the child is distressed. Forms of vascular compression affecting the trachea include innominate artery compression, double aortic arch, and pulmonary artery sling. Vascular rings that result from a retroesophageal subclavian artery and a ligamentum arteriosum are less likely to be associated with airway compromise. Bronchial compression by either the pulmonary arteries or aorta may be significant, but in the absence of associated major cardiac anomalies, it is typically a unilateral problem. The diagnosis of airway compression is best established with rigid bronchoscopy. Thoracic imaging then assists in determining the relevant vascular anatomy. Imaging modalities generally include high-resolution computed tomography (CT) with contrast enhancement and 3D reconstruction, magnetic resonance imaging (MRI), magnetic resonance angiography (MRA), and echocardiography (echo). In some cases, formal angiography is required. Although imaging is used primarily to assess intrathoracic vasculature, excellent images of the airway and the thymus gland can also be obtained.

In a child in whom vascular compression causes airway compromise, CPAP frequently offers a degree of temporary improvement, as segmental tracheomalacia may be present in the region of the vascular compression. In a neonate with acute airway compromise, intubation may be required to stabilize the airway prior to definitive treatment. Prolonged intubation should be avoided because of risk of forming an arterial fistula from erosion of an ETT into the area of compression. Similarly, while tracheotomy will establish an unobstructed airway, there is also an increased risk of an arterial fistula into the airway.

The surgical management of symptomatic vascular compression must be individually tailored to address specific pathology. Strategies for managing innominate artery compression include removing the thymus and consideration for suture-pexing the aorta to the sternum to decrease the compression on the trachea. An alternative procedure, though significantly more invasive, is to reimplant the innominate artery more proximally so that it do not traverse the trachea. If the etiological agent of tracheal compression is a double aortic arch, the ligating and dividing the smaller of the two arches is often sufficient to mitigate tracheal compression. If the etiological factor of tracheal compression is a pulmonary artery sling, the pulmonary artery is transected at its origin, dissected free, and reimplanted into the pulmonary trunk anterior to the trachea. Children with a pulmonary artery sling often have associated complete tracheal rings and a high-index of suspicion for this type of lesion should be high when dealing with this vascular anomaly.

Though the etiological factor causing tracheal compression is corrected, the trachea might still be malacic at the site of compression secondary to decreased cartilage integrity. Therefore, the child may still have symptoms of airway compromise until the airway regains its integrity. Until the airway normalizes, children who are persistently symptomatic may require stabilization with a tracheotomy. The use of intratracheal stents in children with tracheal malacia is fraught with complications and should be considered very carefully prior to use.[21]

TRACHEOMALACIA

Tracheomalacia is the most common congenital tracheal anomaly. Most children are either asymptomatic or minimally symptomatic and most cases involve posterior malacia of the trachealis, with associated broad tracheal rings. Commonly associated abnormalities include laryngeal clefts, TEFs, and bronchomalacia. Presenting symptoms include a honking cough, wheezing, respiratory distress when agitated, and dying spells.[22] Diagnosis is established with rigid or flexible bronchoscopy, while maintaining spontaneous respiration. The key elements of diagnosis include: ascertaining the severity of the malacia; ascertaining the location of the malacia, particularly the possible presence of associated bronchomalacia; and determining whether positive pressure support improves the malacia. Although mild tracheomalacia is watched expectantly and anticipated to improve with time, more severe symptoms warrant intervention.[23] Tracheotomy placement, with the tip of the tracheotomy tube bypassing the malacic segment, remains the most common intervention. Positive pressure support delivered down the tracheotomy tube assists with associated bronchomalacia. An alternative surgical procedure for isolated tracheomalacia is aortopexy, with thymectomy and anterior suspension of the ascending arch of the aorta to the posterior periosteum of the sternum. While alluring, the placement of intratracheal stents is presently discouraged.

COMPLETE TRACHEAL RINGS

Complete tracheal rings are a rare congenital tracheal anomaly, and associated symptoms can range from asymptomatic to severe and life-threatening. Although complete tracheal rings are rare, they are life-threatening. Children with tracheal stenosis, especially in the intrathoracic

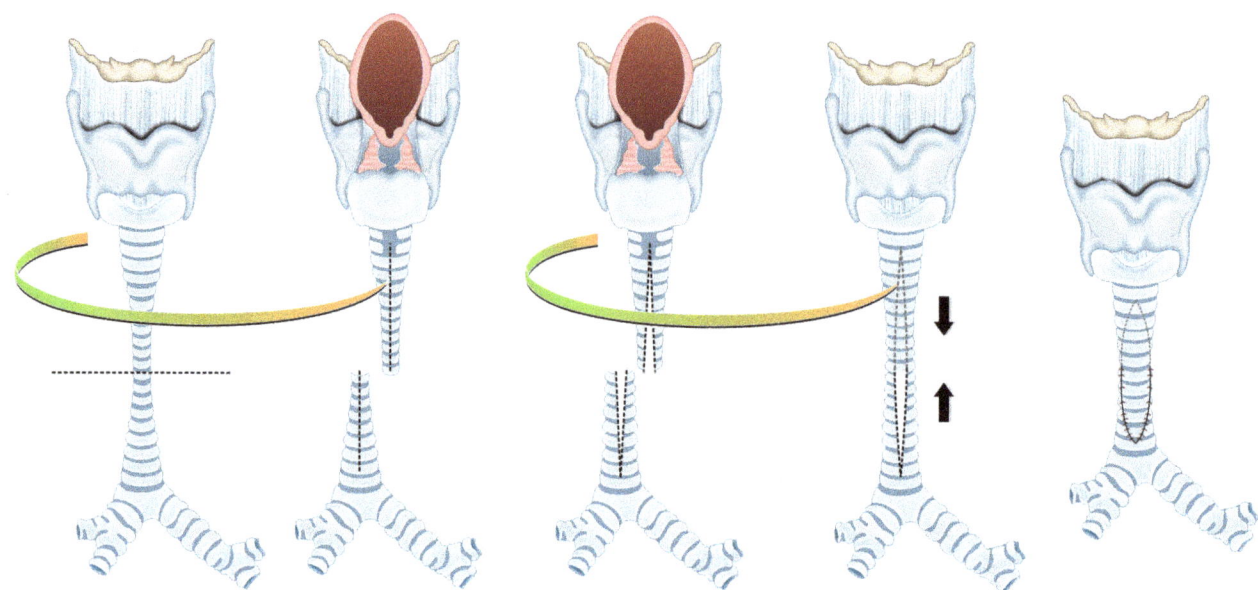

Fig. 6 Schematic representation of a slide tracheoplasty

trachea, have a characteristic biphasic wet-sounding breathing pattern that transiently clears with coughing. While definitive diagnosis is made with rigid bronchoscopy, an initial high-kilovolt airway film or high-resolution chest CT may provide necessary information for anesthesia planning. Airway endoscopy on children with suspected complete tracheal rings should be performed with great caution and critical airway precautions. Airway endoscopy should be performed with the smallest possible telescopes, as any airway edema in the region of the stenosis may turn a narrow airway into an extremely critical airway. During endoscopy, determination of the location, extent, and degree of stenosis are relevant, though the primary goal is to stabilize the airway. Children with complete tracheal rings can have airways as small as 2 mm in diameter, and therefore, standard methods for managing a compromised airway are not applicable. The smallest ETT (2.5 ETT) has an outer diameter of 2.9 mm, and the smallest tracheotomy tube has an outer diameter of 3.9 mm. Therefore, in these children intubation and tracheotomy are not options to bypass the stenosis and stabilize the airway. Extracorporeal membrane oxygenation (ECMO) is often needed to stabilize these children and therefore should be resource available if an airway is to be managed properly in these patients. Over 80% of children with complete tracheal rings have other congenital anomalies, which are generally cardiovascular in origin. As such, investigation should include a high-resolution contrast-enhanced CT scan of the chest and a cardiac echo. Options for surgical repair of complete tracheal rings are wide and differ in efficacy and required surgical skill level. Open surgical techniques include costal cartilage graft augmentation, perichondrial patch, tracheal resection and slide tracheoplasty (Fig. 6).[24-26]

REFERENCES

1. Hartnick CJ, Hartley BE, Lacy PD, et al. Surgery for pediatric subglottic stenosis: disease-specific outcomes. Ann Otol Rhinol Laryngol. 2001;110(12):1109-13.
2. Holinger LD, Green CG. Anatomy. In: Holinger LD, Lusk RP, Green CG (Eds). Pediatric Laryngology and Bronchoesophagology. Philadelphia: Lippincott-Raven; 1997. pp. 19-33.
3. Fearon B, Crysdale WS, Bird R. Subglottic stenosis of the larynx in the infant and child. Methods of management. Ann Otol Rhinol Laryngol. 1978;87(5):645-8.
4. Baxter MR. Congenital laryngomalacia. Can J Anaesth. 1994;41(4):332-9.
5. O'Sullivan BP, Finger L, Zwerdling RG. Use of nasopharyngoscopy in the evaluation of children with noisy breathing. Chest. 2004;125(4):1265-9.
6. Denoyelle F, Mondain M, Gresillon N, et al. Failures and complications of supraglottoplasty in children. Arch Otolaryngol Head Neck Surg. 2003;129(10):1077-80.
7. Holinger LD, Holinger PC, Holinger PH. Etiology of bilateral abductor vocal cord paralysis: a review of 389 cases. Ann Otol Rhinol Laryngol. 1976;85(4):428-36.
8. Miyamoto RC, Parikh SR, Gellad W, et al. Bilateral congenital vocal cord paralysis: a 16-year institutional review. Otolaryngol Head Neck Surg. 2005;133(2):241-5.
9. Brigger MT, Hartnick CJ. Surgery for pediatric vocal cord paralysis: a meta-analysis. Otolaryngol Head Neck Surg. 2004;126(4):349-55.
10. Hartnick CJ, Brigger MT, Willging JP, et al. Surgery for pediatric vocal cord paralysis: a retrospective review. Ann Otol Rhinol Laryngol. 2003;112(1):1-6.
11. Miyamoto RC, Cotton RT, Rope AF, et al. Association of anterior glottic webs with velocardiofacial syndrome (chromosome 22q11.2 deletion). Otolaryngol Head Neck Surg. 2004; 130(4):415-7.

12. Wyatt ME, Hartley BE. Laryngotracheal reconstruction in congenital laryngeal webs and atresias. Otolaryngol Head Neck Surg. 2005;132(2):232-8.

13. Halstead LA. Role of gastroesophageal reflux in pediatric upper airway disorders. Otolaryngol Head Neck Surg. 1999;120(2):208-14.

14. Yellon RF, Goldberg H. Update on gastroesophageal reflux disease in pediatric airway disorders. Am J Med. 2001;111(8A):78S-84S.

15. Hartnick CJ, Liu JH, Cotton RT, et al. Subglottic stenosis complicated by allergic esophagitis: case report. Ann Otol Rhinol Laryngol. 2002;111(1):57-60.

16. Walner DL, Cotton RT. Acquired anomalies of the larynx and trachea. In: Cotton RT, Myer CM 3rd (Eds). Practical pediatric otolaryngology. Philadelphia: Lippincott-Raven; 1999. pp. 515-38.

17. Cotton RT, Gray SD, Miller RP. Update of the Cincinnati experience in pediatric laryngotracheal reconstruction. Laryngoscope. 1989;99(11):1111-6.

18. White DR, Cotton RT, Bean JA, et al. Pediatric cricotracheal resection: surgical outcomes and risk factor analysis. Arch Otolaryngol Head Neck Surg. 2005;131(10):896-9.

19. Gustafson LM, Hartley BE, Liu JH, et al. Single-stage laryngotracheal reconstruction in children: a review of 200 cases. Otolaryngol Head Neck Surg. 2000;123(4):430-4.

20. Hartley BE, Gustafson LM, Liu JH, et al. Duration of stenting in single-stage laryngotracheal reconstruction with anterior costal cartilage grafts. Ann Otol Rhinol Laryngol. 2001;110(5):413-6.

21. Wright CD. Pediatric tracheal surgery. Chest Surg Clin N Am. 2003;13(2):305-14.

22. Rutter MJ, Azizkhan RG, Cotton RT. Posterior laryngeal cleft. In: Ziegler MM, Azizkhan RG, Weber TR (Eds). Operative pediatric surgery. New York: McGraw-Hill; 2003.

23. McNamara VM, Crabbe DC. Tracheomalacia. Paediatr Respir Rev. 2004;5(2):147-54.

24. Rutter MJ, Cotton RT, Azizkhan RG, et al. Slide tracheoplasty for the management of complete tracheal rings. J Pediatr Surg. 2003;38(6):928-34.

25. Cheng W, Manson DE, Forte V, et al. The role of conservative management in congenital tracheal stenosis: an evidence-based long-term follow-up study. J Pediatr Surg. 2006;41(7):1203-7.

26. Chiu PP, Kim PC. Prognostic factors in the surgical treatment of congenital tracheal stenosis: a multicenter analysis of the literature. J Pediatr Surg. 2006;41(1):221-5.

18

Pediatric Dysphagia

J Paul Willging, Aliza P Cohen

INTRODUCTION

In view of improved survival rates of children with a history of prematurity, low birth weight, and complex medical conditions affecting the swallowing process, it is not surprising that the incidence of pediatric dysphagia has increased over the past four decades.[1-4] Given this increase, there is a high likelihood of practitioners encountering dysphagic patients in clinical practice. With this in mind, the aim of the present discussion is to provide clinicians with a basic understanding of the swallowing process and to present an overview of the etiologies of pediatric dysphagia, the recommended diagnostic workup, and current management strategies.

MATURATIONAL CHANGES IN SWALLOWING

Ultrasound studies have shown that the brainstem and cerebral pathways critical to oral sensorimotor function, respiration, and swallowing undergo development throughout the fetal period and that the ability to produce a rhythmic sucking, swallowing, and breathing pattern is generally established at 32 weeks' gestation.[5] Although preterm infants lack the ability to coordinate sucking, swallowing, and breathing, they demonstrate active nonnutritive sucking and swallowing bursts.

The small size and shape of the oral cavity relative to the tongue facilitates early suckling as well as the gradual development of more mature sucking skills during the first 4 months of life. The oral cavity forms a relatively rigid suction chamber with thick buccal fat pads laterally and the palate superiorly. The buccal fat pads provide lateral stability and the tongue fills most of this sucking chamber, contacting all surfaces. The nipple is drawn into the oral cavity, and the lips seal over the nipple anteriorly while the tongue seals against the palate posteriorly. The mid-tongue descends in a piston-like motion, creating a negative pressure in the oral cavity. The creation of negative pressure draws fluid out of the nipple. As infant suckling transitions into mature sucking, lip closure on the nipple increases and tongue movements become vertical with accompanying slight vertical movement of the jaw, resulting in improved sucking efficiency. The changes in range and variation of overall tongue movement are essential for the eventual transition to ingestion of food material other than liquid.

The high position of the infant's larynx functionally separates the respiratory and digestive tracts until 4–6 months of age in term infants by minimizing the overlap of the hypopharyngeal airway and the digestive tract. This position forces a bolus to divert around the epiglottis as the pharynx fills with the bolus and contracts sequentially for swallowing. The proximity of hypopharyngeal structures requires cessation of respiration during swallowing to minimize the risk of aspiration.

With maturity, changes in the swallowing response occur. The prominent buccal pads decrease, the oral cavity enlarges, and the relative size of the tongue decreases—creating more space for both differentiated tongue movements and soft-palate movement. Elongation of the pharynx occurs, as does maturational descent of the larynx. During this gradual descent, support is provided by increased neuromuscular control of the structural elements of the hypopharynx, as opposed to the positional stability provided earlier by the proximity of structures. Maintenance of continued airway protection during swallowing depends on normal neuromuscular development.

As the larynx descends to its adult level, with the cricoid cartilage overlying the C6 or C7 vertebral bodies, the airway is protected by the laryngeal adductor reflex (LAR); this reflex provides closure of the vocal folds, thereby preventing aspiration of bolus contents. Both mechanoreceptors and chemoreceptors within the laryngeal and pharyngeal walls are associated with the LAR. The presence of a bolus passing the supraglottis stimulates the nerve endings of the superior laryngeal nerve (SLN), which sends afferent sensory information though the nodose ganglion to the nucleus solitarius in the brainstem. The glottic closure response is initiated at the nucleus ambiguus, which sends an efferent signal through the vagus nerve to the recurrent laryngeal nerve. This signal results in adduction of the true and false vocal folds to protect the airway. Neurologic impairment or a structural abnormality that interferes with glottic closure can impede this protective mechanism, leaving the child at increased risk of aspiration with feeding.

During maturation of the swallow response, additional anatomic changes occur in conjunction with the development of neuromuscular head and neck control. These changes facilitate the development of the controlled jaw, lip, and tongue movements necessary for the development of oromotor skills. Increased coordination for bolus manipulation and transfer into the hypopharynx initiate a pharyngeal swallow response similar to that in adults. This initial maturational phase typically occurs during the first 6 months of life. During this period, pureed foods are introduced.

At 7–9 months, head control and postural stability are present, providing support for the introduction of solids. The presentation of food boluses with texture stimulates lingual exploration and helps to initiate the lateral tongue movements required for the development of chewing skills. At 10–12 months of age, children generally begin to accept new and varied tastes and textures. This increasing ability, combined with growing independence with self-feeding, reflects ongoing motor development. During the second year of life, oromotor skills for feeding continue to be refined. By 24 months, basic feeding patterns are established. Further refinements in oromotor skills occur gradually as the child continues to mature.

NORMAL SWALLOWING PHYSIOLOGY

The neural control of swallowing comprises input afferent signals, nerve networks, synaptic connections, and responses driven by motor neurons. A sequential discharge of neurons controls muscle activity in the pharynx, larynx, and esophagus. Four neural components of swallowing have been elucidated: (1) afferent sensory fibers contained in the cranial nerves; (2) efferent motor fibers contained in the cranial nerves and the ansa cervicalis; (3) cerebral, midbrain, and cerebellar fibers that synapse in the midbrain; and (4) the paired swallowing centers in the brainstem.[6,7]

Three Phases of Swallowing

The normal swallowing is a synchronized process that entails an intricate series of voluntary and involuntary neuromuscular contractions. This process consists of three well-defined phases, each of which has a specific function. Difficulties in one or more of these phases constitute dysphagia.

The oral phase of swallowing, which is under voluntary neural control, begins with the introduction of food material into the mouth. Coordinated contractions of the tongue and muscles of mastication shape this material into a bolus. The tongue elevates as the bolus is held in its central groove and then moves in a peristaltic fashion against the palate. The posterior propulsion of the bolus by the tongue into the pharynx triggers the onset of the involuntary swallow reflex.

For the most part, the second or pharyngeal phase is involuntary. Pharyngeal swallows are initiated in an ordered sequential pattern in response to stimulation by food or secretions in the pharynx. Tactile receptors in the pharynx provide sensory stimulation to the medullary swallowing center via the trigeminal, glossopharyngeal, and vagus nerves.[8] The medullary swallowing center initiates a swallow by stimulating the nucleus ambiguus and the dorsomedial vagal nucleus. Next, the soft palate closes against the posterior pharyngeal wall to isolate the nasopharynx from the oropharynx as food is propelled posteriorly. The bolus is propelled through the oropharynx by the contraction of the pharyngeal muscles against the base of the tongue. Proprioceptive feedback adjusts the peristaltic activity for different food bolus sizes and consistencies.[9]

Because the pharynx serves as a conduit for food as well as air exchange, precise coordination of breathing and swallowing is necessary during feeding. With the initiation of the swallow, respiration is inhibited and the larynx is pulled superiorly and anteriorly, effectively moving the laryngeal inlet out of the direct path of the bolus. The true and false vocal folds are then closed, and the epiglottis retroflexes over the laryngeal inlet. The secondary effect of laryngeal elevation is that the upper esophageal sphincter is pulled open, and the peristaltic contractions of the pharyngeal constrictor muscles propel the bolus into the esophagus.

The esophagus is a conduit between the pharynx and the stomach, with muscular sphincters at either end in tonic contraction to keep the esophagus closed between swallows. The upper esophageal sphincter relaxes during swallowing and is actively opened by laryngeal elevation to allow the food bolus to enter the esophagus. Peristaltic contractions propel the bolus into the stomach. The lower esophageal sphincter (LES) relaxes to allow passage of the bolus. Tonic contraction of the LES prevents the reflux of gastric contents into the lower esophagus.

MECHANICS OF SWALLOWING

The normal swallowing process protects the lower airway from contamination by oropharyngeal secretions and liquid or solid food materials. Once the bolus is formed, the swallowing process is voluntarily initiated by propelling the bolus posteriorly into the pharynx. As tongue base retraction occurs to deliver the bolus into the pharynx, both the true and false vocal folds begin to close, providing a double layer of closure over the top of the airway. Laryngeal elevation actively pulls the upper esophageal sphincter open in preparation for the descending bolus. After the bolus passes into the esophagus, the larynx descends along with the hyoid, the epiglottis returns to its vertical position, and the true and false vocal cords open to allow resumption of breathing. The soft palate also descends to its resting position, allowing nasal respiration to resume.

Aspiration

Aspiration is the passage of solid or liquid material below the level of the vocal folds; the potential for this to occur is greatest during the pharyngeal phase of swallowing. Aspiration of small volumes of material may be cleared from the airway by normal mucociliary clearance or a cough. Large volumes of aspirated material may, however, reach the distal airway and be only partially cleared, leading to the possibility of developing aspiration pneumonia. Because oral secretions are laden with high concentrations of bacteria from the oral cavity, aspiration of these secretions may lead to chronic lung damage over time.[10]

For children whose strength and endurance is compromised due to developmental, neurologic or other medical conditions, fatigue during feeding can increase the risk of aspiration.[11]

CLINICAL PRESENTATION

Clinical presentation varies widely. Symptoms may range from observable problems such as projectile vomiting, coughing, or choking to silent aspiration, in which no coughing, choking, or other signs of problems are apparent when food or liquid enters the trachea. Neonates may exhibit sucking difficulty or sucking that is unaccompanied by swallowing. They may also have little interest in feeding. Other signs that should arouse a high index of suspicion include delayed or restricted oromotor skills for intake of food or liquid, retaining food in the mouth, coughing and gagging when feeding, nasal reflux

of food or liquid, failure to gain weight, changes in respiratory patterns when feeding or shortly after, or noisy breathing. Dysphagia should also be suspected in children who have repeated episodes of respiratory infections and suffer chronic bronchial congestion and in children with various metabolic diseases and genetic syndromes. Dysmorphic features often indicate the presence of syndromes commonly associated with dysphagia (e.g. Cornelia de Lange syndrome, Pierre-Robin syndrome, velocardiofacial syndrome, and VACTERL association).[12]

ETIOLOGIES

The predominant etiologies of pediatric dysphagia fall within six broad categories, including: (1) structural anomalies, (2) neurologic conditions, (3) cardiorespiratory problems, (4) behavioral issues, (5) developmental problems, and (6) metabolic or inflammatory disorders.[13]

Any structural anomaly from the nasal cavity to the gastrointestinal tract can potentially disrupt swallowing. Children with defects in the oral cavity or oropharynx may experience difficulty in the oral phase, and children with congenital defects of the larynx or trachea may develop feeding difficulties secondary to airway compromise during swallowing. Esophageal abnormalities may interfere with the transport of food material into the distal digestive tract. All of these problems may create discomfort during feeding, leading to feeding refusal and consequent behavioral feeding problems. In children who have undergone reconstructive procedures to correct anatomic anomalies, the behavioral issues may continue to predominate, thereby perpetuating feeding problems.

Neurologic disorders are the most frequently encountered etiology. Neuromotor impairment as a result of cortical dysfunction, brainstem abnormalities, or cervical cord injuries affects the strength and efficiency of the oral and pharyngeal phases of swallowing, the adequacy of coordination of airway protection and swallowing, as well as overall alertness and the postural control required for safe and efficient feeding. In addition, these children often present with esophageal problems that further complicate management.

Cardiorespiratory compromise often affects an infant's ability to initiate or sustain a coordinated suck-swallow-breathe sequence. Feeding often results in accompanying apnea or episodes of bradycardia, thereby affecting feeding endurance and often preventing adequate food intake. Problems with respiratory compromise may result in poor coordination or inappropriate timing of airway protection during swallowing; in turn, these scenarios may result in coughing, choking, or episodes of apnea, bradycardia, chronic noisy breathing, or wheezing, as well as chronic or recurrent pneumonia, bronchitis, or atelectasis.

Behavior-based feeding problems may stem from psychosocial factors such as dysfunctional feeder—child interaction, poor environmental stimulation, conditioned dysphagia (a phobic response resulting from an aversive oral or pharyngeal experience or a painful feeding experience such as choking), or negative feeding behaviors. Behavioral responses may include refusal to eat, rejection of certain foods or textures, and gagging or vomiting. Eliminating the possibility of underlying physiologic factors before focused behavioral treatment is essential.

An evaluation of feeding ability must consider the child's developmental status. Most important, the clinician must be cognizant of the fact that feeding skills mature over time in concert with other developmental milestones.

Metabolic abnormalities such as hereditary fructose intolerance or endocrine problems, and inflammatory processes such as allergies or esophagitis can interfere with the development or maintenance of normal oromotor and feeding patterns.

OVERALL EVALUATION

A Multidisciplinary Approach

Optimally, patients are assessed by a multidisciplinary team comprising physicians as well as professionals from psychology, speech pathology, nutrition therapy, and occupational therapy. The collective aim is to identify physiologic and behavioral factors that may be disrupting the normal feeding and swallowing process. A comprehensive assessment involves an evaluation of the child's overall health status as well as consideration of parental concerns and parent-child interactions. Medical history, physical examination, and clinical observation are the three major components of the assessment.

Medical History

The medical history should identify any possible medical, developmental, neurologic, or surgical etiology that could compromise the normal airway protective mechanism or interfere with the swallowing process.[14,15] Documentation of the child's previous medical and surgical interventions, including periods in which no oral nutrition was received, should be obtained. Given that abnormal oral skills are frequently observed in children who have had feeding withheld during critical periods of development, this information is particularly important. During these critical periods, a specific feeding stimulus must be experienced to promote subsequent oral motor and feeding skills. Beyond these periods, the particular behavior pattern is difficult to learn.[16] Distinguishing between infants who resist feedings because of previous unpleasant experiences and those who have current physiologic problems is fundamental to the provision of appropriate feeding treatment.

Parents should be questioned regarding the child's history of recurrent upper respiratory infections, recurrent pneumonia, upper airway noise, or stridor in relation to feeding. The status of the airway before, during, and after feeding should be explored, as should be a possible correlation between feeding and symptoms such as gagging, coughing, apnea or cyanosis.

Physical Examination

Physical examination should focus on the upper aerodigestive tract. Structures related to the oral cavity should be examined.[17] Attention should be paid to the lip and palate, as clefts can have a significant impact on oral feeding efficiency. The relative size and position of the tongue and mandible can influence the swallow and adequacy of the airway during feeding. The status of the craniofacial skeleton may indicate syndromes associated with oromotor difficulties. The absence of a gag reflex may also signal other neurologic abnormalities. Examination of the chest should focus on the presence of rales and rhonchi. An abdominal examination should also be performed to rule out any associated abnormalities. Patients with a history of coughing or choking associated with feeding and those with a history suggestive of aspiration should undergo flexible laryngoscopy, which can be performed in the office setting without sedation. This procedure can document the mobility of the vocal folds as well as the presence of laryngomalacia or other laryngeal pathology. The general status of the hypopharynx with respect to the amount of retained secretions, tongue position, and sensation can also be ascertained.

Clinical Observation

Oromotor problems may present with specific clinical signs. If lip closure is poor, food materials may spill out of the mouth during feeding. In the presence of decreased orofacial tone, food materials may tend to collect in the anterior or lateral sulci. Improper tongue control may propel food material out of the mouth rather than posteriorly for swallowing. Poor tongue mobility affects chewing patterns and the efficiency of mastication. Poor tongue movements also may be a sign of apraxia of swallowing. A child with a weak suck or poor coordination of the sucking process tends to present with multiple sucks per swallow to compensate for the lack of efficiency. Nasopharyngeal regurgitation may occur with poor timing of velopharyngeal closure during the swallow, or may be caused by muscular weakness or paralysis preventing adequate closure. It also may be suggestive of cricopharyngeal achalasia, as the bolus does not exit the hypopharynx with contraction of the pharyngeal muscles. The bolus remains under pressure and may be expelled into the nasopharynx when the velum descends.

Attention to the position and posture of the child and the mechanics of feeding skills during the ingestion of various textures also provides clues regarding underlying structural or physiologic problems. Underlying neurologic or structural problems may be identified by observing behaviors such as the ability to handle oral secretions, the pace of feeding, escape of food from the mouth, tongue and jaw movements, number of swallows to clear a bolus, noisy airway sounds after swallowing, coordination of suck and swallow, laryngeal elevation, gagging, coughing, or emesis associated with feedings.

Observation of a feeding session by multidisciplinary team members provides insight into the underlying feeding problem. Parent-child interactions and the child's responses to offered food materials are noted. These observations focus on behavior problems, allowing for future structuring of behavioral interventions.

DIAGNOSTIC WORKUP

Radiographic Studies

Videofluoroscopic Swallow Study

Often referred to as the gold standard for evaluating infants and children with swallowing disorders,[18] the videofluoroscopic swallow study (VSS) allows for the noninvasive assessment of the oral, pharyngeal, and esophageal phases of swallowing and the interrelationship of these phases. Additionally, VSS enables the determination of consistencies and conditions for safe swallowing and allows a trial of compensatory and therapeutic techniques to improve the safety and efficiency of swallowing. Patients are positioned for both lateral and anterior/posterior viewing under fluoroscopy and are presented with liquid and solid consistencies mixed with barium. Ideally, the study is performed jointly by a radiologist and a speech pathologist, with parent involvement in the feeding process. Prior to the study, parents or caretakers provide the speech pathologist with information regarding the child's best eating position and preferred method of food presentation. To ensure a successful examination, food materials that the child is accustomed to and can easily manage are initially offered. These food materials then progress to materials that are problematic. When problems are demonstrated, therapeutic interventions can be attempted to improve the safety of swallowing. These interventions may include examining the patient's response to other textures, alternating presentations of liquid and solids, and exploring

the therapeutic efficacy of modifications in bolus volume, nipple or utensil types, the pace of presentation, and body posture.

The most notable downside of the VSS is that it exposes both the patient and the feeder to radiation. Moreover, assessment of compensatory strategies adds to the overall exposure time. As well, adding barium to liquid and food sometimes decreases a child's willingness to drink or eat during the study. Moreover, because adding barium significantly increases viscosity, preparing a true thin liquid is not possible. Lastly, the study is not feasible for patients who take extremely limited amounts of liquid or food orally because the patient must be able to ingest a sufficient amount of contrast in order to obtain adequate imaging.

Esophagram and Upper Gastrointestinal Study

The esophagram and upper gastrointestinal study examine the anatomy and function of the esophagus, stomach, and duodenum. Infants are studied in the supine and lateral positions as barium suspension is either taken from a bottle or injected through a nipple placed intraorally. Dynamic images are obtained as the bolus passes through the oropharynx, into the esophagus, and into the stomach. Careful assessment of a possible tracheoesophageal fistula requires an adequate volume of contrast to distend the esophagus. In patients who cannot swallow an adequate volume of contrast, a tube is passed into the esophagus, providing a means of demonstrating the fistulous tract. Abnormalities such as esophageal strictures, webs, vascular rings, or achalasia may be identified.

Chest X-ray

Chronic aspiration leads to changes in the lung parenchyma that can be seen on plain chest X-rays. Typical findings include hyperinflation, segmental infiltrates, peribronchial thickening, and bronchiectasis. Aspiration events affect the basilar and superior segments of the lower lobes, and the posterior upper-lobe segments. Subtle changes associated with early lung injury cannot be detected radiographically.

High-resolution Computed Tomography

High-resolution computed tomography (HRCT) of the chest provides a means to detect parenchymal changes in the lungs at an earlier stage of development than detected in a plain chest film. Findings commonly associated with chronic aspiration though not specific to it include bronchiectasis, centrilobular opacities, air trapping, and bronchial thickening.

High-resolution computed tomography findings must be interpreted with caution. Indications of chronic change may not reflect current aspiration problems, but rather, may reflect past aspiration events. HRCT of the chest is best used as a baseline measure from which future comparisons can be made.

Fiberoptic Endoscopic Evaluation of Swallowing

Indications for a Pediatric FEES

Deciding who will benefit from fiberoptic endoscopic evaluation of swallowing (FEES) depends on a number of clinical factors.[19] Children who have never fed orally or who accept only limited oral intake are poor candidates for VSS, as it requires oral ingestion of an adequate amount of barium suspension to visualize the swallowing process. In this patient population, FEES allows assessment of structure, function, management of secretions, sensory awareness, and spontaneous swallowing without having to administer food items. Assessment of a patient's ability to manage secretions provides the clinician with insight into the patient's ability to protect the airway. Patients who have had abnormal findings on a VSS also benefit from FEES, as additional and complementary information can be obtained. The study allows an assessment of overall swallowing safety and permits a trial of compensatory strategies, eliminating the concern for prolonged radiation exposure. The routine FEES screening of patients who are candidates for airway reconstruction can identify those at increased risk of aspiration following repair of the airway. In such cases, the family can be made aware of the problem and can be advised regarding the need for postoperative nutritional modifications.

Anesthesia Preparation

Patient cooperation is essential to the success of the pediatric FEES examination. To maximize cooperation, a topical anesthetic is used. Our preferred material is a 1:1 mixture of oxymetazoline and 2% lidocaine or topical lidocaine. To prevent anesthetizing the hypopharynx, it is important to have the child upright with the head in a neutral position. Because the nasal mucociliary clearance of a substance from the nose to the hypopharynx takes longer than 30 minutes, the effect of anesthesia remains localized to the nose and the FEES examination can be performed prior to the onset of potential hypopharyngeal anesthesia.

Alternatively, anesthesia can be obtained by applying a thin layer of 2% topical viscous lidocaine gel to coat the distal end of the endoscope. The lidocaine gel will be absorbed primarily as it passes through the nasal cavity. This is our preferred approach for children younger than 1 year of age, children with complex underling medical conditions (e.g.

congenital heart disease, and severe bronchopulmonary dysplasia) and for those who do not have a tracheotomy in place but who have a tenuous airway.

Passage of the Endoscope

The patient is positioned upright for passage of the endoscope. Infants, children younger than age 8, and those with special disabilities require gentle restraint and are thus positioned in the lap of the parent or caretaker or an assistant. Older children and adolescents often can sit without assistance in the examining chair. Once the endoscope has been passed, positioning alterations can carefully be implemented either to simulate normal positioning during feeding or as a compensatory strategy to improve the swallowing process.

Anatomic Evaluation

Evaluation of upper aerodigestive tract anatomy begins with an assessment of the nasal cavity. Nasal patency should be documented as the endoscope is advanced through the nose. Nasal obstruction can interfere with swallowing function, particularly in infants. The function of the velopharyngeal sphincter is evaluated as the scope is passed through the choanae. Abnormal sphincter closure may be associated with nasopharyngeal reflux during feeding. Incomplete or inefficient velopharyngeal closure also may interfere with the generation of tongue base driving pressure required for bolus propagation into the hypopharynx.

It is important to appreciate that the position of the larynx descends during childhood, reaching its adult location at C6 after puberty. As the larynx descends, there is less separation of the respiratory and digestive tracts. Food materials, liquids, and secretions can therefore pass more readily over the tip of the epiglottis, leading to an increased chance of laryngeal penetration or aspiration.

The pyriform sinuses are assessed for masses and asymmetry that may interfere with the swallowing process. Special attention is paid to the possible presence of laryngeal anomalies, which can interfere with swallowing as well as airway protection. In addition, the degree of pooled secretions at the beginning of the examination should be noted. These secretions may increase throughout the procedure, reflecting an abnormal swallowing process. Secretions that spill into the pyriform sinuses should always be rapidly followed by a clearing swallow, even when the child is upset or crying. Pooled secretions that do not initiate a swallowing response often indicate significant abnormality. Symmetry of pharyngeal contraction during swallowing also should be documented. If structural or functional abnormalities of the supraglottic or glottic larynx are found, they should be described in reference to their impact on the swallowing process and the patient's ability to control secretions.

Components of FEES Assessment

The swallowing assessment is performed with liquids as well as a variety of pureed, smooth, and solid textures as developmentally appropriate. To aid with visualization, the liquid and food items are mixed with green food coloring by the speech pathologist before the study.

The pediatric FEES examination cannot be adequately interpreted without a thorough understanding of the clinical conditions and initial feeding assessment of the patient. All findings obtained from the FEES must be interpreted within the context of this clinical setting.

Pooling of secretions: Pooling of secretions occurs when secretions produced in the oral cavity spill over the tongue base into the hypopharynx and accumulate due to the absence of an adequate swallowing response. This may occur for a variety of reasons, including: an underlying sensory deficit; poor oral motor control; incoordination of swallowing timing; poor pharyngeal clearance; and inadequate relaxation of the cricopharyngeal sphincter. Excessive pooling and poor management of secretions are immediately apparent when the hypopharynx is viewed endoscopically.

Patients with excessive secretions that are not cleared or that increase during the initial part of the examination are at risk for aspiration. In patients with normal hypopharyngeal sensation and pharyngeal clearance mechanisms, secretions do not accumulate in the hypopharynx.

Premature spillage: Premature spillage is the escape of material over the tongue base in the absence of purposeful oral transfer before the initiation of swallowing. Material can enter the vallecula or may overflow and enter the pyriform sinuses. The degree of spillage needs to be evaluated with respect to the ability of the patient to initiate a clearing swallow. Mild delay in the initiation of swallowing can be evidenced by material moving across the tongue base into the vallecular space and into the pyriform sinus region before initiation of the swallow. Premature spillage of a volume sufficient to start filling the pyriform sinuses is of concern, as it may increase the risk of aspiration. If swallowing is not initiated, continued overflow of the bolus into the laryngeal inlet may occur. It is important to note, however, that premature spillage is not always indicative of a pathologic swallow, and may reflect a normal developmental pattern of swallowing. Infants often trigger the swallow from the level of the vallecula without increasing the risk of aspiration.

Laryngeal penetration: Laryngeal penetration is the passage of food material or secretions into the endolarynx. The significance of laryngeal penetration depends on the volume of material entering the larynx and the frequency of penetration events.

Aspiration: As discussed earlier, aspiration is defined as the passage of solid or liquid material below the level of the true vocal folds. It can be visualized on FEES either before or after a swallow; however, it cannot be observed during the height of the swallow, as pharyngeal contraction, laryngeal elevation, and epiglottis retroversion obscure the view of the glottis (whiteout period). Aspiration that occurs during the whiteout period can be deduced by visualizing the events that occur immediately after the swallow, when material is expelled from the airway by a cough, or by identification of stained subglottic structures. The actual volume of aspirated material cannot be estimated by FEES.

Residue: Residue refers to the food material remaining in the hypopharynx after completion of the swallow, thus increasing the risk of aspiration. The amount of residue persisting after the swallow relates directly to the risk of aspiration and the overall safety of swallowing a given food consistency. The patient's awareness of residue is assessed by documenting attempts to clear with additional swallows, throat clearing, or coughing.

Evaluation of Airway Protection

Vocal fold mobility: To prevent aspiration, the distal airway must be adequately protected. This requires intact vocal fold function. The integrity of airway protection can be determined by the FEES. This examination allows direct visualization of vocal fold mobility during phonation and respiration. Bilateral vocal fold paralysis is a significant finding, as it may preclude adequate airway protection. Unilateral vocal fold paralysis can also be problematic. It may be associated with an increased risk of aspiration if the contralateral fold does not cross the midline to oppose the paralyzed vocal fold, closing the glottis.

Fiberoptic Endoscopic Evaluation of Swallowing with Sensory Testing

Performed as an adjunct to FEES, fiberoptic endoscopic evaluation of swallowing with sensory testing (FEESST) offers a tool to further investigate the neural control of swallowing and airway protection.[20] This is assessed by administering an air pulse calibrated for duration and intensity (ranging from 2.5 mm Hg to 10 mm Hg) to the aryepiglottic fold (AE fold) region, and observing the induction of a swallow, a cough, or vocal fold closure. The stimulation threshold required to induce the LAR should be determined for each side of the larynx. We have found that an elevated sensory threshold greater than 4.5 mm Hg strongly correlates with a positive history of aspiration pneumonia.

Dye Studies

In a patient with a tracheotomy tube, signs of an aspiration event can be directly observed. The ingestion of intensely colored food material often stains tracheal secretions when the material is aspirated; adding food coloring may enhance the sensitivity of this test. Suctioning tracheal secretions during or after a meal may reveal traces of the colored material in the suction catheter, indicating that an aspiration event has occurred; however, determining whether the event is secondary to reflux or related to an airway problem during the swallowing process can be difficult. In patients with a feeding tube, dye can be placed directly into the stomach, thereby clarifying the nature of the aspiration. Placing dye within the oral cavity stains oral secretions, providing a means of assessing the patient's ability to protect the airway from salivary contamination.

Nuclear Medicine Scans

Nuclear medicine scans may be used in the assessment of gastric emptying and gastroesophageal reflux. They are also used as a tool for demonstrating aspiration of oral secretions.

Technetium Scan

Technetium scans are useful in the evaluation of children with gastric motility problems. Technetium is mixed with familiar food and administered to the patient. Frequent images are then obtained by a gamma camera for 1 hour; delayed images are obtained for up to 24 hours. Reflux events can be demonstrated by identifying labeled material in the esophagus. The reflux event may deposit gastric contents into the hypopharynx, where it can be cleared through normal pharyngeal contractions or aspirated. The amount of material collecting in the airway is then quantified.

Thallium Scan

Intravenously injected thallium, which is concentrated in the functioning salivary gland tissues, is excreted into the mouth with saliva. This can be used to quantify oral secretions aspirated over time. Images of labeled secretions are obtained with a gamma camera.

Manometry

Although manometric assessment of the upper pharynx and esophagus can provide valuable information regarding esophageal motility, it is technically difficult to carry out in children and is unavailable in most pediatric centers. Generally, it is used only to clarify the physiology of abnormalities noted with barium studies. Additional information about cricopharyngeal tone and relaxation in relation to bolus accommodation can be obtained in children who have difficulty passing a bolus past the upper esophageal segment.

MANAGEMENT APPROACHES

The goal of treatment is to maximize each child's nutritional status in the context of safe and efficient feeding.[21] This frequently involves modifications in the volume, consistency, texture, or temperature of foods and liquids; the use of adaptive oral feeding utensils or equipment (e.g. bottle nipples with varying size, shape, and flow rates) to increase liquid tolerance; or repositioning the head and body to allow for better airway protection or more efficient passage of a food bolus through the oropharynx. For example, tilting the head forward widens the vallecular space, thereby diverting food away from the laryngeal inlet. When appropriate, parents or caregivers also may be provided with exercises to strengthen or improve the coordination of weak muscles of the child's face, tongue, lips, and palate. In patients with a tracheotomy there is a loss of normal subglottic pressure, which may interfere with airway protection. Capping the tracheotomy or placing a speaking valve onto the tracheotomy can normalize this pressure.

Children with psychosocial or behavioral components associated with their dysphagia are generally responsive to behavior therapy. A structured therapeutic program includes techniques such as rewarding successive approximations of targeted behaviors and offering positive reinforcement through praise, access to favorite toys or music, clapping, or any similar age-appropriate reward. Optimally, the gradual advancement of rewarded goals eventually leads to full oral feeding. Behavior therapy is also used to overcome conditioned food refusal (i.e. a learned aversion to feeding) associated with a previous anatomic abnormality that has been corrected.

For many children with neurologic or anatomic abnormalities, safe oral feeding is extremely difficult or impossible. Deciding whether to pursue efforts at oral feeding requires judicious consideration of the potential risks of aspiration and chronic lung disease versus the convenience and emotional rewards of oral feeding. Supplementing a child's nutrition by nasogastric or gastrostomy feedings may be either essential or prudent in terms of the child's overall development and well-being.

REFERENCES

1. Arvedson JC. Assessment of pediatric dysphagia and feeding disorders: clinical and instrumental approaches. Devel Disabil Res Rev. 2008;14:118-27.

2. Lefton-Greif MA. Pediatric dysphagia. Phys Med Rehabil Clin N Am. 2008; 19:837-51.

3. Newman LA, Keckley C, Petersen MC, et al. Swallowing function and medical diagnoses in infants suspected of dysphagia. Pediatrics. 2001;108:E106.

4. Hawdon JM. Bequregard N, Slattery J, et al. Identification of neonates at risk of developing feeding problems in infancy. Dev Med Child Neurol. 2000;42:235-9.

5. Miller JL, Sonies BC, Macedonia C. Emergence of oropharyngeal, laryngeal, and swallowing activity in the developing fetal upper aerodigestive tract: an ultrasound evaluation. Early Hum Dev. 2003;71:61-87.

6. Miller AJ. Deglutition. Physiol Rev. 1982;62:129-84.

7. Dodds WJ, Stewart ET, Logemann JA. Physiology and radiology of the normal oral and pharyngeal phases of swallowing. Am J Roentgenol. 1990;154:953-63.

8. Kahrilas PJ. Pharyngeal structure and function. Dysphagia. 1993;8:303-7.

9. Miller AJ. The search for the central swallowing pathway: the quest for clarity. Dysphagia. 1993;8:185-94.

10. Boesch RP, Daines C, Willging JP, et al. Advances in the diagnosis and management of chronic pulmonary aspiration in children. Eur Respir J. 2006;28:847-61.

11. Friedman B, Frazier JB. Deep laryngeal penetration as a predictor of aspiration. Dysphagia. 2000;15:153-8.

12. Cooper-Brown L, Copeland S, Dailey S, et al. Feeding and swallowing dysfunction in genetic syndromes. Dev Disabil Res Rev. 2008;14:147-57.

13. Burklow KA, Phelps AN, Schultz JR, et al. Classifying complex pediatric feeding disorders. J Pediatr Gastroenterol Nutr. 1998;27:143-7.

14. Derkay CS, Plant RL. Dysphagia. In: Bluestone CD, Stool SE, Alper CM, et al. (Eds). Pediatric Otolaryngology, Vol 2, Fourth edition. Philadelphia: Saunders; 2003. pp. 11128-37.

15. Levy Y, Levy A, Zangen T, et al. Diagnostic clues for identification of nonorganic vs organic causes of food refusal and poor feeding. J Pediatr Gastroenterol Nutr. 2009;48:355-62.

16. Illingworth RS, Lister JL. The critical or sensitive period, with special reference to certain feeding problems in infants and children. J Pediatr. 1964;65:839-48.

17. Garg BP. Dysphagia in children: an overview. Semin Pediatr Neurol. 2003;10:252-4.

18. Logemann JA. Approaches to management of disordered swallowing. Baillieres Clin Gastroenterol. 1991;5:269-80.

19. Willging JP. Benefit of feeding assessment before pediatric airway reconstruction. Laryngoscope. 2000;110:825-34.

20. Willging JP, Thompson DM. Pediatric FEESST: Fiberoptic endoscopic evaluation of swallowing with sensory testing. Curr Gastroenterol Rep. 2005;7:240-3.

21. Prasse JE, Kikano GE. An overview of pediatric dysphagia. Clin Pediatr. 2009;48:247-51.

Effects of Swallow Therapy in Oropharyngeal Dysphagia

Divya Chandrasekhar

INTRODUCTION

Working with adults with dysphagia is a challenging and rewarding part of the practice of speech-language pathology. The ultimate aim of swallow rehabilitation is to improve and restore the impaired swallow physiology of an individual, so as to maximize participation in social events. Swallow rehabilitation is usually patient-specific. It varies according to the diagnosis, underlying cause, alteration in the anatomy and physiology of swallow mechanism, patient's mental status and motivation, and medical prognosis.

The best treatment for swallowing is swallowing! (Logemann, 1999).[1] Generally, management of swallowing disorders are either by compensatory strategies or therapeutic approaches. Compensatory strategies include postural changes,[1] and modification of bolus volume and consistency, as well as rate of food presentation. These strategies are designed to eliminate the symptoms of swallowing problems, but may not directly change the swallow physiology. It is generally used in the acute and/or severe phases of recovery. An example is the chin-tuck posture. This reduces the bolus spillage into the hypopharynx before the swallow. Therapeutic strategies are rehabilitative which are intended to restore or improve the actual swallowing physiology. It includes oral sensory stimulation, oromotor exercises, swallow maneuvers, maxillofacial prosthesis, medication and surgical procedures. An example is laryngeal adduction exercise which is intended to improve laryngeal valving. In general, rehabilitative strategies are recommended for patients with greater potential for swallow recovery and for patients who have the physical, cognitive, and psychological resources to perform, learn, retain, and use the strategies independently.

Many of these techniques may be used in combination with one another, and the basic rule of application is to use that approach which works best with the individual patient.

This chapter describes swallow therapy techniques used clinically. They are described under the headings of overview, goal and rationale, instruction/procedural steps, candidacy, contraindications if any and relevant literature regarding the efficacy of the techniques. Practical suggestions and cautions gained from clinical practice are also illustrated.

INDIRECT THERAPEUTIC STRATEGIES

Posture

Body Posture

One of the first rules for safe oral feed is determining the best body posture for an individual (Fig. 1). In general, an upright posture is advised to take advantage of the effects of gravity in propelling the bolus through the pharynx more quickly and the laryngeal protective responses do not get affected when swallowing occurs in the upright sitting posture.[2] In addition, upright posture makes it harder for the refluxed material to re-enter the pharynx after swallowing.

However, in individuals with impaired trunk and/or head control through stroke, TBI, or other acquired neurological or physical injury, measures must be taken to allow head and/or trunk support to occur. This may involve progressively reclining the chair/bed to an angle that best allows the body to be supported and reduce the physiological load during eating. Dorsey (2002) found that upright positioning (70–90°) in individuals with severe disabilities was associated

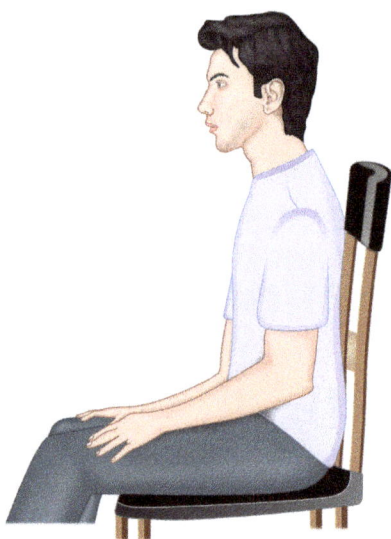

Fig. 1 Body posture

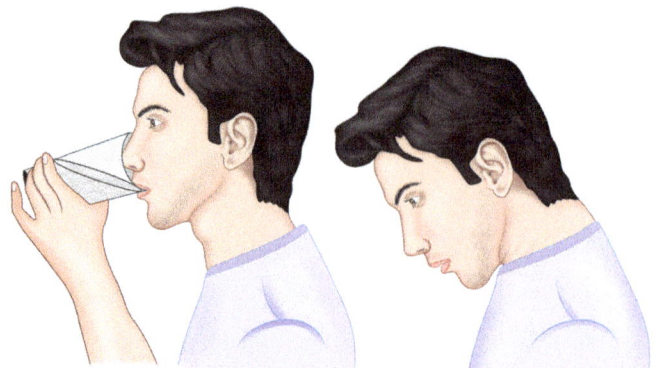

Fig. 2 Chin tuck posture

with aspiration.[3] However, 60–35° positioning showed reduction in aspiration.

Head posture

Overview: Logemann (1983) developed various head posture strategies with an understanding that a change to the swallowing physiology is possible when there is a change to the anatomical alignment of the structures during swallowing.[4]

Various head postures which are used with dysphagic patients are as follows:
- Chin tuck
- Head rotation
- Head tilt
- Neck extension.

Chin tuck posture: It is one of the widely used head postures (Fig. 2).
- *Rationale:* In chin tuck posture, airway is maximally protected. (i.e. larynx is brought further under the base of the tongue so as to physically bring it away from the bolus). In addition, tongue base is afforded a closer position to the pharyngeal walls and pushes epiglottis posteriorly.[5]
- *Instruction:* Patient is asked to position his chin toward the chest and look down toward the knees during swallow.
- *Candidacy:* The chin tuck has been used when there is a delay in triggering pharyngeal swallow or if there is reduced posterior movement of the tongue base.[6]
- *Contraindications:* Patients with compromised respiratory system may find it difficult to use chin tuck effectively as extreme flexion of the head can collapse the airway.[7]

Individuals with weak pharyngeal constrictor muscles could be at risk for post-swallow residue and aspiration as head flexion loosens the pharyngeal constrictors making them potentially less effective in propelling the bolus through the pharynx.[8]

Individuals with impaired laryngeal excursion may also be at disadvantage, as chin tuck may inhibit laryngeal elevation, which is a key mechanical movement in effecting epiglottic closure.

Head rotation:
- *Rationale:* The head turn effectively closes off the weaker side and physically encourages the bolus down the stronger side (Fig. 3). This technique also has the effect of pulling the cricoid cartilage further away from the posterior pharyngeal wall, which reduces the resting pressure on upper esophageal sphincter (UES) muscles.[5]
- *Instruction:* Patient is instructed to turn his or her head to the weaker side to the full extent of comfort, whereas the trunk should remain in neutral position.
- *Candidacy:* Individuals with unilateral weakness or who have undergone reconstruction of the pharynx may benefit from this technique. This technique has been shown to be beneficial with unilateral UES dysfunction and unilateral vocal cord palsy.
- *Contraindication:* Head rotation is not advisable if there are multiple structures involved in different side. For instance, when there is a combination of left unilateral pharyngeal weakness along with right sided weakness of tongue, head rotation is not recommended.

Head tilt:
- *Rationale:* Head tilt posture uses the effect of gravity to move the bolus in the desired direction (Fig. 4).
- *Instruction:* The patient is instructed to tilt the head toward the stronger side during swallowing.
- *Candidacy:* Individuals with unilateral oral weakness or pharyngeal weakness may benefit from head tilt to stronger side during swallow.
- *Contraindication:* It is contraindicated if oral and pharyngeal weaknesses are not on the same side.

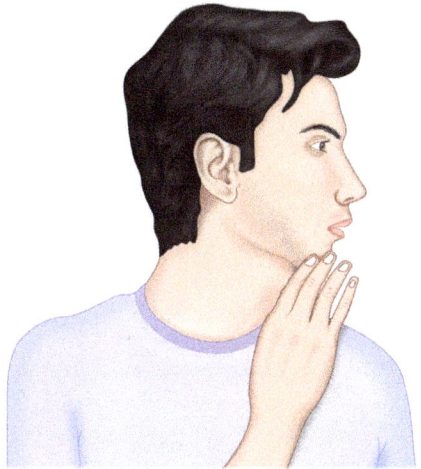

Fig. 3 Head rotation

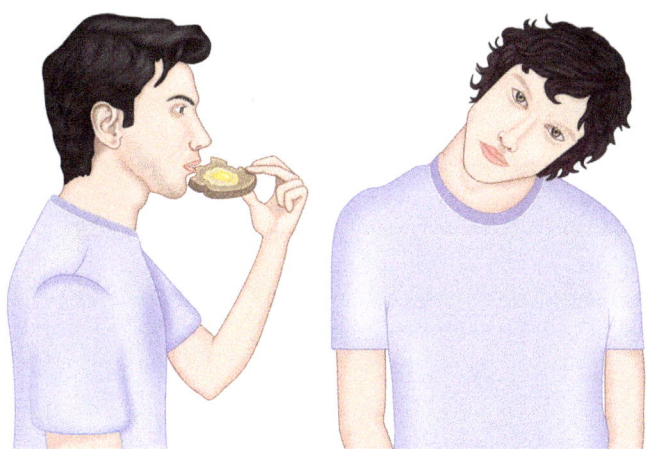

Fig. 4 Head tilt posture

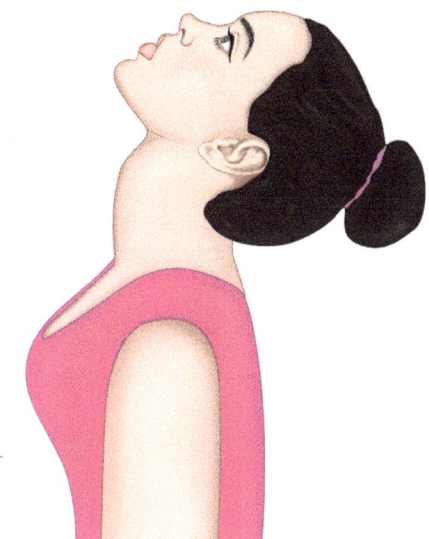

Fig. 5 Neck extension

Neck extension:
- *Rationale:* This technique uses gravity to clear the bolus.[5]
- *Instruction:* In neck extension, the patient is instructed to sit in an upright position and when ready to transfer the bolus from oral cavity to pharynx, to extend the neck backward and lift the chin upward (Fig. 5).
- *Candidacy:* Neck extension is recommended for patients with velopharyngeal incompetence and nasal regurgitation. In addition, it is effectively used for individuals with impairments in the oral transfer phase, with symptoms of post-swallow oral residue and bolus transfer problems, e.g. labial resection, anterior tongue and floor of mouth resection, hemiglossectomy, and glossectomy.
- *Contraindications:* Caution needs to be taken while adopting this technique, as neck extension may inhibit laryngeal elevation and opening of UES muscle. Therefore,

patient must be taught to adopt neck extension only for transfer phase from oral to pharyngeal cavities and then quickly resume an upright posture. Also it is advisable to use it with individuals with excellent cognitive skills and auditory comprehension.

- *Efficacy studies:* Logemann et al. (1994) studied chin tuck postural technique on patients with oral resection and found that they were effective in at least 60% of the patients at 1 mL and 3 mL volumes. If the patient first aspirated at a 3 mL volume, the posture was effective in 80% of the patients for 5 mL boluses. All patients were able to swallow 10 mL boluses from cup using the posture without aspiration. Clinically, we have found that chin tuck has major role in airway protection. In unilateral oral and pharyngeal weaknesses, head rotation to weaker side has proven to be beneficial. Therefore, selection of appropriate head posture should be patient specific, which is based on requisite cognitive skills and physical reserve to use them. Careful thought should also be given to the indications and contraindications of the techniques.[9,10]

Bolus Consistency

Overview

One of the most important compensatory acts is to change the type or texture of food and/or fluid the dysphagic individual receives. Clinicians are aware, for example, that a thickened fluid is more cohesive than a thin liquid bolus and travels more slowly than a thin liquid bolus. Cohesiveness and slower transit generally equate to better oropharyngeal control of the bolus.

Table 1 Type of food and fluid recommended by speech pathologists for individuals with dysphagia

Consistency	Examples	Clinical application
Ice chips	Ice cubes	Sensory deficit (delay in oral and pharyngeal swallow)
Thin liquids	Milk, juice, and water	Inefficient oral transit/total glossectomy
Thick liquids	Honey, milk shakes, and soups	Unilateral laryngeal dysfunction/subtotal glossectomy
Puree	Pudding, pastries, custard, pureed pasta, pureed fruit, mousse, and yoghurt,	Reduced pharyngeal contraction, unilateral laryngeal dysfunction
Semisolid food	Muffin, dalia, mashed potato, banana, well-cooked soft pasta, soft-cooked eggs, and cooked rice if sticky	Delay in triggering pharyngeal swallow
Soft solid food	Bread, cheese soft cookie, cooked vegetables, rice dishes, and cooked fruits	Cricopharyngeal dysfunction
Hard chewy, crunchy food	Green salad, raw vegetables, roti, hard crusted bread, rolls, hard fruit, nuts, and candies	Normal oral and pharyngeal function
Mixed consistencies	Soup with food bits, apple or raw fruit, and cereal with milk	Normal swallow function

During intervention, the speech pathologist will begin with bolus consistencies that are predicted to be easier and then move to harder consistencies. Table 1 briefly describes the types of food and fluid that are recommended by speech pathologists for individuals with dysphagia.

Each of the bolus consistencies should be tried in increasing volumes before they are considered safe for swallowing. Order of bolus volume suggested by Langmore, 2001 are as follows:[11]

- Less than 5 mL, if the patient is medically fragile and/or pulmonary clearance is poor
- 5 mL (1 teaspoon)
- 10 mL
- 15 mL (1 tablespoon)
- 20 mL (heaping tablespoon)
- Single swallow from cup or straw
- Consecutive swallows from cup or straw
- Consecutive swallows of food and liquid, self-selected.

Efficacy Studies

Bhattacharyya et al. (2003) suggests thicker food consistencies to be safer for oral intake in patients with unilateral vocal fold paralysis due to decreased risk of laryngeal penetration and aspiration.[12] Clave et al. (2006) confirmed that increasing the bolus viscosity from liquids to nectar and pudding for patients with either nonprogressive brain diseases or neurodegenerative diseases significantly improved both the efficacy and the safety of swallowing by reducing aspiration and penetration.[13] With clinical experience, we have found in Medanta, The Medicity that in head and neck patients involving oral tongue and floor of mouth resections, thin liquid were easier for swallow, whereas in stroke patients, soft semisolid food were least aspirated and thin liquids were introduced later during the course of intervention.

DIRECT THERAPEUTIC STRATEGIES

Oral Sensory Stimulation

Normally, when the food is presented, it stimulates the sensory receptors of touch, taste, and temperature. These receptors will transmit the sensory information by afferent pathways to higher cortical, subcortical, and brainstem swallowing centers, where the sensory information will be processed and a command to swallow will be generated. It is noticed that in weak or delayed swallow reflex, oral sensory stimulation has shown to improve the speed and strength of swallow.[11]

Figure 6 represents different types of orosensory stimulation used for patients with dysphagia.

Ice Chip Maneuver

- *Rationale:* Ice chip represents a cold, solid food bolus that stimulates thermal, chemoreceptors, and tactile receptors in the mouth. It can be manipulated with the tongue in preparation of swallow. The swallow itself can be executed with purpose, if cortical and subcortical neural circuits are functioning and the motor pathways are able to carry the command to the appropriate musculature.
- *Instruction:* The patient is instructed to take the ice chip and encouraged to prepare the bolus for several seconds. Then he/she is asked to swallow the ice chip carefully and forcefully, "all at once".
- *Candidacy:* Ice chip is recommended for weak and delayed onset of swallow as in anterior tongue resection and in stroke patients; premature spillage, for example as in tongue base resection reduces pharyngeal contraction. If ice chip triggers a swallow and has noticeable effect on clearing secretions that were in hypopharynx or larynx prior to swallow, this is a strong prognostic marker

because it suggests that the swallow may be adequately strong and just may need to be stimulated.

- *Contraindications*: In severe swallowing impairment, if ice chip is aspirated and does not stimulate cough, even after 2–3 swallows, the maneuver may be terminated till the patient stabilizes medically.
- *Efficacy studies*: Thermal stimulation using ice chip maneuver has shown to be beneficial in improving the awareness of residue in the oral cavity, mistimed or delayed swallow initiation, namely premature spillage to the pharynx.[14] It is further supported by Rosenbek et al. (1991) and Hwang et al. (2007) that ice chip maneuver reduced of stage transition and total swallow duration.[15-17]

Oromotor Exercises

Oromotor exercises have been commonly accepted and practised by speech language pathologists. These exercises target lips, tongue, face, palate, pharynx, larynx and are designed to improve the mobility, strength, and control for swallowing.

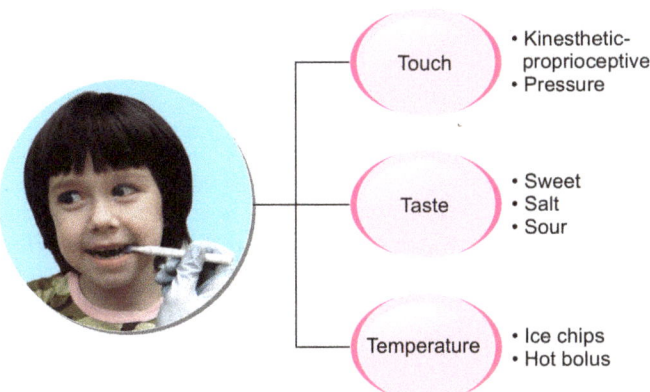

Fig. 6 Different types of orosensory stimulation

Lip Closure Exercise

- *Rationale*: Lip closure range of motion and strengthening exercises are assumed to improve oral containment, oral pressure and ability to manipulate and propel material from oral cavity into the pharynx.
- *Candidacy*: Lip exercises are used in conditions of facial palsy or labial resection, where there is difficulty in taking food off a spoon, or having trouble sucking from a straw and for oral containment.
- *Instruction*: Patient is instructed to:
  - Purse your lips and protrude as far forward as possible and hold
  - Pull your lips back into a wide smile and hold
  - Smack your lips together forcefully (Figs 7A and B).

Range of Motion Exercise

- *Rationale*: Tongue range of motion exercises are designed to improve bolus manipulation and propulsion from oral cavity into the pharynx, and to prevent premature spillage.[18,19]
- *Candidacy*: Range of motion exercises are recommended in patients with anterior and lateral tongue resection, patients who have undergone hemiglossectomy and neurological involvement also benefit from these exercises.
- *Instructions*:
  - Forward/backward movement:
    - Stick your tongue out of your mouth as far as possible and hold. Try to keep your tongue in the middle while you do this
    - Pull your tongue back as far as you can in your mouth, as if you are trying to scratch the back wall of your throat with the back of your tongue
    - Lift the tip of your tongue to the roof of your mouth. Move the tip back as far as you can, keeping the tip on the roof of your mouth.

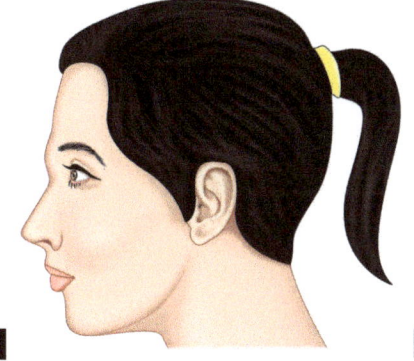 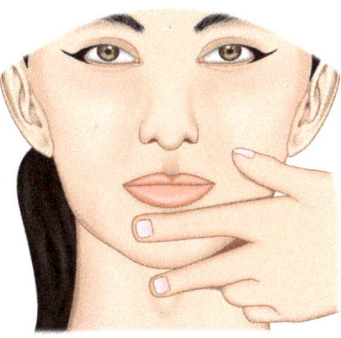

Figs 7A and B Lip closure exercise

– *Side-to-side movement:*
  ♦ Put the tip of your tongue in your right cheek as far back as you can and hold it. Repeat with tip of tongue in left cheek
  ♦ Smile. Put the tip of your tongue in the corner of your lips on the right, then move it to the left.
– *Base of tongue movement and strength:* The following is a set of exercises, which strengthens the tongue base volume and function:
  ♦ Pull the back of your tongue as far back as you can in your mouth. Pretend you are trying to scratch the back wall of your throat with the back of your tongue. Hold the tongue in this position for several seconds
  ♦ Pretend to gargle as it elicits base of tongue and pharyngeal wall movement
  ♦ Pretend to yawn as it helps reduce amount of food residue in the upper throat
  ♦ Repeat these words ending with "k." Make a hard, forceful "k" each time you say a word. For example, walk talk work pack pike peek.

Oromotor exercises (stretching and strengthening) described by Van der Molen et al. (2011) are diagrammatically represented and explained in Figures 8 and 9.[20]
- *Stretch exercises*: Repeat every exercise session (Figs 8A to E) for *three times*.
- *Strength exercise*: Repeat every exercise session (Figs 9A to C) for *five times*.

Head Lifting Exercise

This exercise was described by Shaker et al., 1997.
- *Rationale*: Head lifting exercise also known as Shaker exercise, strengthens the suprahyoid and infrahyoid muscles, which helps in laryngeal elevation and cricopharyngeal opening.
- *Candidacy*: It is recommended for patients with dysfunction of UES and cricopharyngeal muscle.
- *Instruction*:
  – Lie flat on your back with no pillow under your head
  – Lift your head to look at your toes
  – Keep your shoulders flat on the floor or bed
  – Hold that position for 60 seconds
  – Release
  – Repeat twice.
- *Efficacy studies*: Veis et al. (2000) analyzed several stretch exercises and concluded that the gargle task elicited the greatest tongue base retraction in a group of subjects with suspected dysphagia (e.g. head/neck cancer, progressive and sudden onset neurologic damage, Parkinson's disease, stroke, and muscular dystrophy).[21] Robbins et al.

(2007) studied the effects of an isometric lingual exercise of tongue and the hard palate and found significant improvement in swallowing function and dysphagia-specific quality-of-life measures, with reported changes in their social life and dietary intake.[22]

Shaker et al. (2002) analyzed the effect of head raising exercise program on patients with diverse etiology (neurological pathology, post-pharyngeal radiotherapy, cardiovascular disease) and abnormal UES opening and suggested that shaker exercise showed significant therapy effects.[23] These include improvement in the anteroposterior diameter of the sphincter opening and the anterior laryngeal excursion, decrease of postdeglutitive residue, and resolution of aspiration. Scores on a seven-point swallowing competency scale (functional outcome assessment of swallowing score) showed positive changes as well.

Swallow Maneuvers

Swallow maneuvers are voluntary controls that can be used during swallow to change selected aspects of neuromuscular control. They have immediate positive effects on the swallow. In addition, if used habitually, they may strengthen or permanently increase the range of motion of the involved structures and muscles.

Supraglottic Swallow

Supraglottic swallow was described by Logemann, 1983.[4]
- *Rationale*: Supraglottic swallow is a maneuver that is designed to achieve adduction of true vocal cords before and during the swallow, thus protecting the airway from aspiration.
- *Candidacy*: This maneuver can be used for weak or incomplete vocal cord adduction secondary to tumor involvement, surgical resection or neurologic insult to the laryngeal branch of CN X (i.e. superior laryngeal nerve and right and left recurrent laryngeal nerves).
- *Instruction*: The patent is asked to follow these steps in the order mentioned here:
  ♦ The patient is instructed to inhale and then adduct the true vocal folds by humming
  ♦ The hum is abruptly cut off and the patient is asked to hold the breath and tense the neck
  ♦ The bolus is swallowed while the breath is held and the neck is tensed
  ♦ Immediately after the swallow a throat clearing maneuver/coughing is performed. This forces any residual bolus left in the pharynx into oral cavity.

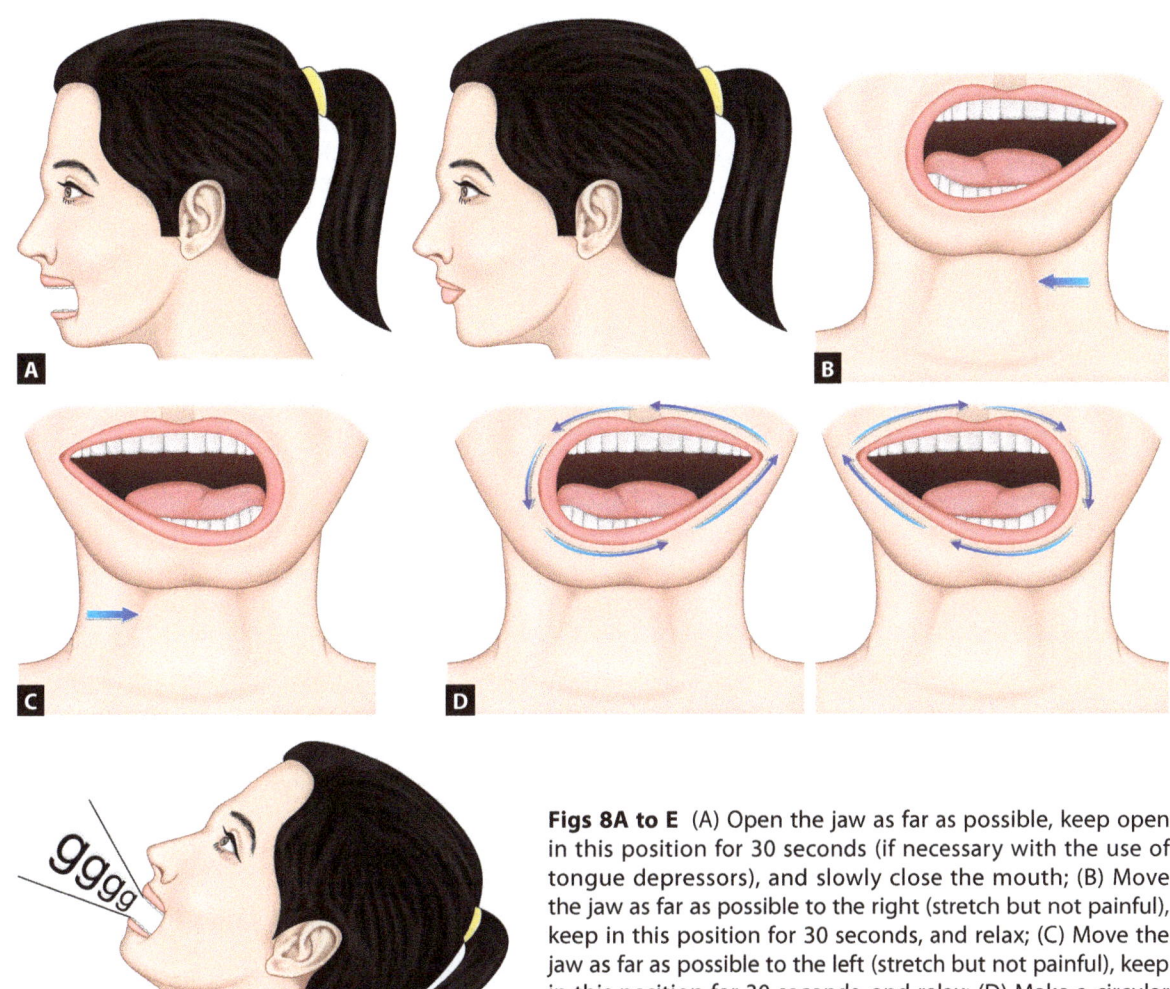

Figs 8A to E (A) Open the jaw as far as possible, keep open in this position for 30 seconds (if necessary with the use of tongue depressors), and slowly close the mouth; (B) Move the jaw as far as possible to the right (stretch but not painful), keep in this position for 30 seconds, and relax; (C) Move the jaw as far as possible to the left (stretch but not painful), keep in this position for 30 seconds, and relax; (D) Make a circular movement with the jaw (stretch but not painful), and relax after completing one circle; (E) Gargle with tongue pulled back (as far as possible), keep on gargling for 10 seconds, and relax

Super Supraglottic Swallow

Super supraglottic swallow was described by Martin et al., 1993; Logemann, 1986.[24]

- *Rationale*: This maneuver is a modification of supraglottic maneuver. This variation is designed to provide maximal and sustained airway protection, where not only will the true vocal cords adduct, but also the false cords contact and arytenoids tilts forward sometimes touching petiole of the epiglottis.
- *Candidacy*: Super supraglottic swallow is advised for weak and reduced laryngeal closure, like vocal cord palsy.
- *Instruction*: The patent is asked to follow these steps in the order mentioned here:
  - Put the bolus in the mouth
  - Hold your breath
  - Swallow it all at once
  - Immediately after the swallow a throat clearing maneuver/coughing is performed.

Mendelsohn Maneuver

This maneuver was described by Kahrilas et al., 1991.[25]

- *Rationale*: This technique is assumed to increase hyolaryngeal elevation and thereby prolonging the UES opening.
- *Candidacy*: It is used if you have food sticking in your throat which might fall into your airway due to impaired laryngeal elevation and cricopharyngeal dysfunction.
- *Instruction*: Place your fingers lightly on your neck to feel how the larynx/voice box lifts as you swallow. You will notice that at the very peak of the swallow, the larynx

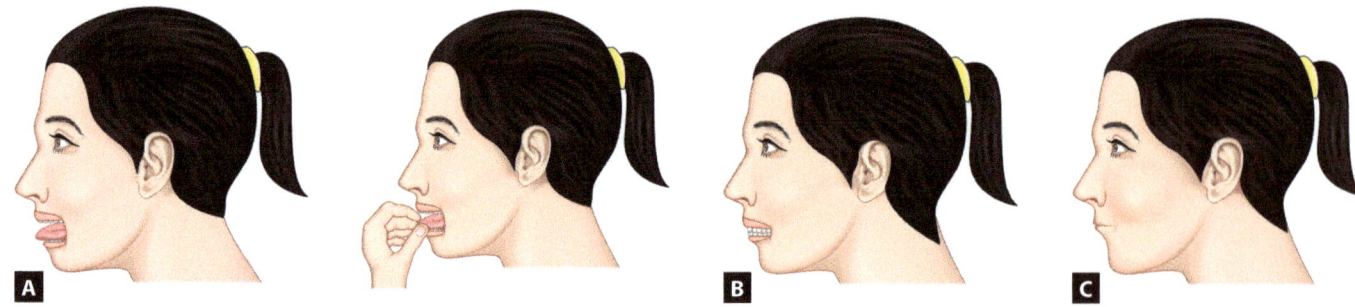

Figs 9A to C (A) Stick out your tongue slightly. Alternative: hold the tongue between the teeth (or fingers), swallow with the tongue stuck out or held between the teeth/fingers; (B) Bite forcefully on teeth, tense the tongue, and neck muscles, and swallow; (C) Inhale and tightly hold your breath, bear down, keep holding your breath and bearing down as you swallow, and cough when you are finished

is lifted to its highest point in the neck, and when the swallow is finished, the larynx falls down again.

– Swallow with your fingers lightly on your larynx
– When you feel your larynx get to its highest point, hold it up by pushing your tongue hard against the roof of your mouth and keeping it there. (The base of the tongue is attached to the hyoid bone, which is attached to the larynx, and that is why pushing the tongue up keeps the larynx up)
– Keep the larynx lifted for a count of five.

Effortful Swallow

Effortful swallow was described by Kahrilas et al. (1993).[26]

- *Rationale*: The effortful swallow is aimed at increasing the force of tongue propulsion and contact against the posterior pharyngeal wall.
- *Candidacy*: This strategy is recommended for patients with ineffective swallow with incomplete bolus clearance, e.g. in facial palsy, lateral tongue resection, where there is reduced posterior tongue movement.
- *Instruction*: The patient is asked to squeeze all of your mouth and throat muscles as hard as possible (as if trying to swallow a ping-pong ball) and then swallow.
- *Efficacy studies showing combined effects of the maneuvers*: It is very interesting to note that although each of the maneuvers were designed to have a specific and respective effect on the swallow, research has determined that in fact, each has multiple effects on the swallow, some of which go beyond the intended effects. For example, the supraglottic swallow was designed to achieve voluntary closure at the level of true vocal cords before swallow, however, when this maneuver is implemented, laryngeal elevation may also be increased with prolonged UES opening.[8,27] Bulow and colleagues (1999) reported similar extended effects of effortful swallow, showing larynx and hyoid bone elevation earlier in relation to bolus flow. Finally, Mendelsohn maneuver in addition

to hyolaryngeal elevation and UES opening, sometimes, show timely onset and better tongue base retraction to the posterior pharyngeal wall and effective airway closure.[28]

CONCLUSION

The ultimate goal of dysphagia rehabilitation is to restore the patient's swallowing ability as near normal as possible. Determination of the treatment strategy should be unique to a given patient, based on requisite cognitive skills and physical reserve to use them. As evident from research, combination of various therapeutic techniques may be required to treat the swallowing difficulty in an individual. For example, in a patient who has undergone hemiglossectomy, a combination of compensatory and rehabilitative strategies may be used, i.e. sensory stimulation, with changes in bolus consistency, adoption of neck extension, with super supraglottic swallow maneuver yields best possible swallow.

Temporary replacement or supplement to oral feeding like nasogastric tube feeding may be required to allow for adequate nutrition during the recovery or during chemotherapy in head and neck patients to minimize the risk of aspiration. During the process of swallow rehabilitation, tube feedings may be adjusted according to the amount of oral intake, with the goal of removing the tube and relying solely on oral feeding. It is therefore advantageous if multidisciplinary team members comprising of head and neck surgeon, speech language pathologist, and a dietician to work closely during this transition period to ensure proper nutritional maintenance and patient compliance.

REFERENCES

1. Logemann JA, Rademaker AW, Pauloski BR, et al. Effects of postural change on aspiration in head and neck surgical patients. Otolaryngol Head Neck Surg. 1994;110(2):222-7.
2. Barkmeier J, Bielamowicz S, Tekeda N, et al. Laryngeal activity during upright vs. supine swallowing. J Appl Physiol (1985). 2002;93(2):40-5.

3. Dorsey LD. Effects of reclined supported postures on management of dysphagic adults with severe developmental disabilities. Dysphagia. 2002;17(2):180.

4. Logemann JA. Evaluation and Treatment of Swallowing Disorders, 1st edition. Austin, TX: Pro-Ed Publishers; 1983.

5. Logemann JA. Role of the modified barium swallow in management of patients with dysphagia. Otolaryngol Head Neck Surg. 1997;116(3):335-8.

6. Lazarus CL. Management of swallowing disorders in head and neck cancer patients: optimal patterns of care. Semin Speech Lang. 2000;21(4):293-309.

7. Wolf LS, Glass RP. Feeding and Swallowing Disorders of Infancy. Tuscon: Therapy Skill Builders; 1992.

8. Bülow M, Olsson R, Ekberg O. Videomanometric analysis of supraglottic swallow, effortful swallow, and chin tuck in healthy volunteers. Dysphagia. 1999;14(2):67-72.

9. Logemann JA, Gibbons P, Rademaker AW, et al. Mechanisms of recovery of swallow after supraglottic laryngectomy. J Speech Hear Res. 1994;37(5):965-74.

10. Logemann JA, Pauloski BR, Colangelo L, et al. Effects of a sour bolus on oropharyngeal swallowing measures in patients with neurogenic dysphagia. J Speech Hear Res. 1995;38(3):556-63.

11. Langmore SE. Endoscopic evaluation and treatment of swallowing disorders. NY: Thieme, Library of Congress Cataloguing-in-Publication Data; 2001.

12. Bhattacharyya N, Kotz T, Shapiro J. The effect of bolus consistency on dysphagia in unilateral vocal cord paralysis. Otolaryngol Head Neck Surg. 2003;129(6):632-6.

13. Clave P, De Kraa M, Arreola V, et al. The effect of bolus viscosity on swallowing function in neurogenic dysphagia. Aliment Pharmacol Ther. 2006;24(9):1385-94.

14. Lazzara GI, Lazarus C, Logemann JA. Impact of thermal stimulation on the triggering of the swallowing reflex. Dysphagia. 1986;1:73-77.

15. Rosenbek JC, Robbins J, Fishback B, et al. Effects of thermal application on dysphagia after stroke. J Speech Hear Res. 1991;34(6):1257-68.

16. Hwang CH, Choi KH, Ko YS, et al. Pre-emptive swallowing stimulation in long-term intubated patients. Clin Rehabil. 2007;21(1):41-6.

17. Rosenbek JC, Roecker EB, Wood JL, et al. Thermal application reduces the duration of stage transition in dysphagia after stroke. Dysphagia. 1996;11(4):225-33.

18. Daniels SK, Brailey K, Foundas AL. Lingual discoordination and dysphagia following acute stroke: analyses of lesion localization. Dysphagia. 1999;14(2):85-92.

19. Dworkin J, Hartman D. Progressive speech deterioration and dysphagia in amyotrophic lateral sclerosis: case report. Arch Phys Med Rehabil. 1979;60(9):423-5.

20. van der Molen L, van Rossum MA, Burkhead LM, et al. A randomized preventive rehabilitation trial in advanced head and neck cancer patients treated with chemoradiotherapy: feasibility, compliance, and short-term effects. Dysphagia. 2011;26(2):155-70.

21. Veis S, Logemann JA, Colangelo L. Effects of three techniques on maximum posterior movement of the tongue base. Dysphagia. 2000;15(3):142-5.

22. Robbins J, Kays SA, Gangnon RE, et al. The effects of lingual exercise in stroke patients with dysphagia. Arch Phys Med Rehabil. 2007;88(2):150-8.

23. Shaker R, Easterling C, Kern M, et al. Rehabilitation of swallowing by exercise in tube-fed patients with pharyngeal dysphagia secondary to abnormal UES opening. Gastroenterology. 2002;122(5):1314-21.

24. Martin BJ, Logemann JA, Shaker R, et al. Normal laryngeal valving patterns during three breath-hold maneuvers: a pilot investigation. Dysphagia. 1993;8(1):11-20.

25. Kahrilas PJ, Logemann JA, Krugler C, et al. Volitional augmentation of upper esophageal sphincter opening during swallowing. Am J Physiol. 1991;260(3 Pt 1):G450-6.

26. Kahrilas PJ, Lin S, Logemann JA, et al. Deglutitive tongue action: volume accommodation and bolus propulsion. Gastroenterology. 1993;104(1):152-62.

27. Ohmae Y, Logemann JA, Kaiser P, et al. Effects of two breath-holding maneuvers on oropharyngeal swallow. Ann Otol Rhinol Laryngol. 1996;105(2):123-31.

28. Lazarus C, Logemann JA, Gibbons P. Effects of maneuvers on swallowing function in a dysphagic oral cancer patient. Head Neck. 1993;15(5):419-24.

20

Laryngeal Management in Sleep Apnea Patients

Claudio Vicini, Filippo Montevecchi, Mohamed Rashwan,
Marco Barbieri, Valeria Roustan, Fabiola Incandela, Giorgio Peretti

INTRODUCTION

Obstructive sleep apnea hypopnea syndrome (OSAHS) is a growing clinical concern as it is the most prevalent sleep disorder in the adult population affecting 11.4% of men and 4.7% of women. While the gold standard treatment for OSAHS remains continuous positive airway pressure (CPAP), patients who are unable to tolerate it need another treatment option. Inside the diagnostic protocol to define the sites of obstruction in the upper airway, drug-induced sedation/sedated or sleep endoscopy (DISE) is a crucial maneuver, especially to define a laryngeal involvement in the origin of the apneas. The purpose of this chapter is to describe how to define a possible involvement of the larynx in sleep apnea patient and how to surgically manage this anatomical area.

DRUG-INDUCED SEDATION ENDOSCOPY

Drug-induced sedation/sedated or sleep endoscopy is a fiber-optic examination of the upper airway under controlled sedation to determine the exact site(s) of upper airway collapse in patients with sleep disordered breathing.

Quantifying the location and mechanism of upper airway collapse with DISE in an apneic patient can potentially be used to tailor surgical treatments and improve surgical outcomes.

In 1991, Croft and Pringle[1] described an original way to study obstructive sleep apnea (OSA) patients, by "sleep nasendoscopy", a procedure designed to observe the upper airway under pharmacologically induced sleep. The technique, however, has been labeled with controversies, which have been subsequently and adequately addressed.

The main criticism would seem to be that natural physiological sleep is different from sleep-induced during DISE. Numerous studies have subsequently looked at sleep architecture during sedation to demonstrate similarities. The depth of sedation was questioned as differing degrees of obstruction would be observed depending on how deep the sedation was. This was rectified by utilizing bispectral index (BIS) monitoring (BIS®, Medtronic Minneapolis, MN, USA) instead of simple clinical judgment (patient's capability to react to different verbal and tactile stimuli). Inter- and intraobservational variations may exist and studies have demonstrated good correlation. This has become of increasing interest in the medical community, as evidenced by the increasing number of articles concerning its use and by its ever increasing practice worldwide.

In 2014, a European Position Paper[2] defined DISE as Drug-Induced Sedation Endoscopy instead of Drug-Induced Sleep Endoscopy, considered more appropriate to define the pharmacological condition as "sedation" instead of "sleep".

Our Experience

We started DISE in November 2005 in selected patients, using Propofol® (by bolus technique and then by infusion pump) with an anesthesiologist in the operating room. Since 2009 we have been following the same basic protocol as published in 2010[3] and according to the options recently validated in the European Position Paper on DISE,[2] that is:

- *Patient selection for DISE:*
  - Polysomnography (PSG) findings do not match awake endoscopic findings (sleep studies/awake endoscopic mismatch)
  - Suspected isolated supraglottic obstruction

- Surgical failures
- Suspected stridor related to multisystemic atrophy
- *Setting:*
  - Operating room
  - ENT (ear, nose, and throat) and anesthesia team
  - No topical decongestion or topical anesthesia
  - No systemic drying agent (i.e. atropine, glycopyrrolate)
  - Quite and dark room
- *Technical equipment:*
  - Standard monitoring [arterial oxygen saturation (SaO_2), electrocardiogram (ECG), blood pressure]
  - TCI® (Target control infusion)—not available in USA
  - BIS®
  - Video and audio recordings
  - Simultaneous cardiorespiratory monitoring in selected cases (e.g. Embletta®, Natus Incorporation, Canada)
- *Patient positioning and diagnostic maneuvers:*
  - Standard supine primary position (with or without pillow)
  - Transnasal fiber-optic endoscopy (in selected cases transoral also)
  - Mandibular advancement, mouth open/close comparison
- *Drug:* Propofol®
- *Observation window:*
  - At least two or more cycles (snoring, collapse) for each segment of the upper airway
  - *Cycle definition:* A complete and stable sequence of snoring—obstructing hypo/apnea—oxygen desaturation—breathing
  - BIS® level around 60 or desaturation level close to the previously registered lowest O_2 saturation at the sleep study
- *Target events:*
  - *Snoring:* Pharyngeal and/or laryngeal vibration
  - *Apnea-hypopnea:* Partial or complete pharyngeal obstruction and collapse pattern (lateral, anteroposterior, circumferential)
  - Epiglottic trap-door phenomenon or different pattern of collapse
  - Laryngeal stridor
- *Classification system:*
  - Nose oropharynx hypopharynx and larynx (NOHL) classification system as described[4]
- *Contraindications:*
  - *Absolute:* ASA 4, pregnancy, allergy to Propofol®
  - *Relative:* Morbid obesity.

Drug-induced Sedation Endoscopy Why?

In 2010, we published[5] a retrospective study on 250 consecutive patients making a comparison between awake and DISE findings. In this study, we found significant differences between hypopharyngeal degree and pattern of obstruction (59% and 49%, respectively) and we discovered up to 30% of cases demonstrated laryngeal obstruction by DISE; it was classified as *primary* if the collapse was produced by intrinsic instability of the larynx or *secondary* if the tongue base or the lateral wall were responsible for the supraglottic collapse. Endoscopic findings are essential to guide the surgical decision making. It has to be acknowledged that awake endoscopy may frequently underestimate the degree of the hypopharyngeal and laryngeal obstruction.

Drug-induced sedation endoscopy, in our experience, remains one of the best tools for evaluating upper airway obstructions for those patients considering surgical intervention.

SURGICAL TREATMENT OPTIONS

It is crucial to divide two main categories of epiglottis involvement: *primary epiglottis* and *secondary epiglottis*. In the first pattern (primary), the epiglottic collapse itself causes obstruction over the larynx. In the second pattern (secondary), the epiglottic collapse is secondary to tongue base collapse. In case of primary epiglottis, the transoral laryngoscopy (TOL) technique by means carbon dioxide (CO_2) laser is the main treatment. We will describe a new surgical technique addressed for treating exclusively the epiglottis. In case of secondary epiglottis, the latest technology we can use is the da Vinci Robot (Intuitive Incorporation). Da Vinci tongue base reduction (TBR) and supraglottoplasty (SGP) is devised in order to provide similar functional outcomes of the classic open approach described by Chabolle and colleagues (1999)[6] as well as all the potential benefits of a completely transoral robotic surgery (TORS) approach. The da Vinci system three-dimensional (3D) high-definition (HD) visualization, wristed instrumentations and intuitive movement help to provide the ultimate, precise and endoscopic approach for TBR and SGP. A really reduced invasiveness, a significant efficacy and relatively limited surgical time are the keys of these procedures.

Surgical Treatment of the Primary Epiglottis

For this surgical procedure a Lumenis® CO_2 laser and a microscope Zeiss S7® are used. The surgical equipment includes: a MicroFrance 124 laryngoscope (for the exposure of the supraglottic region), a suspension system (prototype developed in collaboration with MicroFrance), angled aspiration tube and forceps (MicroFrance, Laryngoforce® II).

- The patient lies supine in the bed in the Boyce-Jackson's position; the eyes are protected by wet bandage and the superior teeth by a silicone device. We choose the smallest efficient tube (MicroFrance, Laser Shield® 2 endotracheal tube) for the transoral intubation. The skin of the neck is disinfected using alcoholic solution.

- The exposure of the supraglottis, obtained by a Sataloff vallecula laryngoscope (124, MicroFrance), is to be considered adequate when the tongue base, the entire valleculae, and the epiglottis are visualized. The position of the hyoid bone is marked on the skin as a landmark for the following surgical steps.

- CO_2 laser, set on ultrapulse mode, at 3 Watts of output power at a 400 mm working distance, is used to vaporize the mucosa overlying the valleculae and the tongue base outlining two raw areas on the base of the tongue and on the lingual surface of the epiglottis leaving a rim of 2–4 mm of healthy mucosa along the entire profile of the suprahyoid epiglottis. The cicatricial retraction during the healing process determines an iatrogenic synechia attracting the epiglottis to the tongue base. The surgical field is, during the operation, mostly bloodless thanks to the capacity of the CO_2 laser to coagulate vessels with a diameter less than 0.5 mm. For wider vessels a cauterizing monopolar forceps is routinely adopted and surgical clips are also strongly recommended. In case of hypertrophy of the lingual tonsils, a resection of the lymphatic tissue may be combined. A cottonoid, soaked in saline solution, is applied postoperatively to remove the char and clean the raw surface facilitating the endoscopic evaluation for detecting any residual intact mucosal island causing retention cysts after the healing process when the two surfaces stick to each other.

- To ensure a perfect seal of the pexy 2 Premilene sutures embrace the hyoid bone guided by means of two catheters 16-G (Gauge) and 18-G, respectively. The first suture is bent in the middle to form a sort of handle; the handle is then inserted inside the 16-G needle to exit from the tip and fixed with a "Klemmer" forceps. The assistant passes the so prepared catheter through the anterior neck, in a suprahyoid position, along the midline to avoid big vessel and nerve injuries until it reaches the internal aspect of the glossoepiglottic vallecula. This procedure is monitored from the inside, by the first operator, under microscopic control. The needle is then pushed down to penetrate the epiglottis, while the first surgeon holds the cartilage with two clamps. Once done the first operator retrieves the loop out of the mouth and ensures it with a Klemmer forceps.

- The second suture, inserted into the 18-G catheter, passes the neck beneath the hyoid. One end of the wire is fixed outside the neck, while the second one follows the way of the handle out of the mouth.

- The surgeon inserts the free end of the wire within the loop and holds it with one hand. The assistant retracts the terminal part of the loop, with a firm movement, allowing the second suture to exit the neck.

- The suture is passed through a Silastic sheet on the anterior neck to protect the skin from scarring, then through a surgical button. Before tying the suture a small amount of Tissucol® is injected in the glossoepiglottic vallecula using a Duplocath® catheter.

- At the end of the procedure the patient is awakened and extubated.

- A soft and cold diet is administered from the day after surgery.

- The patient is discharged after 48 hours of observation.

- Antibiotics and analgesics (paracetamol is preferable) are recommended for 1 week. A small medication can be applied to cover the fixing stich.

- The patient is controlled 7 day, 21 day, 90 day and 180 day after surgery.

- The stitch is removed after 21–30 days under endoscopic control in an office-based procedure, no anesthesia is required.

- A PSG is performed in the 6th month.

The aim of the surgical procedure we proposed is to provide a stable support to the epiglottis without interfering with its function during swallowing.

In patients suffering from OSAs the primary collapse of the epiglottis is due to the high negative intrathoracic pressure that generates during obstructive events in contrast to the one that characterizes laryngomalacia. According to our experience, to obtain satisfactory results, it is not sufficient to apply a surgical procedure conceived for laryngomalacia, but it is mandatory to give a durable stabilization of the cartilage. We achieve this goal by modifying Monnier's glossoepiglottopexy with a strong nonabsorbable stich fixed to the skin of the neck through a plastic device.

The role played by the epiglottis in preventing the inhalation on the bolus is double: on one end it offers a physical closure of the glottis folding over the vocal cords to stop the ingested and on the other its sensitive receptors (distributed in the laryngeal surface, aryepiglottic folds, arytenoids and posterior commissure) stimulate the so-called "glottis closure reflex". This reflex is coordinated by the X cranial nerve, the vagus, and more precisely by its superior laryngeal branch and it provides the adduction of the vocal folds during deglutition avoiding the entrance of the bolus in the airways. To maintain these two functions unchanged, two technical precautions have to be taken into consideration: (1) it is necessary to leave a 3–4 mm rim of healthy cartilage and mucosa along the whole profile of the epiglottis to address food to the piriform sinuses; and (2) the mucosa of the supraglottis (except the lingual aspect of the epiglottis) and the glottis has to be preserved in order to allow the activation of reflex. It is even obvious that an impaired laryngeal function has to be considered a contraindication.

Surgical Treatment of the Secondary Epiglottis

Mild-to-severe OSAHS patients [Apnea-Hypopnea Index (AHI) > 20], usually with Excessive Daytime Sleepiness [Epworth Sleepiness Scale (ESS) > 10], significant obstruction at Tongue Base (Cormack-Lehane grading > 2)[7] and/or supraglottic area prolapse endoscopically demonstrated are the ideal application for TORS procedure, provided that a sufficient oropharyngeal exposure is possible (inter-incisive distance > 2.5 cm).

Tongue-base exposure is achieved in the standard TORS approach with a combination of tongue body traction with strong sutures and tongue body displacement by Storz® Davis-Meyer Mouth Gag. A complete set of tongue blades of different sizes with integrated suction tubes (for smoke and blood) is of paramount importance. FK® Mouth Gag is available on the table but usually is not necessary for TBR in most cases but sometimes may be useful for SGP. A small size blade proved to be the most suitable tool in most cases, especially in the first steps of BOT (base of tongue) approach.

Only two robotic 5 mm EndoWrist® arms are used for each patient: a Maryland Dissector 400143/420143 for grasping and dissection of tissues and a Monopolar Cautery with Spatula Tip 400142/400160 for dissection and coagulation.

Transoral robotic surgery approach in OSAHS surgery includes two different surgical procedures usually combined in the same patient (Vicini and Colleagues 2010 and 2012):[8,9]
1. Tongue base reduction (TBR)
2. Supraglottoplasty (SGP).

Tongue Base Reduction

Tongue base reduction is basically a different application and a proper modification of the tongue base resection described by O'Malley and colleagues in 2006.[10] The goal of tongue base reduction (TBR) is to enlarge the oropharyngeal section in the anterior wall area as well as classically palatine tonsils removal and lateral pharyngoplasty address the more common lateral oropharyngeal wall obstruction. As in the lateral oropharyngeal wall, in tongue base area there is surgically safe superficial layer composed of lymphoid tissue easy to remove and surgically dangerous deep muscular layer composed of muscles covering great vessels (lingual artery and its dorsal branches) and functionally crucial nerves (hypoglossal nerve and lingual nerve).

The endpoint of TBR may be probably achieved when the obtained surgical view shifts from a Cormack-Lehane Grade IV to a Grade II, or far less commonly, to a Grade I. In all but few cases lymphoid tissue as well as tongue base muscle must be removed in order to clear the so-called Retrolingual Space or Posterior Airway Space (PAS).

The more lymphatic hyperplasia, the less muscular tissue violation. Conversely, if lingual tonsil is no more than a thin layer, a more aggressive muscular resection is required in order to get the Cormack-Lehane Grade II goal. The mean volume of removed tissue is of about 15 cc, but sometimes the overall volume may be over 50 cc. Surgical steps are quite standardized in a precise and may be logic sequence, and may be sequentially applied in most of the approached cases:

- Midline split of the two lingual tonsils from foramen cecum down to identify epiglottic tip and vallecula. The section is carried out by Monopolar Cautery and get in depth the junction between tonsil and muscle. Sometimes difficult to identify in extreme lingual tonsil hyperplasia, foramen cecum is the key point for starting the dissection. This point must be stressed because it locates the upper limit of the resection, helping the surgeon to spare circumvallate papillae area and taste function, and in the same time giving to the surgeon a reasonable location of the midline. At the end of this first step lingual tonsil is completely split in midline, and a deep groove joining foramen cecum to midline glossoepiglottic area at the lymphoid-muscle junction in depth is our goal.
- Superior (sulcus terminalis), lateral (amigdaloglossus sulcus), and inferior (glossoepiglottic sulcus) borders of the right lingual tonsil are identified and possibly marked by cautery.
- In case of mild-to-moderate lingual tonsil hyperplasia the right lingual tonsillectomy is performed "en block" up to down keeping the section close to the muscular plane.
- Left lingual tonsillectomy is completed in the same way after side inversion of the robotic tools.
- The surgical field is now inspected in order to evaluate the residual degree of obstruction. If Cormack-Lehane Grade more than 2 is measured, additional resection in true muscle area is required.
- The key of this step is to remove a sufficient amount of muscle in order to open the PAS as well as to avoid any possible injury to XII cranial nerve, lingual nerve, and lingual artery.

Supraglottoplasty

Supraglottoplasty is very often carried out after TBR in the same patient and during the same operation. The key of supraglottoplasty (SGP) is to fix the inward inspiratory collapse of floppy and/or redundant tissue in epiglottis, aryepiglottic folds, and arytenoids area.

The extra time required for laryngeal step after TBR is usually less than 15 minutes. The most common choice in supraglottic area includes the following basic steps:

1. Vertical midline splitting of suprahyoid epiglottis; the section is carried out along the midline, following the medial glossoepiglottic fold, from the tip down to spare at least 5 mm over the deep vallecular plane (a sufficient strip of cartilage is left for preventing aspiration).
2. An horizontal section on both side is done in a plane joining the vertical section in midline and running laterally immediately over the pharyngoepiglottic fold, in order to leave a lateral fold preventing aspiration, and in order to avoid possible bleeding from the superior laryngeal vessels.
3. During the postoperative scarring of the vallecular and perivallecular area a progressive adhesion and stabilization of the residual epiglottis to the tongue base is observed.

After the robotic assisted step, if necessary, palate and/or nose may be addressed in a conventional way inside a single step multisite procedure.

POSTOPERATIVE MANAGEMENT

After a 1-hour stay in the recovery room, the patient is transferred directly to the ENT ward or in the intensive care unit for the first night. Morphine in sustained release form is used for analgesia for the first 3–5 days. A liquid diet is permitted on the 2nd day and solid diet is resumed after a week. Average hospital stay is about 4 days.

In our experience, complications were rare and transient. No conversion to open technique was needed. No complications related to robot instrumentation occurred. A few cases of self-limiting delayed bleeding in the first 1–3 weeks were treated by simple observation. Transient hypogeusia occurred in some patients, but this resolved within a few weeks. Average level of dysphagia was fairly low, as measured by MDADI (MD Anderson Dysphagia Inventory), a dysphagia-specific quality-of-life questionnaire.[11] In a multicentric study published in 2014[12] we have summarized our results in a group of 243 patients out of our overall series of 242 TORS for OSAHS. A significant reduction of AHI and ESS was achieved as well as a statistical improvement of Lower Oxygen Saturation and Quality-of-Life (SF-36 score), without any significant reduction of body mass index.

CONCLUSION

Laryngeal surgery by means of TORS or CO_2 laser should be considered as an additional option for treating OSAHS related to obstruction in both the tongue base and supraglottic larynx. New technologies and new surgical techniques are improving the diagnosis and the possibility to treat anatomic areas very difficult to manage in the past years.

REFERENCES

1. Croft CB, Pringle M. Sleep nasendoscopy: a technique of assessment in snoring and obstructive sleep apnoea. Clin Otolaryngol Allied Sci. 1991;16(5):504-9.
2. De Vito A, Carrasco Llatas M, et al. European position paper on drug-induced sedation endoscopy (DISE). Sleep Breath. 2014;18(3):453-65.
3. De Vito A, Agnoletti V, Berrettini S, et al. Drug-induced sleep endoscopy: conventional versus target controlled infusion techniques—a randomized controlled study. Eur Arch Otorhinolaryngol. 2011;268(3):457-62.
4. Vicini C, De Vito A, Benazzo M, et al. The nose oropharynx hypopharynx and larynx (NOHL) classification: a new system of diagnostic standardized examination for OSAHS patients. Eur Arch Otorhinolaryngol. 2012;269(4):1297-300.
5. Campanini A, Canzi P, De Vito A, et al. Awake versus sleep endoscopy: personal experience in 250 OSAHS patients. Acta Otorhinolaryngol Ital. 2010;30(2):73-7.
6. Chabolle F, Wagner I, Blumen MB, et al. Tongue base reduction with hyoepigottoplasty: a treatment for severe obstructive sleep apnea. Laryngoscope. 1999;109(8):1273-80.
7. Cormack RS, Lehane J. Difficult tracheal intubation in obstetrics. Anaesthesia. 1984;39(11):1105-11.
8. Vicini C, Dallan I, Canzi P, et al. Transoral robotic tongue base resection in obstructive sleep apnoea-hypopnoea syndrome: a preliminary report. ORL J Otorhinolaryngol Relat Spec. 2010;72(1):22-7.
9. Vicini C, Montevecchi F, Tenti G, et al. Transoral robotic surgery: Tongue base reduction and supraglottoplasty for obstructive sleep apnea. Operat Tech Otolaryngol Head Neck Surg. 2012;23(1):45-7.
10. O'Malley BW Jr, Weinstein GS, Snyder W, et al. Transoral robotic surgery (TORS) for base of tongue neoplasms. Laryngoscope. 2006;116(8):1465-72.
11. Eesa M, Montevecchi F, Hendawy E, et al. Swallowing outcome after TORS for sleep apnea: short- and long-term evaluation. Eur Arch Otorhinolaryngol. 2015;272(6):1537-41.
12. Vicini C, Montevecchi F, Campanini A, et al. Clinical outcomes and complications associated with TORS for OSAHS: a benchmark for evaluating an emerging surgical technology in a targeted application for benign disease. ORL J Otorhinolaryngol Relat Spec. 2014;76(2):63-9.

Index

Page numbers followed by *f* refer to figure and *t* refer to table.

A

Abductor cord paralysis 117
Abductor muscle 4
Abductor spasmodic dysphonia 40
Accentuated rhythms 63
Accessary cartilages 3
   corniculate 3
   cuneiform 3
Acidification tests 33
Acoustic 14
Acquired immunodeficiency syndrome 106
Acublade 116
Acyclovir 109
Adductor muscles 4
Adductor spasmodic dysphonia 40
Adequate energy 9
Adult laryngotracheal stenosis 121
   causes of 122
Adult larynx 8
Aerodigestive tract, effects of reflux in 30
Aerodynamic measures 9, 15
Aging voice 50, 61
   rejuvenation of 51
Airflow open quotient 15
Airway evaluation 92
Airway protection, evaluation of 148
Airway space, posterior 163
Allergic rhinitis, drugs in 66
Allergy 101
Alpha interferon 106, 107
American Academy of Otolaryngology–head
       and neck surgery 111
American Broncho-esophagological
       Association 111
American Society of Pediatric
       Otolaryngology 103
Amyloidosis 121
Amyotropic lateral sclerosis 41, 51
Anastomosis 127
   dehiscence of 129
Androgen-containing drugs 65
Anesthesia 91
   preparation 147
Anesthetic considerations 104
Anesthetic techniques 105*t*
Angiolytic lasers 105
Angiotensin-converting enzyme 66
   inhibitors 66
Antacids 66
Anticoagulants 67
Antigen-presenting cells 108

Antihistamines 47
Antihistaminics 66
Anti-inflammatory/analgesics 67
Antireflux therapy 109, 131
Apnea-hypopnea index 163
Aryepiglottic fold 6
   left 23*f*
Arytenoid adduction 75, 81, 82*f*
Arytenoid cartilage 82*f*
Arytenoid procedures 74
Arytenoidectomy 89
Arytenoids 1, 3
Aspiration 144
Assessing breath support 46
Asthma 101
Atrophied cord 23*f*
Auditory feedback 56
Auditory-perceptual evaluation 14
Autologous adipose injection 73
Autonomic nervous system 67
Avulsion laryngeal nerve 41

B

Bad breathing techniques 45
Balloon dilator 124*f*
Balloon tracheoplasty 93
Barium studies 32
Basic fibroblast growth factor 52
Bernoulli effect 134
Beta blockers 65
Bispectral index 160
Blood thinners 67
Body mass index 35
Body posture 151, 152*f*
Bogdasarian and Oslon classification 123
Bolus consistency 153
Botox 83
   injection 96
Botulinum toxin 40, 40*f*
Breath, holding 58*f*
Breathing
   correct abdominal 63
   exercises 63
   techniques, good 45
Bronchial asthma 29
Bronchiectasis 29
Bronchitis 101
   chronic 29
Bronchoalveolar lavage 33
Buccal burning 29

C

Calcinosis 28
Calcium hydroxyapatite 54
Carbon dioxide
   laser 117, 117*f*, 118*f*
      excision 105
      lumenis system 116*f*
Carbonic anhydrase III 28
Carcinoma lung 24*f*
Cardiorespiratory 144
Cardiorespiratory adverse events 102
Carotid endarterectomy 69
Cartilages 1
   of larynx 2*f*
   paired 1, 3
   unpaired 1, 2
Cartilaginous portion 85
Central nervous system 23, 51
   pathology 51
Cerebrovascular disease 67
Cervarix 110
Cervical vertebra 1
Chant talk 56
Charcot-Marie-tooth 69, 70
Chewing 56
Childhood hoarseness 84
Chin tuck 152
   posture 152*f*
Chronic disease 104
Cidofovir 106
Circumlaryngeal massage 62*f*
Clopidogrel 67
Clostridium botulinum 40, 43
Coblator cordotomy 77*f*
   intraoperative 76*f*
Cohen grading system 123
Cold
   abscess 122
   steel 105
Collagen vascular disorders 122
Commissure hypertrophy, posterior 34
Complete tracheal rings 139
Concomitant infection 102
Confidential voice therapy 63
Congenital subglottic stenosis 19, 19*f*
Conjugated linoleic acid 111
Connective tissue disorder 121
Consensus auditory-perceptual evaluation
       of voice scale 14
Cooper's approach 60
Cordotomy 89

Cornelia de Lange syndrome 144
Coronal minimum intensity projection 18*f*
Coronal section of larynx 2*f*
Coronary artery disease 67
Corticosteroids 65
    use of 65
Costal cartilage, harvesting of 127*f*
Cough
    chronic 29, 30, 96, 101
    drugs for 66
    suppressants 66
Coughing 146
Cricoarytenoid
    fixation 92
    fixity 92
    joint 5, 6*f*
        dislocation 25, 25*f*
        fixation 88
    lateral 4, 41
    muscle
        lateral 4*f*
        posterior 4, 5*f*
    posterior 72
Cricoid 2
    cartilage anteriorly 127*f*
    fractures 25
    lamina, anterior 137*f*
Cricothyroid joint 5, 26
    dislocation 26
Cricothyroid membrane 40
Cricothyroid muscle 5, 70
    action of 5*f*
Cricotracheal ligament 3
Cricotracheal resection 124, 127, 128
    cautions of 129
    complications of 129, 130
    steps 128*f*
Croup 19, 29, 101
Crunchy food 154
Cuneiform cartilage 8
Cyclooxygenase-2 inhibitors 109
Cyst 18, 20, 86
Cystic lesion 25*f*
Cysts of neck 122
Cytoplasmic inclusions 101

D

da Vinci robots 119
da Vinci tongue base reduction 161
Dendritic cell vaccination 111
Dental/gingival strictures, loss of 29
Deoxyribonucleic acid 100
Digital manipulation 56
Di-hematoporphyrin ether 108
Diphtheria 121
Distal tracheoesophageal fistula 19*f*
Diuretics 68
Drug-induced sedation 160
    endoscopy 160, 161
Drugs acting 67

Dye studies 149
Dying spells 139
Dysarthria 63
Dysphagia 101, 143
Dysphonia
    acute 47
    in children 85
    in singers
        acute 47
        chronic 48
Dyspnea 101
Dysport 40
Dystonia 39

E

Ear, nose, and throat (ENT) 27, 85, 116, 161, 164
Early cancer larynx 12*f*, 118*f*
Effortful swallow 158
Eicosapentaenoic acid 111
Elderberry 68
Electrical pacing 76
Electrocardiogram 161
Electrolaryngograph 15
Electrolaryngographic voice evaluation 14
Eliminating vocal abuse 57
Endoknot 89
Endolaryngeal mucus, thick 34
Endoscope, passage of 147
Endoscopic arytenoidectomy 89
Endoscopic bilateral injection
            laryngoplasty 53, 54
Endoscopic dilatation 124
Endoscopic laser thyroarytenoid
            myoneurectomy 43
Endoscopic management 124
Endoscopic microdebrider 125
Endoscopic procedures, limitations of 125
Endotracheal intubation 8
Endotracheal tube 136
End-to-end anastomosis 129
Enzyme-linked immunosorbent assay 30
Epidermal growth factor receptor 110
Epidermolysis bullosa 121
Epiglottis 3, 84
    mucosa 6
    primary 161
    residual 164
    secondary 161
    surgical treatment of
        primary 161
        secondary 163
Epiglottitis 19
Epithelial resistance 28
Epworth sleepiness scale 163
Erythema 34
Esophageal
    acid clearance 28
    atresia 19*f*
    dysmotility 28

    sphincter 143
        lower 27, 144
Esophagitis 136
Esophagobronchial reflux 29
Esophagoscopy 32
Esophagram 146
Etiology vocal fold paralysis 69
Exhalation 46
Expansion surgeries, external 126
Extensive laryngeal papillomatosis 103*f*
Extensive tracheal papillomatosis 102*f*
Extracorporeal membrane oxygenation 140
Extraesophageal reflux 27
Extralaryngeal spread 102

F

Facilitating approaches 56
False vocal cords 1
FEES assessment, components of 148
Fiber laser, use of 102*f*
Fiberoptic endoscopic evaluation of
            swallowing 147, 148
    with sensory testing 148
Flange laryngoscope 117*f*
Flexible endoscopy 32
Flexible laryngoscope 10
Fluent speech 9
Food and Drug Administration 67, 106
Food and fluid, type of 154*t*
Foreign body 26
    inhalation 85
Friedrich design 81*f*
Functional dysphonia 87

G

Galen's anastomosis 7
Galli-Curci nerve 6
Gamma-aminobutyric acid 35
Gardasil 110
Gastroesophageal reflux 136
    disease 27-36, 129
        symptoms 35
    drugs for 65
Gastrointestinal disturbances 66
Genetic aspects 103
Geniohyoid 5
Geriatric dysphonia 50
Geriatric voice dysfunction 50
Globus sensation 29
Glomus tumors 21
Glottal airflow 15
    alternating 15
Glottic closure 10
Glottic stenosis, posterior 88
Glottis 1, 134*f*
    level of 18*f*
Granulocyte macrophage colony
            stimulating factor 107

H

Haemophilus influenzae 19
Hair-cutting 103
Half-swallow boom method 59
Hard chewy 154
Head-lifting exercise 156
Head rotation 153*f*
Head tilt 152
    posture 153*f*
Heat-shock protein 108
Helicobacter pylori 31, 35
Hemangioma 21
Hemostasis 120
Hepatic growth factor 52
Herbal medicines 67
Histamine receptor antagonists 66
Histocompatibility complex, major 103
Hoarseness 29, 34, 85
Holistic voice therapy 59
Human communicating nerve 7
Human immune deficiency virus 69
Human leukocyte antigen 103
Human papilloma virus 21, 99, 100
    infection 101, 103
        biology of 100
Human papillomavirus-16 genome 100*f*
Humming 59
Hyaluronic acid 51, 73, 94
Hydroxyestrone 108
Hyoepiglottic ligament 3
Hyperemia 34
Hyperkinetic facets 71
Hypertrophic thymus 122
Hypokinetic disorder 71
Hypopharyngeal structures 142
Hypopharynx 146

I

Ice chip maneuver 154
Ice chips 154
Immunological aspects 103
Implant medialization 74
Indirect therapeutic strategies 151
Indirect voice therapy 56
Indole-3-carbinol 108
Infant's larynx 142
Inferior thyroid artery 7
Inflammatory causes 23
Inflammatory disease, chronic 122
Infrahyoid epiglottis 1
Infrahyoid muscles 5
Inhalation-phonation 57
Initiating voice, problems with 63
Injection laryngoplasty 73
Intensive care unit 127
Interarytenoid muscle 4, 6
Intermittent dysphonia 85
Intrinsic laryngeal muscles 4

Intrinsic ligaments 3
Isolated tracheal stenosis 123
Isshiki's work 80

J

Jostle sign 92
Juvenile laryngeal papillomatosis 85

K

Keratosis 117
Kymography 12

L

Lamina propria, superficial 53
Lano classification 122
Laryngeal adduction exercises 58
Laryngeal adductor reflex 143
Laryngeal anatomy 1
Laryngeal biopsy 95
Laryngeal blades 106
Laryngeal block, superior 92*f*
Laryngeal cancer 29
    early 118
Laryngeal cartilages 2, 3
Laryngeal clefts 18, 137
    posterior 137
Laryngeal edema 129
    diffuse 34
Laryngeal electromyography 13, 72
Laryngeal elevation 146
Laryngeal framework surgery 80
    advantages of 80
Laryngeal innervation 6
Laryngeal joints 5
Laryngeal ligaments 3
Laryngeal management 160
Laryngeal manual therapy 62
Laryngeal mechanism 61
Laryngeal mucosa 8
Laryngeal muscles 61
    extrinsic 5
Laryngeal musculature 4
Laryngeal nerve
    anatomy of superior 6*f*
    block 7
        superior 92*f*
    superior 5-7, 70, 143
Laryngeal obstruction 18
    in pediatric age group 18
Laryngeal papillomatosis 87
Laryngeal pathology, benign 17
Laryngeal penetration 148
Laryngeal polyp 117*f*
Laryngeal position 8
Laryngeal procedures 91
    office-based 91
Laryngeal reinnervation 75

Laryngeal reposturing maneuvers 62
Laryngeal resistance 15
Laryngeal spasm 29
Laryngeal stenosis 29
Laryngeal surface of aryepiglottic fold 1
Laryngeal surgery 164
Laryngeal ventricle 20
    left 23*f*
Laryngeal web 88, 136
Laryngitis 29
    acute 85
    chronic 29, 36, 85
Laryngocele 18, 20, 20*f*
    mixed 20*f*
Laryngology, lasers in 116
Laryngomalacia 8, 18, 119, 134
Laryngopharyngeal reflux 27-29, 29*t*, 30, 31,
        34, 35, 66, 85, 96, 109
    drugs for 65
    severe 32*f*
Laryngoscope 93
Laryngospasm 28, 51
Laryngotracheal fissure 126*f*
Laryngotracheal reconstruction 124
    steps of 126*f*
Laryngotracheal stenosis 93, 119, 121, 122
    classification of 122
    early stage 124*f*
    techniques for 126
Laryngotracheal trauma, external 122
Laryngotracheobronchitis 19
Laryngo-tracheo-esophageal cleft 18
Laryngotracheoesophageal clefts, types
    of 138*f*
Laryngovideostroboscopy 32
Larynx 2, 50, 57, 84, 92, 152, 154, 155, 157,
        158, 160, 161, 164
    anatomy of 1, 1*f*
    benign tumors of 18, 20
    development of 84
    effect of reflux on 30
    embryological development of 84
    malignant lesions of 85
    mass lesions of 20
    movements of 57
    position of 7
    techniques in study of 17
Laser procedures for airway,
        office-based 94
Laser safety protocol 116
Laser surgery, office-based 119
Laser with robotic systems 119
Laser-assisted procedure 125
Lateralization procedure 89
Lawn mowing 103
Lee Silverman voice
    therapy 52
    voice treatment 63, 64
Leukoplakia 117
Lifestyle modification 34
Ligaments, extrinsic 3

Light-emitting diode 33
Lip closure exercise 155, 155*f*
Lipomas 21
Liquids
    thick 154
    thin 154
Local anesthesia, procedures under 80
Loudness, change of 56
Lymph nodal mass 24*f*

M

Manometry 149
    studies 33
Manual circumlaryngeal
    techniques 62
    therapy 62
Maternal condyloma acuminata 102
Maturational changes in swallowing 142
Maximum phonation duration 46
McCaffrey classification 122
Medialization laryngoplasty 72
Medialization silastic prosthesis 75*f*
Mediastinal neoplasms 70
Medical therapy 40
Medical treatment 35
Mendelsohn maneuver 157
Mesenchymal tumors 21
Metastatic lymphadenopathy 24*f*
Microdebrider 106
Microphones 14
Microtrauma 49
Midzone of laryngeal surface of
        epiglottis 87
Minimal glottal airflow 15
Minimum intensity projection 18
Mitomycin C 125, 130
Mouth ulcers 29
Mucosal wave 10
Mucus, drugs for thick 66
Multichannel intraluminal impedance 33
    monitoring 33
Multiple sclerosis 51, 58
Mumps vaccine 108
Muscle
    contraction 62*f*
    stretching 61*f*
    tension
        dysphonia 62
        patterns 71
Myer-cotton
    grading system 19
    staging 122
Myoclonus 51

N

National Institute of Allergy and Infectious
        Diseases 107
Neck 81*f*
    extension 152, 153, 153*f*

incision, horizontal 128
    muscles, tension in 63
    trauma 69
Necrotic lymph nodes 24*f*
Neodymium: Yttrium-aluminum-
        garnet 116, 119
Neoplasms
    benign 122
    malignant 122
Netterville's silastic preformed implant 82*f*
Neurolaryngology 51
Neuromuscular junction 51
Neuronox 40
Nonacid reflux 28
Nonepithelial tumors, benign 21
Nonrecurrent laryngeal nerve 7
Nonresponders, management of 35
Nose oropharynx hypopharynx 161
Nuclear medicine scans 149

O

Obstructive pulmonary disease, chronic 29
Obstructive sleep apnea 160
    hypopnea syndrome 160
Obvious skin lesions 103
Omohyoid 5
Open mouth approach 59
Open reading frames 100
Open surgical methods 125
Oral
    cavity and pharynx 29
    muscles, tension in 63
    sensory stimulation 154
Oromotor exercises 155, 156
Oropharyngeal dysphagia 151
Orosensory stimulation, types of 155*f*
Ossified thyroid cartilage, continuity of 25*f*
Otalgia 29
Otitis 29
    media with effusion 27, 30

P

Palatopharyngeus 5
Palsy, cause of left 24*f*
Paradoxical vocal cord movement
        disorder 93
Paragangliomas 21
Paresis 69
Parkinson's disease 51, 58
Peak glottal airflow 15
Pediatric
    dysphagia 142
    FEES 147
    laryngopharyngeal reflux 30
    larynx 84
    versus adult upper airway anatomy 133
    voice disorders 84
Pepsin, role of 28
Perceptual evaluation of voice 14

Peripheral vascular disease 67
pH monitoring 33
Pharyngoepiglottic fold 164
Pharyngoesophageal scintigraphy 33
Pharynx 142-144, 151-153, 155, 156
Phenylephrine 67
Phonation 46
    resistance training exercise 52
Phonatory exercises 63
Phonatory flow rate, mean 15
Phonosurgery, lasers in 116
Photodynamic therapy 106, 107
Physical activity 35
Physical examination 145
Pierre-Robin syndrome 144
Pitch changes 63
Pitch limiting voice treatment 64
Pitch, change in 85
Pneumonia 29
Polyps 86, 117
Polysomnography 160
Positive airway pressure, continuous 133,
        160
Postintubation subglottic stenosis 20*f*
Postnasal drip 29
Post-traumatic hematoma and fracture 25*f*
Potassium titanyl phosphate 94, 105, 116
Pre-epiglottic space 19
Premature spillage 148
Preoperative counseling 93
Presbyphonia 50, 54
Presenting symptomatology 101
Professional vocalist 52
Prokinetic agents 66
Pronunciation, correct 47
Prophylactic vaccination 109
Prosody 14
Prostaglandin 111
Proton pump inhibitor 30, 66
Pseudoephedrine 67
Pseudosulcus 34
Pseudo-supraglottic swallow 58
Psychotropic agents 67
Puberphonia 71, 87
Pull down maneuver 62
Pulmonary collapse 29
Pulmonary fibrosis 29
Pulsed-dye laser 105
Pushback maneuver 62

Q

Quadrangular membrane 3

R

Radiation therapy 118
Radionuclide studies 33
Range of motion 62
    exercise 155
Raynaud's phenomenon 28

Recurrent laryngeal nerve 7, 23, 39, 70
  block 7
  injury 129
  sectioning 41
Recurrent nerve avulsion 41
Recurrent pneumonia 101, 145
Recurrent respiratory papillomatosis 21, 87,
    99, 105, 109-111, 117
  resources 111
Red flag 71
Redirected phonation 59
Reflux finding score 34t
Reflux symptom index 14, 31, 34
Reflux, direct 28
Reinke's edema 71
Relapsing polychondritis 121
Respiration 63
Respiratory distress 103
Respiratory papillomas 87f
Respiratory papillomatosis 21f, 87f
Restenosis 129
Retinoids 109
Retrotracheal abscess 122
Rhinosinusitis, chronic 31
Ribavirin 109
Robotic scanner 116f

S

Salivary pepsin 34
Salpingopharyngeus 5
Sandifer syndrome 29
Sarcoidosis 121
Sclerodactyly 28
Scleroma 121
Sellick's maneuver 2
Semisolid food 154
Sex hormones 65
Shoulder breathing 46
Silastic medialization implant 74f
Silent reflux 27
Singing voice 45
  assessment of 47
  care of 45
Sinusitis, chronic 29
Sleep apnea patients 160
Sleep endoscopy 160
Sleep nasendoscopy 160
Sleep surgery 119
Slow-twitch fibers 51
Smoke evacuator 117f
Soft solid food 154
Spasmodic dysphonia 39, 40, 51
  surgery for 41
Speech language pathologists 59, 73
Spine surgery 69
Spinocerebellar atrophy 70
Squamous cell carcinoma 118
Stenosis
  primary 121
  secondary 121

Stenosis, causes of
  primary 121
  secondary 122
Sternocleidomastoid 23
Sternohyoid 5
Sternothyroid 5
Steroids in acute laryngeal conditions 65
Stroboscopy 10
  advantages of 10
  instrumentation for 10
  limitations of 10
  mechanism of 10
Stylohyoid 5
Stylopharyngeus 5
Subglottal pressure 15
Subglottic hemangioma 22f
Subglottic stenosis 29, 121, 133, 136
Subglottis 1, 2, 134f
Submucosal hemorrhage 47-49
Submucosal paraganglioma 22f
Submucosal schwannoma 22f
Substantia nigra 51
Sulcus vocalis 11f, 85, 89
  bilateral 89f
Super supraglottic swallow 157
Supraglottic swallow 156
Supraglottis 1, 19, 134f
Supraglottoplasty 161, 163
Suprahyoid
  epiglottis 1, 164
  muscle 5
Surgical steps 41
Surgical techniques 105
Surgical treatment 35, 103
Survivin 110
Sustained vowels 9
Swallow maneuvers 156
Swallowing physiology, normal 143
Swallowing, mechanics of 144
Swallowing, three phases of 143
Symptomatic voice therapy 56
Syphilis 121
Systemic illness like hypothyroidism 85

T

Tactile perceptual evaluation 14
Taste, loss of 29
Technetium scan 149
Telangiectasia 28
  polyp right vocal cord 86f
Tense dysphonia 51
Tensor muscle 5
Thallium scan 149
Therapeutic strategies, direct 154
Therapeutic vaccination 108
Throat 34
  clearing 29
Thyroarytenoid 40, 51, 72
  muscle 4
    action of 4f

myomectomy 43
Thyrohyoid 5
  ligament, medial 3
  membrane 3, 8, 20f
Thyroid 2, 65
  cartilage 42f
    fracture of 24
  diseases 122
  membrane 40
Thyroidectomy 69
Thyroplasty 41, 80, 82, 83
  type II 42f
Titanium vocal fold medializing implant 81,
    81f
Tongue
  base reduction 163
  carriage 48
    posterior 48
    superior 48
Topical steroid sprays 66
Torticollis 29
Trachea 92
Tracheal papillomas, used for 87f
Tracheal papillomatosis 102f
Tracheal resection 129
  steps of 130f
Tracheoesophageal fistula 138
Tracheoesophageal puncture 95
  secondary 95
Tracheomalacia 139
Tracheostomy 77, 102
  in recurrent respiratory
    papillomatosis 102
Tracheotomy tube 149
Transcricothyroid approach 95
Transesohophageal puncture 96f
Transnasal esophagoscopy 91, 96
Transoral
  approach 95
  laser
    microsurgery 118
    resection 12f
  robotic surgery 161
  route 94
Transthyrohyoid approach 95
Transthyroid cartilage approach 95
Transverse arytenoid muscle, action of 4f
Transverse cordotomy 76, 76f
Transverse laser cordotomy, posterior 117
Trauma 18, 24
Tuberculosis 121
Tuberculous lymphadenopathy 24f
Tumor 23
  neck 122
  necrosis factor-alpha 111

U

Unsedated office-based laser surgery 119
Upper esophageal sphincter 27, 28, 152
Upper gastrointestinal study 146

Upper respiratory
   infection 69
   tract 134*f*
      anatomical 133
      infection 101

V

VACTERL association 144
Vagal reflux 28, 29
Vascular compression 139
Vascular endothelial growth factor-a 110
Vascular lesions 119
Vascular malformation, low flow 21, 22*f*
Vasoconstrictors 66
Velocardiofacial syndrome 136, 144
Ventricular obliteration 34
Vibrating edge, medial 80
Vibrating force 45
Vibratory margin 46
Videofluoroscopic swallow study 146
Videokymographic images 11
Videokymography 10
Videostroboscopy 32
Visual assessment 10
Visual perceptual evaluation 14
Vitamin C 47
Vocal complains 50
Vocal cord
   cysts 85, 89*f*, 117
   examination of 86*f*
   granuloma 88
   injection 94
      superficial 96
   keratosis of 118*f*
   length of 84
   lesions, benign 85
   mucus retention cyst of 11*f*

muscle 41
nodule 13*f*, 20
   bilateral 86*f*
palsy, causing left 24*f*
paralysis 18, 23, 23*f*, 134
   bilateral 135
polyp 20, 119
ulcers 29
Vocal folds 5*f*, 73*f*, 74*f*
   abduction of 4*f*, 5*f*
   cyst 89
   edema 34
   examine 86*f*
   fixation 77*f*
   immobility 69
      causes of unilateral 70*f*
      left 73*f*
      management, bilateral 75
      management, unilateral 72
      surgical causes of bilateral 70*f*
   laminar structure, change in 85
   mobility 148
   paralysis 88
      bilateral 71
      pressure for unilateral 57
      unilateral 71
   paresis 69, 71, 85
Vocal function exercises 52, 61
Vocal hygiene 48
Vocal loading, tests of 9
Vocal nodule 85, 101
Vocal performance, patient questionnaire
      of 14
Vocal polyp 86
Vocal tract 9
Voice 9
   activity 14
   analysis 32
   and medicines 65

disorders 84
evaluation 9
   problems in 9
handicap index 13, 43
material 9
outcome survey 14
practitioners 54
production 45
symptom scale 14
test battery 9
testing in detail 10
therapeutic approaches 56
therapist 40, 56, 63, 73, 86
therapy
   direct 56
   physiological 59
   resonant 60, 60*f*
Voice-related quality of life 14, 52, 118
Volume scanners 17
Vowel play 63

W

Wegener granulomatosis 121

X

Xylocaine 92, 93
Xylometazoline 48

Y

Yawn-sigh approach 57
Yellow jasmine 67

Z

Zenker's diverticulum 96